Non–Operating Room Anesthesia

Mark S. Weiss, MD

Assistant Professor of Anesthesiology and Critical Care
Director of Inpatient Anesthesia Endoscopy Services
Perelman School of Medicine
Hospital of the University of Pennsylvania
Philadelphia, Pennsylvania

Lee A. Fleisher, MD

Robert D. Dripps Professor and Chair of Anesthesiology and Critical Care
Professor of Medicine
Perelman School of Medicine
Senior Fellow, Leonard Davis Institute of Health Economics
University of Pennsylvania
Philadelphia, Pennsylvania

ELSEVIER
SAUNDERS

1600 John F. Kennedy Blvd.
Ste 1800
Philadelphia, PA 19103-2899

NON–OPERATING ROOM ANESTHESIA ISBN: 978-1-4557-5415-1

Copyright © 2015 by Saunders, an imprint of Elsevier Inc.

Notices

Knowledge and best practice in this field are constantly changing. As new research and experience broaden our understanding, changes in research methods, professional practices, or medical treatment may become necessary.

Practitioners and researchers must always rely on their own experience and knowledge in evaluating and using any information, methods, compounds, or experiments described herein. In using such information or methods they should be mindful of their own safety and the safety of others, including parties for whom they have a professional responsibility.

With respect to any drug or pharmaceutical products identified, readers are advised to check the most current information provided (i) on procedures featured or (ii) by the manufacturer of each product to be administered, to verify the recommended dose or formula, the method and duration of administration, and contraindications. It is the responsibility of practitioners, relying on their own experience and knowledge of their patients, to make diagnoses, to determine dosages and the best treatment for each individual patient, and to take all appropriate safety precautions.

To the fullest extent of the law, neither the Publisher nor the authors, contributors, or editors assume any liability for any injury and/or damage to persons or property as a matter of products liability, negligence or otherwise, or from any use or operation of any methods, products, instructions, or ideas contained in the material herein.

Library of Congress Cataloging-in-Publication Data

Non–operating room anesthesia / [edited by] Mark S. Weiss, Lee A. Fleisher.
       p. ; cm.
  Includes bibliographical references and index.
  ISBN 978-1-4557-5415-1 (hardcover)
  I. Weiss, Mark S. (Mark Steven), editor. II. Fleisher, Lee A., editor.
  [DNLM: 1. Anesthesia--standards. 2. Process Assessment (Health Care)--methods. WO 200]
  RD81
  617.9'6--dc23
                                                                    2014014682

Executive Content Strategist: William Schmitt
Content Development Specialist: Lisa Barnes
Publishing Services Manager: Jeff Patterson
Project Manager: Clay S. Broeker
Design Direction: Louis Forgione
Cover Designer: Elaine Kurie

Printed in China

Last digit is the print number: 9 8 7 6 5 4 3 2 1

This book is dedicated:
to Lee Fleisher for his trust and friendship.
to my aunt, Lillian Brick, who is my sunshine.
to my mother, Minnette Weiss, who has always been so supportive.
to my father, Frederick Weiss, who was always there to guide me.
to my sons, Isaac, Noah, and Henry David.

And this book is dedicated to the love of my life, Paulette Marie Lambert.
MSW

This book is dedicated to my wife, Renee, and my children,
Jessica and Matthew, for supporting me in my career
while ensuring that I understand what is truly important.
LAF

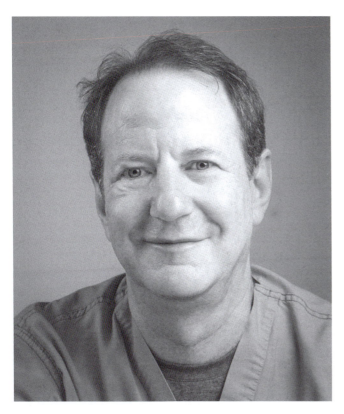

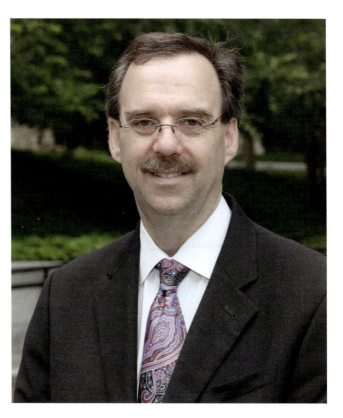

Mark S. Weiss, MD, is an Assistant Professor of Anesthesiology and Critical Care at the University of Pennsylvania's Perelman School of Medicine. He received his medical degree from the University of Cincinnati and completed his residency training at Yale University. His focus is on perioperative management of high-risk patients, with an emphasis on non–operating room anesthesia (NORA). He is currently the director of Inpatient Endoscopy Services at the University of Pennsylvania.

Lee A. Fleisher, MD, is the Robert D. Dripps Professor and Chair of Anesthesiology and Critical Care and a Professor of Medicine at the University of Pennsylvania's Perelman School of Medicine. He received his medical degree from the State University of New York at Stony Brook, from which he received the Distinguished Alumni Award in 2011. His research focuses on perioperative cardiovascular risk assessment and reduction and the measurement of quality of care, and he has received numerous federal, industry, and foundation grants related to these subjects. He is President of the Association of University Anesthesiologists. He is a member of the Consensus Standards Advisory Committee of the National Quality Forum and of the Administrative Board of the Council of Faculty and Academic Specialties of the Association of American Medical Colleges. In 2007, he was elected to membership of the Institute of Medicine of the National Academy of Sciences.

Contributors

Rose Campise-Luther, MD, FAAP
Assistant Professor
Pediatric Anesthesiology
Medical College of Wisconsin
Milwaukee, Wisconsin

Thomas Cutter, MD, MAEd
Professor
Department of Anesthesia and Critical Care
University of Chicago
Chicago, Illinois

Christina D. Diaz, MD
Assistant Professor
Pediatric Anesthesiology
Medical College of Wisconsin
Milwaukee, Wisconsin

Karen B. Domino, MD, MPH
Professor
Department of Anesthesiology and Pain Medicine
University of Washington School of Medicine
Seattle, Washington

Richard E. Galgon, MD, MS
Assistant Professor
Department of Anesthesiology
University of Wisconsin School of Medicine and Public
    Health
Madison, Wisconsin

Esther D. Garazi, MD
Department of Anesthesia
Perioperative and Pain Medicine
Stanford University School of Medicine
Stanford, California

Gregory G. Ginsberg
Professor of Medicine
Director of Endoscopy
Gastroenterology Division
Hospital of the University of Pennsylvania
Philadelphia, Pennsylvania

Basavana G. Goudra, MD, FRCA, FCARCSI
Assistant Professor
Department of Anesthesiology and Critical Care Medicine
Hospital of the University of Pennsylvania
Philadelphia, Pennsylvania

Caitlin J. Guo, MD, MBA
Assistant Professor
Department of Anesthesia
New York University Medical Center
New York, New York

Anil Gupta, MD, FRCA, PhD
Associate Professor
Department of Anesthesiology and Intensive Care
Institution for Medicine and Health
Örebro, Sweden

Manon Hache, MD
Assistant Professor
Department of Anesthesiology
Columbia University Medical Center
New York, New York

Eric A. Harris, MD, MBA
Associate Professor of Clinical Anesthesiology
Department of Anesthesiology, Perioperative Medicine,
    and Pain Management
University of Miami, Miller School of Medicine
Miami, Florida

Jennifer E. Hofer, MD
Assistant Professor
Department of Anesthesia and Critical Care
University of Chicago
Chicago, Illinois

E. Heidi Jerome, MD
Associate Professor
Department of Anesthesiology and Pediatrics
Columbia University Medical Center
New York, New York

Max Kanevsky, MD, PhD
Assistant Professor of Anesthesia
Division of Cardiovascular Anesthesia
Stanford University School of Medicine
Stanford, California

Meghan Lane-Fall, MD, MSHP
Assistant Professor of Anesthesiology and Critical Care
Department of Anesthesiology and Critical Care
University of Pennsylvania
Philadelphia, Pennsylvania

Kelly Lebak, MD
Anesthesiologist
MetroHealth Medical Center
University of Wisconsin—Madison
Madison, Wisconsin

Jeffrey Lee, MS, MD
Assistant Professor
Anesthesiology
University of Wisconsin—Madison
Madison, Wisconsin

Mark A. Leibel, MD
Assistant Professor
Department of Anesthesiology
University of Wisconsin School of Medicine and Public Health
Madison, Wisconsin

Larry Lindenbaum, MD
Assistant Professor
Department of Anesthesiology and Critical Care Medicine
Medical College of Wisconsin
Milwaukee, Wisconsin

Alex Macario, MD, MBA
Professor
Department of Anesthesiology, Perioperative and Pain Medicine
Vice-Chair for Education
Program Director, Anesthesia Residency
Stanford University School of Medicine
Stanford, California

Jeff E. Mandel, MD, MS
Assistant Professor of Anesthesiology and Critical Care
Perelman School of Medicine
University of Pennsylvania
Philadelphia, Pennsylvania

Ramon Martin, MD, PhD
Staff Anesthesiologist
Department of Anesthesiology, Perioperative and Pain Medicine
Brigham and Women's Hospital
Assistant Professor
Anesthesia
Harvard Medical School
Boston, Massachusetts

Julia I. Metzner, MD
Associate Professor
Department of Anesthesiology and Pain Medicine
University of Washington
Seattle, Washington

Roger A. Moore, MD
Clinical Associate Professor of Anesthesiology and Critical Care
Chair Emeritus, Deborah Heart and Lung Center
Perelman School of Medicine
Hospital of the University of Pennsylvania
Philadelphia, Pennsylvania

Melissa L. Pant, MD
Clinical Associate
Department of Anesthesia and Critical Care
University of Chicago
Chicago, Illinois

Mark C. Phillips, MD
Assistant Professor and Medical Director, Advanced GI Endoscopy Anesthesia
Department of Anesthesiology
University of Alabama at Birmingham School of Medicine
Birmingham, Alabama

Christopher D. Press, MD
Department of Anesthesiology, Perioperative and Pain Medicine
Stanford University School of Medicine
Stanford, California

Johan Raeder, MD, PhD
Professor
Faculty of Medicine
NOR Consultant
Department of Anaesthesiology
Oslo University Hospital
Oslo, Norway

W. Kirke Rogers, MD
Associate
Department of Anesthesiology
The University of Iowa Roy J. and Lucille A. Carver College of Medicine
Iowa City, Iowa

Daniel Rubin, MD
Assistant Professor
Department of Anesthesia and Critical Care
University of Chicago
Chicago, Illinois

John P. Scott, MD
Assistant Professor
Department of Anesthesiology and Pediatrics
Medical College of Wisconsin
Milwaukee, Wisconsin

Jack S. Shanewise, MD
Professor of Anesthesiology
Columbia University Medical Center
New York, New York

Preet Mohinder Singh, MD
Assistant Professor
Department of Anesthesiology and Critical Care Medicine
Postgraduate Institute of Medical Education and Research
Chandigarh, India

Scott Springman, MD
Professor
Anesthesiology
University of Wisconsin—Madison
Madison, Wisconsin

Lena S. Sun, MD
E.M. Papper Professor of Pediatric Anesthesiology
Department of Anesthesiology and Pediatrics
Columbia University Medical Center
New York, New York

BobbieJean Sweitzer, MD
Professor of Anesthesia and Critical Care
Department of Anesthesiology and Critical Care
University of Chicago
Director
Anesthesia Perioperative Medicine Clinic
Professor of Medicine
Department of Medicine
University of Chicago
Chicago, Illinois

Pedro P. Tanaka, MD, PhD
Department of Anesthesiology, Perioperative and
    Pain Medicine
Stanford University School of Medicine
Stanford, California

Jonathan W. Tanner, MD, PhD
Assistant Professor of Clinical Anesthesiology and Critical
    Care
Department of Anesthesiology and Critical Care
Perelman School of Medicine
University of Pennsylvania
Philadelphia, Pennsylvania

John M. Trummel, MD MPH
Assistant Professor
Department of Anesthesiology
Dartmouth-Hitchcock Medical Center
Lebanon, New Hampshire

Sophia van Hoff, MD
Resident
Department of Anesthesiology
Dartmouth-Hitchcock Medical Center
Lebanon, New Hampshire

Lindsay L. Warner, BS
Mayo Medical School
Mayo Clinic
Rochester, Minnesota

Mary Ellen Warner, MD
Associate Professor of Anesthesiology
Mayo Clinic
Rochester, Minnesota

Nafisseh S. Warner, MD
Mayo School of Graduate Medical Education
Mayo Clinic
Rochester, Minnesota

Mark S. Weiss, MD
Assistant Professor of Anesthesiology and Critical Care
Director of Inpatient Anesthesia Endoscopy Services
Perelman School of Medicine
Hospital of the University of Pennsylvania
Philadelphia, Pennsylvania

Foreword

Anesthesiology has witnessed incredible advances over the past 3 decades. Improved patient safety has been a driving force for our advancements in medical technology, in the expansion of our pharmacological armamentarium, and in the development of innovative anesthetic techniques. The reward for these improvements is better patient outcomes and the ability to provide complex surgical interventions to patients that would have been impossible to perform without the anesthetic advancements. There has never been a better time for anesthesiologists to take the sickest and most debilitated of patents of all ages through the most highly invasive and stressful procedures in such a safe and effective manner. In the 21st century, and significantly due to advances in anesthetic care, surgery has also had an increased focus on out-of-operating room procedures, necessitating continued anesthesia innovation for the environment outside the operating room. Just a few decades ago, it was rare that anesthesiologists were called to provide care outside the typical operating room setting; when doing so, it was usually limited to emergent or highly unusual circumstances. Indeed, training programs primarily focused on providing the highest quality and safest care under the controlled environment of an operating room arena, where supplies, equipment, and personnel were readily available to support most medical complications. The "comfort zone" for nearly all anesthesiologists did not extend far past the sterile corridors of the operating room.

Once the acknowledgment is made that out-of-operating room anesthetic care has to be provided, guidelines for the delivery of that care must be established. As previously stated, providing anesthesia out of the operating room typically falls outside the training and comfort zone of most anesthesiologists. There are few comprehensive guidelines, protocols, or educational materials tailored to the specific needs of these types of anesthetics. Also, the environment and the techniques are unfamiliar to many anesthesiologists. Education and information are critical for both reducing physician anxiety and for standardizing the procedures and practices for care outside the operating room.

Recent reports filed with the Anesthesia Quality Institute indicate that many of the anesthetics today are delivered outside of traditional operating room locations. At the Hospital of the University of Pennsylvania, the increase in anesthetics delivered outside the operating room has grown over the past decade from a minimal number of cases yearly to a time today when over 30% of the anesthetics are given in nontraditional locations. Many anesthesia departments are unprepared psychologically and educationally to meet the increasing demand for out-of–operating room care. There are significant manpower, economic, educational, and patient safety factors that need to be explored in order to operationalize an effective out-of–operating room care plan. However, if an anesthesia department is to continue to be viable in this changing surgical and procedural environment, it is imperative that the departments and anesthesia groups take a cooperative approach, rather than an obstructive attitude, in partnering with those physicians performing the procedures.

In this book, Drs. Mark Weiss and Lee Fleisher have provided an important tool to address both the challenges and opportunities for anesthesiologists in providing non–operating room anesthesia (NORA) care. As NORA continues to consume more of the time and effort of anesthesia departments, NORA training should become an integral part of anesthesia residency programs. However, until anesthesiologists do receive formal education in NORA, I believe this book will go a long way in expanding the comfort zone of anesthesiologists to out-of–operating room locations. As minimally invasive procedures rapidly increase, it is certain that the practice of anesthesia will significantly expand in nontraditional environments and that our services will be vital for the smooth flow of patient care in all out-of–operating room settings.

Roger A. Moore, MD
**Clinical Associate Professor of
Anesthesiology and Critical Care,
Hospital of the University of Pennsylvania
Past President, Society of Cardiovascular
Anesthesiologists
Past President, American Society
of Anesthesiologists**

Preface

The past several years have seen advances in medical technology that allow physicians to treat a patient with minimally invasive procedures. With increasing frequency, these procedures are being performed outside the traditional operating room environment. Non–operating room anesthesia (NORA) cases now comprise as many as 70% of the cases being reported to the Anesthesia Quality Institute. In spite of the exponential increase in NORA caseloads, very little attention has been paid to this subspecialty area and even less with regard to developing guidelines, protocols, and educational materials tailored to the specific needs of providing anesthesia in these settings.

This book is meant to serve as an educational resource in regard to issues of setup, quality control, patient care and safety, and economic viability that are specific to NORA. The contributing authors are all outstanding clinicians who have developed expertise that relates to NORA.

It is hoped that the information presented will facilitate improved patient care and provide a resource for the inclusion of NORA training within residency training programs.

This is, in many ways, an important part of the future of anesthesia.

There are many people who have worked hard to make this project possible. We would first like to thank the professionals at Elsevier who have been so wonderful to work with: Lisa Barnes, William Schmitt, Clay Broeker, and the entire staff. We would like to thank Amy Meros, Administrative Coordinator in the department, who has been patient and tireless in helping to bring this manuscript together. Finally, we would like to thank the authors and contributors to this book for the many hours it takes to write a chapter.

Mark S. Weiss, MD
Lee A. Fleisher, MD

Contents

SECTION 1 PREPARATION FOR NON–OPERATING ROOM ACTIVITIES, 1

1 Engineering Excellence in Non–Operating Room Anesthesia Care, 2
MEGHAN LANE-FALL and MARK S. WEISS

Achieving Excellence in Health Care, 2
Proactive Versus Reactive Approach to Problems, 3
Proactive Approaches: Anticipating Problems, 3
Reactive Approaches: What Happens When Something Goes Wrong, 5
Moving from "Good to Great" : Organizational Approaches to Excellence, 6
Conclusion, 6

2 Designing Safety and Engineering Standards for the Non–Operating Room Anesthesia Procedure Site, 8
KELLY LEBAK, SCOTT SPRINGMAN, and JEFFREY LEE

Initial Planning, 8
Ergonomics, 9
Movement, 10
Tasks, 10
Communication, 10
Lighting, 10
Noise Control, 10
Temperature Control, 10
Power Management, 11
Ventilation, 12
Materials Management, 12
Individual Non–Operating Room Anesthesia Sites, 12
Hybrid Operating Rooms, 14
Conclusion, 15

3 Room Setup, Critical Supplies, and Medications, 18
MARK C. PHILLIPS

Room Setup, 18
Critical Supplies, 24
Safety Issues in Non–Operating Room Anesthesia Locations, 24
Medications, 26
Allergic Reactions, 28
Benzocaine Spray and Methemoglobinemia, 28
Malignant Hyperthermia, 29
Conclusion, 29

4 The Role of the Non–Operating Room Anesthesiologist, 30
E. HEIDI JEROME, MANON HACHE, and LENA S. SUN

Oversight of Non–Operating Room Anesthesia, 30
Levels of Sedation and Anesthesia, 31
Organizing Safe Practice, 32
Equipment, 33
Personnel, 33
Conclusion, 34

SECTION 2 GENERAL MANAGEMENT PRINCIPLES, 35

5 Continuous Quality Improvement for Non–Operating Room Anesthesia Locations, 36
JULIA I. METZNER and KAREN B. DOMINO

Quality, 36
Selecting Indicators, 36
Validity of Continuous Quality Improvement Indicators in Anesthesiology, 37
Methods to Improve Quality of Care: Quality Improvement Model Descriptions, 38
Critical Incidents, 38
Sentinel Events, 38
Root Cause Analysis, 39
Human Factors Analysis, 40
Quality and Safety Improvement Efforts Outside the Operating Room, 41
Conclusion, 42

6 Critical Monitoring Issues for Non–Operating Room Anesthesia, 43
JOHN P. SCOTT

Basic Monitors, 43
Temperature, 45
Advanced Monitors, 46
Site-Specific Monitoring Considerations, 47
Conclusion, 48

7 Intravenous Anesthesia and Sedation Outside the Operating Room, 50
ANIL GUPTA and JOHAN RAEDER

Sedation, Sedation and Analgesia, and Anesthesia, 51
Drugs Used for Sedation and Anesthesia, 52
Monitoring During Total Intravenous Anesthesia and Analgesia, 56

Side Effects and Complications, 56
Recovery and Discharge, 57
Total Intravenous Anesthesia for Specific
  Patients, 58
Conclusion, 59

SECTION 3 PRACTICES
AND PRINCIPLES, 61

8 *Practice Procedure,* 62
ERIC A. HARRIS

Patient Selection, 62
Pitfalls of Non–Operating Room Anesthesia, 63
Risks and Safety of Non–Operating Room
  Anesthesia, 65
The Future of Non–Operating Room Anesthesia, 67

9 *Preoperative Evaluations,* 70
JENNIFER E. HOFER, MELISSA L. PANT and BOBBIEJEAN SWEITZER

Preoperative Assessment, 70
Coexisting Diseases, 73
Preoperative Testing, 78
Perioperative Medications, 78
Fasting Guidelines, 80
Conclusion, 80

10 *Anesthesia in the Catheterization Laboratory:
Valves and Devices,* 82
JACK S. SHANEWISE

Hemodynamic Monitoring, 82
Transcatheter Aortic Valve Replacement, 83
Transcatheter Aortic Valve Replacement Procedural
  Complications, 85
Transapical Closure of Mitral Prosthesis Paravalular
  Regurgitation, 87
Left Atrial Appendage Closure Device, 88
Mitral Valve Edge-to-Edge Clip Repair, 88
Conclusion, 88

11 *Anesthesia for Electrophysiology Procedures,* 91
JONATHAN W. TANNER, ROGER A. MOORE, and MARK S. WEISS

Role of the Anesthesiologist in the Electrophysiology
  Laboratory, 91
Considerations in the Electrophysiology
  Laboratory, 92
The Physiology of Cardiac Arrhythmias, 100
Catheter-Based Ablations, 102
Device Implantation, 107
Lead Extractions, 108
Noninvasive Programmed Stimulation, 109
Postoperative Care and Pain Management, 109
Conclusion, 110

12 *Anesthesia for Cardioversion,* 113
MAX KANEVSKY

Preoperative Assessment, 113
Intraoperative Management, 114
Postoperative Course, 115
Conclusion, 115

13 *High-Frequency Ventilation for Respiratory
Immobilization,* 117
JEFF E. MANDEL

Uses of High-Frequency Ventilation for Respiratory
  Immobilization, 117
Types of Ventilators, 118
Physics of High-Frequency Jet Ventilation, 121
Entrainment, 121
Carbon Dioxide Elimination, 122
Breath Stacking, 122
Monitoring of High-Frequency Jet Ventilation, 123
Humidification of Inspired Gas, 124
Hemodynamic Effects of High-Frequency Jet
  Ventilation, 124
The Physiology of Apnea, 124
Anesthetic Management, 124
Future Directions, 124

14 *Anesthesia for Upper Gastrointestinal
Endoscopy,* 126
BASAVANA G. GOUDRA, JONATHAN W. TANNER, PREET MOHINDER
SINGH, and GREGORY G. GINSBERG

Patient Populations Presenting for Upper
  Gastrointestinal Endoscopic Procedures, 126
Preprocedure Evaluation, 126
Anesthetic Drugs for Gastrointestinal
  Endoscopy, 127
Airway Management, 128
Conduct of Anesthesia for Upper Gastrointestinal
  Endoscopy, 129
Monitoring, 130
Complications, 130
Future, 130

15 *Anesthesia for Colonoscopy,* 132
ESTHER D. GARAZI, CHRISTOPHER D. PRESS, and PEDRO P. TANAKA

History of Anesthesia for Gastrointestinal
  Endoscopic Procedures, 132
General Considerations, 132
Complications, 135
Conclusion, 135

16 *Anesthesia in the Bronchoscopy Suite,* 137
MARK A. LEIBEL, W. KIRKE ROGERS, and RICHARD E. GALGON

Interventional Bronchoscopic Techniques, 137
Preoperative Evaluation, 139
Management of Anesthesia: Pharmacology, 140
General Anesthesia, 142

Management of Anesthesia: Airway Choice,   143
Management of Anesthesia: Oxygenation and
    Ventilation,   145
Management of Anesthesia: Other
    Considerations,   146
Management of Complications,   147
Conclusion,   148

17 *Adult Anesthesia in the Radiology Suite,*   151
DANIEL RUBIN and THOMAS CUTTER

Radiopaque Contrast,   151
Radiation Safety,   152
General Considerations,   153
Visceral Procedures,   154
Vascular Procedures,   155
Neurological Procedures,   156

18 *Pediatric Anesthesia in the Radiology Suite,*   161
CHRISTINA D. DIAZ and ROSE CAMPISE-LUTHER

Pediatric Anesthesia in Remote Locations,   161
Preoperative Considerations,   161
Specific Areas of Radiology Procedures,   164
Conclusion,   169

19 *Anesthesia Concerns in the Magnetic Resonance
Imaging Environment,*   171
RAMON MARTIN

Training and Personnel,   171
The Magnetic Resonance Imaging Suite,   171
Patient Selection,   172
Remote Monitoring,   172
Devices in Magnetic Resonance Imaging,   172
Anesthetic Concerns With Computerized Axial
    Tomography,   174
Remote Monitoring,   174
Bore of the Computed Tomography,   174
Contrast Dye Anaphylactic Response,   174
Summary,   174

SECTION 4 FINANCIAL CONSIDERATIONS,   177

20 *Scheduling Anesthesia Services Outside
the Operating Room,*   178
RAMON MARTIN

Associated Background Issues,   178
Knowledge of the Procedure,   179
The Schedule,   179
Summary,   182

21 *Financial and Operational Analysis
for Non–Operating Room Anesthesia,*   183
CAITLIN J. GUO and ALEX MACARIO

Market Analysis,   183
Competitive Landscape,   184
Comparative Advantages,   185
Financial Considerations,   185
An Example Analysis,   186
Operational Infrastructure,   187
Conclusion,   189

22 *Anesthesia and Competitive Strategies,*   190
JOHN M. TRUMMEL and SOPHIA VAN HOFF

Practice Patterns in Non–Operating Room
    Sedation,   190
Propofol Use by Nonanesthesiologists,   191
Safety of Propofol in the Non–Operating Room
    Setting,   192
Economic Considerations,   194
Policy Considerations and Guidelines for the
    Use of Propofol,   195
Moderate Sedation,   196
Other Modalities,   196
Conclusion,   197

SECTION 5 THE FUTURE OF NON–OPERATING ROOM ANESTHESIA,   199

23 *Development of Future Systems,*   200
LARRY LINDENBAUM

Evolution of Automated or Computer-Assisted
    Systems,   201
Conclusion,   203

24 *Novel Staffing Coverage for Anesthesia Outside
the Operating Room,*   205
MARY ELLEN WARNER, LINDSAY L. WARNER, and
NAFISSEH S. WARNER

Complexity as the Norm,   205
Personnel for Anesthesia Services,   206
How are Practice Models Determined?   207
Novel Anesthesia Models for Outside the Operating
    Room,   208
Conclusion,   209

*Appendix: Relevant American Society
    of Anesthesiologists Guidelines,*   211

Index,   247

Downloadable File Contents

CHAPTER 1

Table 1-1: Non–Operating Room Anesthesia Safety Checklist

Box 1-1: Sample Protocol for Cardioversion with Non–Operating Room Anesthesia

CHAPTER 2

Table 2-1: Minimum Size of Non–Operating Room Anesthesia Site

Table 2-2: Minimum Number of Outlets Recommended in Various Hospital Locations

Table 2-3: Magnetic Resonance Imaging Suite Zones

Table 2-4: Timeline for Design and Implementation of a Non–Operating Room Anesthesia Site

CHAPTER 3

Figure 3-1: American Society of Anesthesiologists Statement on Nonoperating Room Anesthetizing Locations.

Table 3-1: Magnetic Resonance Suite Zones

Box 3-2: Airway Supplies Checklist

Box 3-3: Safety Considerations in Non– Operating Room Anesthetizing Locations

Box 3-4: Treatment of Anaphylaxis and Anaphylactoid Reactions

CHAPTER 5

Table 5-1: Quality Improvement Checklist for Locations Other Than the Operating Room

Figure 5-1: Continuous quality improvement (CQI) process uses a plan-do-study-act approach.

Table 5-2: Anesthesia Quality Institute Recommended Quality Indicators

Figure 5-2: Postanesthesia care patient satisfaction survey.

CHAPTER 6

Table 6-1: Continuum of Depth of Sedation: Definition of General Anesthesia and Levels of Sedation and Analgesia

Table 6-2: American Society of Anesthesiologists Physical Status Classification

CHAPTER 7

Table 7-1: American Society of Anesthesiologists Definitions of General Anesthesia and Levels of Sedation and Analgesia

Table 7-2: Ramsay Sedation Scale

Table 7-3: Modified Observer's Assessment of Alertness/Sedation Scale

Table 7-4: Propofol and/or Remifentanil Sedation Doses

Table 7-5: Modified Aldrete Scoring System

Table 7-6: Post-Anesthetic Discharge Scoring System

CHAPTER 9

Table 9-1: American Society of Anesthesiologists Physical Status Classification

Figure 9-1: Patient medical history

Table 9-2: Metabolic Equivalents of Functional Capacity Measured 1 Through 12

Box 9-1: Elements of the Airway Examination

Figure 9-2: Cardiac evaluation algorithm.

Box 9-2: Cardiac Conditions for Which Endocarditis Prophylaxis Is Indicated

Box 9-3: Endocarditis Prophylaxis Indications

Box 9-4: Summary of Recommendations from the 2007 Science Advisory and the 2007 American College of Cardiology and American Heart Association

Box 9-5: Potential Problems with Cardiovascular Implantable Electronic Devices During Surgical Procedures

Table 9-3: Preoperative Testing Guidelines for Procedures Performed Outside the Operating Room

Figure 9-3: STOP BANG questionnaire.

Box 9-6: Preoperative Medication Management

CHAPTER 10

Figure 10-4: Key anesthesia elements for transcatheter aortic valve replacement.

CHAPTER 11

Table 11-1: Common Electrophysiology Cases and Estimated Anesthesia Times

Box 11-1: Air Bubble Precautions With Right-to-Left Shunting of Blood

Table 11-2: Drugs Commonly Used in Electrophysiology Procedures

Box 11-2: Common Bradyarrhythmias and Tachyarrhythmias

Protocol for Anesthesia for Ablation of Atrial Fibrillation

Table 11-3: Potential Complications of Catheter Ablation of Atrial Fibrillation

Protocol for Anesthesia for Defibrillator Implantation

Protocol for Anesthesia for Lead Extraction

Protocol for Anesthesia for Noninvasive Programmed Stimulations

CHAPTER 13

Figure 13-8: Axial dispersion of gas in an airway.

Figure 13-9: When two adjacent lung units are ventilated at high rates, flow is dominated by resistance.

Figure 13-10: The Venturi effect

Figure 13-11: Entrainment

Figure 13-12: Thoracic volume measured by respiratory inductance plethysmography under high-frequency jet ventilation.

CHAPTER 14

Table 14-1: Comparison of Drugs for Anesthesia for Upper Gastrointestinal Endoscopy

Box 14-1: Common Indications for Upper Gastrointestinal Endoscopy Procedures

Box 14-2: Complications Related to Sedation for Upper Gastrointestinal Endoscopy

CHAPTER 15

Box 15-1: Guidelines for Anesthesiology Assistance During Gastrointestinal Endoscopy

Table 15-1: Continuum of Depth of Sedation

Box 15-2: Predictors of Difficult Mask Ventilation and Difficult Intubation

Table 15-2: Favorable Sedative Effect Profile of Common Sedative Agents

CHAPTER 16

Table 16-1: Anesthesia for Interventional Bronchoscopic Techniques

Box 16-1: Desirable Qualities for Supraglottic Airways To Be Used During Flexible Bronchoscopy

Box 16-2: Undesirable Qualities for Supraglottic Airways To Be Used During Flexible Bronchoscopy

Table 16-2: Characteristics of Common Supraglottic Airways Deemed Adequate for Use During Diagnostic and Therapeutic Flexible Bronchoscopy

Box 16-3: Emergency Cricothyroidotomy

CHAPTER 17

Box 17-1: Classification of Severity of Reactions to Contrast Media

Figure 17-1: Distribution of scatter radiation from a lateral C-arm with the radiation source on the same side as the anesthesiologist.

CHAPTER 18

Table 18-1: Normal Range of Vital Signs in the Pediatric Patient

Table 18-2: Endotracheal Tube Sizes

Table 18-3: American Society of Anesthesiologists Nil Per Os Guidelines

Table 18-4: Common Hypnotic Drugs, Dosages, Duration, and Properties

Box 18-1: Pediatric Anesthesia Preoperative Checklist for Outside the Operating Room

Box 18-2: Joint Commission Sentinel Event Alert: Preventing Accidents and Injuries in the MRI Suite

Box 18-3: Magnetic Resonance Imaging Checklist

Box 18-4: Computed Tomography Checklist

Box 18-5: Radiation Therapy Checklist

Box 18-6: Interventional Radiology Checklist

Box 18-7: Nuclear Medicine Checklist

Box 18-8: Magnetoencephalography Scan Checklist

CHAPTER 19

Table 19-1: Magnetic Resonance Imaging Zones

Table 19-2: Degrees of Deflection and Force for Commonly Used Devices

CHAPTER 20

Table 20-1: Daily Schedule of Coverage for Outside the Operating Room

Figure 20-1: Anesthesia services agreement for outside the operating room.

CHAPTER 21

Figure 21-1: Chart of population 65 years of age and over by age: 1900 to 2050.

Table 21-1: Predicted Anesthesia Professional Participation Rates (%) for Colonoscopy and Esophagogastroduodenoscopy by Year

Figure 21-2: Total cost as a function of volume, including fixed and variable costs.

Figure 21-3: Cost volume profit analysis.

Figure 21-4: Cost volume analysis for variable coverage.

Figure 21-5: Underused hours reflect how early the room finishes.

Table 21-2: Sample Weekly Schedule for Procedures Outside the Operating Room

CHAPTER 22

Table 22-1: Continuum of Depth of Sedation: Definition of General Anesthesia and Levels of Sedation and Analgesia

CHAPTER 24

Box 24-1: Agreements and Arrangements Necessary for Procedures and Anesthesia Services Outside the Operating Room

Box 24-2: Potential Triage Criteria in a Gastroenterological Endoscopy Center Using a Nurse Sedation Model

Preparation for Non–Operating Room Activities

SECTION OUTLINE

1 *Engineering Excellence in Non–Operating Room Anesthesia Care*

2 *Designing Safety and Engineering Standards for the Non–Operating Room Anesthesia Procedure Site*

3 *Room Setup, Critical Supplies, and Medications*

4 *The Role of the Non–Operating Room Anesthesiologist*

1 Engineering Excellence in Non–Operating Room Anesthesia Care

MEGHAN LANE-FALL and MARK S. WEISS

The past two decades have seen advances in medical technology that now allow physicians to treat a patient with noninvasive or minimally invasive procedures. Patients who would have been subjected to sternotomy, thoracotomy, major vascular surgery, or laparotomy just a few years ago may now be treated more effectively, more economically, and more comfortably by nonsurgical intervention in specialized areas outside of the operating room. These procedures are changing medicine, and the specialty is learning to change with it. Anesthesia cases occurring in non–operating room locations make up approximately 30% of all cases in the Department of Anesthesiology and Critical Care at the University of Pennsylvania, following a nationwide trend.[1]

Indeed, we are witnessing the development of a new subspecialty: Non–Operating Room Anesthesia (NORA). NORA cases are frequently challenging procedures that involve compromised patients deemed poor candidates for more invasive procedures. NORA cases may additionally involve sharing, or sometimes ceding, the airway to the proceduralist, as in interventional pulmonology. In the NORA procedure room, both people and the airway are managed. NORA practitioners are ideally able to manage a high volume of rapid-turnover cases and attend to the needs of patients, proceduralists, and staff.

In NORA settings, the room, the procedure, and the staff are all highly specialized to perform a specific task. The locations where these procedures are done are often designed for a specific subspecialty, such as gastroenterology or electrophysiology; anesthesia services are sometimes an afterthought, although incorporating plans for anesthesia services is occurring more frequently as new space is developed. In contrast, operating rooms are generally designed to accommodate a variety of case types, with interchangeable staff. Staff roles such as the circulating nurse or scrub technician are usually quite structured. Such standardization leads to a consistency that produces an acceptable level of care at minimum and a standard of excellence at best. The same standardization is not necessarily present in the NORA room, which may compromise the provided quality of care.

If NORA rooms are not held to the same set of standards as the operating room, how do you provide consistently superior care? Consistent success in NORA, as in the operating room, may be achieved by adhering to the structural and organizational standards addressed in this and other chapters. This chapter will focus on the organizational aspects of designing—or engineering—excellence in NORA. Such aspects include protocols, checklists, communication during the procedure and during transfer of patient care, quality improvement methods, and continuing education. The following chapters will discuss structural aspects of engineering safety in the physical plant, where seemingly mundane questions such as "Where does the anesthesia machine go?" or "How many electrical outlets are needed?" become very important when designing a NORA area.

The deliberate pursuit of excellence in NORA is important because this venue represents the future of anesthesia. Complex procedures on sicker patients, many of which would be canceled or postponed in a traditional operating room setting, will become more common. It is important to hold remote NORA locations to the same high standards of quality as those of the operating room. Engineering a high standard of excellence will lead to the ultimate goal—improvements in both quality and safety for the patient receiving NORA.

Achieving Excellence in Health Care

The seminal report in 2000 by the Institute of Medicine (IOM) titled *To Err is Human: Building a Safer Health System* sparked the modern movement to improve patient safety and increase health care quality.[2] One year later, the IOM published *Crossing the Quality Chasm: A New Health System for the 21st Century*, in which six aims for health care improvement are advanced. According to the report, care should be safe, effective, patient-centered, timely, efficient, and equitable.[3] Cases in NORA settings are well poised to meet these goals, because shorter, less-invasive procedures may enable more rapid discharge and return to preprocedure function.

Nevertheless, it is important to consider how NORA systems may be engineered to optimize the likelihood of desirable patient outcomes. This chapter explores proactive and reactive approaches to operating in high-stress, high-stakes environments. To explore proactive systems design, we draw examples from medical and nonmedical settings. As part of this discussion, we consider organizational structures that promote safe care and effective communication among teams. Next, we present several protocols that have been useful in guiding NORA care at our institution.

Even though effective organizations take steps to prevent adverse incidents, problematic events still occur. It is therefore vital that organizations have a defined approach to reacting to adverse events, including errors and near-misses. We consider how anesthesia and perioperative providers respond to these events within NORA settings and describe how to use these opportunities to improve care.

Proactive Versus Reactive Approach to Problems

It is imperative that individuals and organizations engaged in high-risk activities develop an approach to dealing with problems, including errors, near-misses, and adverse events. Health care has historically taken a reactive stance to problems by waiting to enact fixes until a pattern of adverse events such as wrong-side surgeries, medication errors, and health care–associated infections emerges. Health care organizations are learning how to anticipate reasonably expected problems, which allows them to engineer systems to avoid a bad outcome before it can happen. We first describe the discipline of human factors engineering, explaining how principles from this field can inform perioperative systems design. Next, we explore the rise of protocols and checklists in perioperative medicine and discuss how these tools can prevent adverse events.

Proactive Approaches: Anticipating Problems

HUMAN FACTORS ENGINEERING

Human factors engineering (HFE; also known as human factors and ergonomics) is a discipline that considers individuals' physical and mental/cognitive limitations in task development and evaluation. The use of color-coding, such as yellow-striped epidural infusion tubing, and pin-index safety systems are two examples of HFE applied to the respective problems of inadvertent medication administration and medical gas mix-ups.

HFE is especially important in the selection of devices employed in clinical care. Undesirable device features may prompt users to create workarounds that compromise safety features. Poorly designed user interfaces can predispose to malfunction or error. Lin et al[4] showed patient-controlled analgesia pumps with cumbersome interfaces contributed to adverse events, including overdose. In NORA settings, devices are used by practitioners from multiple disciplines. The training, needs, and expectations of these users should be considered in the selection of monitors, drug-dispensing systems, airway support equipment, and other shared devices.

PROTOCOLS AND CHECKLISTS

Despite concerns about diminishing clinical autonomy and the rise of "cookbook medicine," robust evidence demonstrates that the use of protocols and checklists in certain clinical settings decreases error and improves clinical outcomes. Perhaps the most well-known recent example is the work done by Atul Gawande and the Safe Surgery Saves Lives study group that used presurgical checklists to standardize care and serve as a safety check (an example is provided in Table 1-1).[5] This group demonstrated that use of checklists was associated with decreased morbidity and mortality in eight international hospitals. Peter Pronovost's work[6] has similarly demonstrated a decrease in complications—specifically, central line–associated bloodstream infections—when checklists are used before central line insertion. Use of a daily goals sheet in the intensive care unit improved health care team communication and decreased length of stay.[7]

Table 1-1   Non–Operating Room Anesthesia Safety Checklist

Before Induction of Anesthesia	Before Procedure Start	Before Patient Leaves Procedure Room
Has the patient confirmed his or her identity, site (if applicable), procedure, and consent? □ Yes	Confirm all team members have introduced themselves by name and role.	Nurse verbally confirms: The name of the procedure Completion of instrument counts (if applicable) Specimen labeling (read specimen labels aloud, including patient name) Whether any equipment problems need to be addressed
Is the site marked? □ Yes □ Not applicable	Confirm the patient's name and procedure	
Is the anesthesia machine and medication check complete? □ Yes	Has antibiotic prophylaxis been given within the last 60 minutes? □ Yes □ Not applicable	To the proceduralist, anesthetist and nurse: What are the key concerns for recovery and management for this patient?
Does the patient have a: Known allergy? □ No □ Yes Difficult airway or aspiration risk? □ No □ Yes, and equipment and assistance are available Risk for >500 mL blood loss (7 mL/kg in children)? □ No □ Yes, and two intravenous lines or central access and fluids planned	Anticipated critical events: To proceduralist: What are the critical or nonroutine steps? How long will the case take? What is the anticipated blood loss? To anesthetist: Are there any patient-specific concerns? To nursing team: Has sterility (including indicator results) been confirmed? Are there any equipment issues or concerns?	
Is the pulse oximeter on the patient and functioning? □ Yes	Is essential imaging displayed? □ Yes □ Not applicable	

Modified from World Health Organization Safe Surgery Saves Lives Surgical Safety Checklist. http://www.who.int/patientsafety/safesurgery/en/.

Protocols and guidelines can be especially helpful in infrequently encountered situations. In our institution, a core group of anesthesiologists provides care for patients receiving NORA. However, it is common for NORA locations to be staffed by someone who is not in this core group during evenings and weekends. Guidelines for particular NORA settings, such as for endoscopy and electrophysiology, were designed to ensure uniformity of care (Box 1-1). Ideally, protocols provide guidance without unnecessarily constricting providers' ability to customize care plans for individual patients.

It is important to note that safety gains seen with checklist or protocol implementation are not always uniform. In any organization, cultural interactions (e.g., the relationship and reporting structures of the various providers) are present that determine how effectively any intervention is executed. Identifying champions of and potential barriers to implementation are important first steps in adopting changes in practice, including protocols.[8]

HEALTH CARE FAILURE MODE AND EFFECT ANALYSIS

In engineering, failure mode and effect analysis (FMEA) is used to examine error-prone processes, allowing identification and prioritization of "failure modes"—situations in which errors can be expected to occur. FMEA was adapted by the U.S. Department of Veteran Affairs for application to health care, which resulted in the creation of health care FMEA (HFMEA).[9] Medication administration and blood

transfusion are two processes that have been deconstructed using the HFMEA approach.

HFMEA is a rigorous multistep process, as follows:

1. Define the topic
2. Assemble a multidisciplinary team
3. Graphically describe (map) the process
4. Define failure modes
5. Analyze hazards (including assignment of severity and probability scores)
6. Make recommendations, define action steps, and determine outcome measures

The HFMEA process as originally described requires significant time and engagement from all involved participants. At least eight meetings are suggested in the original paper,[9] with five of them devoted to the definition of failure modes and analysis of hazards.

In 2010, Nagpal et al[10] published a report of HFMEA applied to communication during the perioperative period. Excluding the intraoperative phase, the team found four major steps subject to information transfer and communication errors:

1. Preoperative assessment and optimization
2. Transfer and preprocedural teamwork
3. Postoperative handoff
4. Daily ward care

Each of these steps was divided into subprocesses, and each subprocess had one or more failure modes, specific manners in which failure occurs. For example, preoperative assessment

---

Box 1-1   Sample Protocol for Cardioversion with Non–Operating Room Anesthesia

1. Evaluate the patient for anesthesia (airway, cardiac function, allergies, etc.) and fill out the anesthesia assessment form.
2. Verify patient identity and procedure.
3. Make sure consent for the procedure and anesthesia have been obtained.
4. Check NPO status (solids 6 hours, clear liquids 2 hours). If not NPO, discuss with the cardiologist whether the risk for aspiration is outweighed by the risk for postponing the cardioversion. If not, postpone until patient status is NPO; if so, proceed with the head of the bed elevated and apply cricoid pressure while the patient is unconscious and consider succinylcholine and intubation.
5. Place routine monitors.
   a. Electrocardiogram: If sinus rhythm is observed, cancel the procedure.
   b. Pulse oximeter: Make it audible.
   c. Blood pressure: Place cuff on limb that does not have intravenous line or pulse oximeter and start automatic measurement every minute.
6. Make sure patient has a free-flowing intravenous line.
7. Make sure necessary supplies are available.
   a. Yankauer suction
   b. Airway supplies (bring a "tackle box" from the electrophysiology anesthesia workroom; a list of suggested contents is taped inside the lid).
   c. Emergency medications (including epinephrine, atropine, succinylcholine, phenylephrine, and ephedrine)
8. Denitrogenate the patient with 100% oxygen mask and bag.

9. If using a non–central venous line, pretreat the vein with 1 mg/kg IV lidocaine* unless the patient is allergic to it.
10. If the patient is allergic to propofol, soybeans, or eggs or has a left ventricular ejection fraction <25%, induce with etomidate 0.1 mg/kg IV; otherwise, use propofol 1 mg/kg IV.
11. If the patient becomes hypotensive, notify the cardiologist, consider intravenous fluid and phenylephrine, and use etomidate rather than further propofol.
12. If the patient responds to tapping his or her forehead or shouting his or her name, tell the patient to take deep breaths, then give propofol 0.4 mg/kg or etomidate 0.04 mg/kg and reassess.
13. Check for loss of eyelash reflex; if not, give propofol 0.4 mg/kg or etomidate 0.04 mg/kg and reassess.
14. Support the patient's airway as needed.
15. Tell the cardiologist that he or she may proceed.
16. Check for pulse and check blood pressure.
17. If the patient is bradycardic, ask the cardiologist if he or she wants you to administer atropine.
18. If cardioversion is unsuccessful, ask the cardiologist if he/she will attempt again. If so, go back to step 11.
19. Check that the patient moves all extremities on command when awake.
20. Give report to the cardiology nurse.
21. Be sure that the front pages of the anesthesia record and of the anesthesia assessment form get on the patient's chart.
22. Return the "tackle box" to the EP anesthesia workroom, and do not leave medications, syringes, or needles lying around.

*See also Davis, MF. Lidocaine for the prevention of pain due to injection of propofol. *Anesth Analg* 74:246-249, 1992; based on 2013 protocol at the Hospital of the University of Pennsylvania.
IV, Intravenously; *NPO,* nil per os (nothing by mouth).

and optimization had 12 subprocesses, including "request and check radiological investigations" (five failure modes) and "prescribe medications and bowel preparation" (nine failure modes). Assigning severity and probability scores to the 132 failure modes within the four steps and 29 subprocesses enabled the team to prioritize 41 of the failure modes as high risk. For example, two high-risk failure modes within the subprocess "check special investigation results" (e.g., echocardiography or pulmonary function test) were noted as "checked investigation results but action not taken" and "checked investigation results but action delayed." High-risk failure modes were further evaluated by using decision trees to determine each mode's criticality and deciding whether adequate control measures were in place. Those modes deemed critical that "did not have effective control measures in place and [were] not easily detectable were prioritized for further action."[10]

The use of the full HFMEA approach has been called into question because it is so time-consuming.[11] However, time invested in process mapping and exploring failure modes before incidents occur may ultimately save time and money and prevent harm to patients in the long run.

THE DAILY HUDDLE

Throughout the day in the NORA room, rapidly changing short cases with challenging patients are seen. This requires clear communication among the staff to facilitate the room order, tend to the needs of individual procedures, and address patient care issues. A proactive preoperative measure incorporating both human factors principles and protocols is the preoperative briefing, also known as a "huddle." The huddle may take place before the day's schedule begins, before individual cases, or after induction of anesthesia.[12] Patient cases are reviewed by the attending anesthesia staff, proceduralists, and nursing staff. At any time during the huddle, a team member may inform the group about special needs or concerns, such as transportation, specialized equipment, or staffing issues that may require advance arrangements to maintain the efficiency of room flow.

The daily huddle is a scheduled meeting, but it is also important to meet periodically and review progress or problem areas of mutual concern to the health care team. Such meetings are appropriate at regularly scheduled intervals to review issues that arise, such as staffing, continuing education, scheduling, or supply logistics. It is also appropriate to meet after a particularly difficult patient or unsatisfactory outcome to review process and procedures, in a constructive and nonthreatening manner, so that the actions that led to a particular outcome can be analyzed and lessons can be learned from these situations. The goal of these meetings is the same—to freely share information that will enable NORA team members to perform their jobs better, which ultimately leads to improved care of the patient.

Reactive Approaches: What Happens When Something Goes Wrong

Adverse events may still occur despite health care organizations designing systems to anticipate and prevent them.

In this circumstance, it is also important to have a system capable of responding to adverse events, understanding why they occurred, and trying to prevent them from recurring. In this section, we describe various approaches to dealing with adverse events.

BACKUP CLINICAL SUPPORT

Poor outcomes from unrecognized clinical deterioration prompted hospitals to develop rapid response teams (RRTs; also known as medical emergency teams). These teams are meant to respond to patients experiencing some form of physiological compromise, such as respiratory distress or hemodynamic instability. Use of RRTs has been shown to decrease rates of cardiac arrest and improve patient outcomes.[15]

What is the role of RRTs in NORA settings? NORA locations commonly have both anesthetist-staffed cases and those in which moderate, or "conscious," sedation is administered. Patients receiving moderate sedation at times become deeply sedated or transition into general anesthesia with subsequent ineffective respiration or hemodynamic compromise. Anesthetists may be available for rescue, but RRTs may serve as a backup system if an anesthesia practitioner is not immediately available.

PROVISION FOR UNPLANNED ADMISSION

Many patients receiving NORA are undergoing outpatient procedures, but procedural findings or complications occasionally necessitate hospital admission. Different considerations apply when NORA is administered in free-standing nonhospital facilities versus in a hospital, but provisions must be made in either case for dealing with unplanned admissions. Proceduralists and NORA staff should develop protocols or guidelines for dealing with unplanned admissions, accounting for transport and monitoring needs.

EVENT REPORTING SYSTEMS

Requirements differ across states on adverse events in health care that may be subject to mandatory reporting. In addition to mandatory reporting, many health care organizations have voluntary reporting systems that allow them to collect information about adverse events, near-misses, problems with professionalism, or other issues of interest to facility administrators. These reporting systems may be anonymous or confidential. Although staff should be encouraged to discuss adverse events with their supervisors, event report systems allow staff to report systems problems they may not want to discuss. Staff sometimes fear retaliation for a real or perceived error, and these reporting systems may allow the capture of events that would otherwise go undetected. Underreporting may occur even when event reporting systems are in place, because of lack of staff familiarity with the systems or fear of retaliation.

ROOT CAUSE ANALYSIS

Root cause analysis (RCA) is a tool used to examine why a particular adverse event occurred. A fundamental principle underlying RCA is that every adverse event has multiple causes. In James Reason's "Swiss Cheese" model of error,

needs and preferences. One aspect to consider is a second set of outlets in addition to the set for the interventionalist for different room setups and future needs, because adding or changing outlet locations in the future is costly.[8] The gas delivery method should be chosen as early as possible in the design process because the locations of outlets can be dictated by room infrastructure and ventilation equipment.[8]

In addition to the ASA identified ergonomic considerations, infrastructure, including ventilation and materials management, should be addressed in the planning phase of NORA room design.

Ventilation

Along with temperature control, which has already been discussed, room ventilation also includes control of humidity, anesthetic gases, and physical and microbiological pollutants that need to be adequately regulated.[6] Development and organization of ventilation should be guided by specifications from multiple institutions, including the National Institute for Occupational Safety and Health (NIOSH), ASHRAE (American Society of Heating, Refrigerating and Air Conditioning Engineers), Centers for Disease Control and Prevention (CDC), and American Institute of Architects (AIA).[6] The ASA has specific guidelines on these topics in design of a traditional operating room, but not specifically in NORA sites. A conservative design should maintain operating room standards in NORA sites. The design team should refer to local and regional standards for specific requirements.

NORA sites can be ventilated via a recirculating or nonrecirculating system or a combination of the two.[6] Inside air is recirculated back into the NORA site in a recirculating system. If all air brought to the inside of a NORA site is outside air, then it is a non-recirculating system. If a recirculating system is used, a high-efficiency particulate air (HEPA) filter should be built into the air return duct[6]; it can remove 99.97% of all particles larger than 0.3 μm from the air that passes through.[15] To limit exposure of NORA site personnel to waste anesthetic gases and leaks from anesthesia delivery or scavenging systems, NIOSH and the CDC recommend that the ventilation system change air in the operating room at least 15 times, with a minimum of three fresh air changes per hour.[8]

Careful humidity control in NORA sites is important. Too much humidity results in uncomfortable conditions for both the patient and staff, and too little humidity leads to increased evaporation from the body, potential loss of body heat, and damage to the respiratory tract.[6] ASHRAE states operating room humidity should be between 30% and 60%.[2] To have precise control over temperature and humidity, the ASA recommends that a facility have a heating and cooling system with a single-point control system specifically designed and made for operating rooms and that is routinely calibrated.[6]

Proper infection control depends on appropriate room ventilation, because flora from the patient and staff are distributed as airborne particles.[6] The particles dilute as air flows through the room, but this turbulent flow increases the spread of the particles throughout the room; thus lowvelocity, positive-pressure flow with a HEPA filtration system minimizes airborne particles throughout the room.[6]

The AIA operating room standard for air flow is use of a nonaspirating diffuser, also known as a unidirectional flow diffuser, in which air flows with very low velocity unidirectionally downward from the ceiling, with minimal entrainment of room air, over the patient and the interventional team.[2] The air is then returned through low sidewall grills approximately 8 inches above the room floor.[2] The goal is to provide for steady flow of clean air throughout the room.[2]

Materials Management

Thought should be given to the materials chosen for NORA sites in the beginning stages of planning and budgeting because they can affect space needs (e.g., use of rolling carts versus equipment booms, a compact mobile anesthesia machine versus one that remains in the NORA site, an interventional table or bed that is fixed to the floor versus a mobile one). High-quality equipment may be initially expensive, but it may be more efficient over the long term.[3] As much storage space as possible should be incorporated in the NORA site because efficiency is lost if personnel constantly have to leave the area to get supplies. Built-in storage space is preferred, but it should be determined on individual needs and budget.

As in operating rooms, the floors, walls, and ceilings in NORA sites should be seamless because maintaining an easily cleanable environment demands hard surfaces throughout. Operating room walls with tiles are now becoming obsolete; the trend is to have stainless-steel sheets extending up 42 to 48 inches from the floor to protect the wall from impact from rolling equipment, although this can be difficult in MRI locations. Unlike in private dwellings, the floor and walls should not meet at right angles because this is difficult to clean; instead, the floor material should extend up the wall for 4 to 6 inches.[3] Openings for ventilation, medical gases, and lighting in a ceiling must be gasketed.[2] TJC and individual state departments of health should be consulted on regional requirements.

Individual Non–Operating Room Anesthesia Sites

The specific NORA sites of radiation therapy, MRI, and hybrid operating rooms will be discussed because these areas have specific attributes that affect room design.

RADIATION THERAPY

Radiation therapy areas are often very far from the main operating room because of the use of strong radiation; therefore a dedicated area for preparation and recovery of patients requiring anesthesia services should be available.[12] Fixed equipment and rotating treatment arms may impede on ease of management of ventilator tubing, lines, and cords, and a slightly larger area may be considered to allow for easy turning of beds and patient access. High-dose radiation precludes the continual presence of anesthesia personnel at bedside; thus a clear view and monitoring capabilities from the control room needs to be implemented in design of this area.[12] Noise may interfere with audio monitoring of pulse and saturation monitors, and thus remote monitoring may be needed. A clear path to the patient, free of equipment and cables, is recommended in the event of an emergency. Radiation protection is needed in these areas, and room designs should prevent the escape of radioactive photons and neutrons to other areas of the facility. This is ensured by baffling all openings into the room such as doors, ducts, and other penetrations.[2]

MAGNETIC RESONANCE IMAGING

The MRI suite poses significant challenges for the anesthesiologist because of the presence of the strong magnetic field. Patient access and adequate monitoring may be severely limited by noise from the magnet and the shape and structure of the magnet.[13] The ASA has guidelines for anesthetic care in MRI that can help direct room design[13]:

1. The line of sight must be clear to the patient and monitors (direct observation or a video camera), in either zone III or zone IV.
2. Anesthetic delivery equipment should be located in a place where there is easy control of anesthesia depth. If an MRI-safe anesthesia machine is not available, inhalational anesthetics may be administered from an anesthesia machine located in zone III using an elongated circuit through a wave guide, or if a total intravenous anesthetic is used, it can be administered by using an MRI-safe pump located in zone IV or an MRI-unsafe pump in zone III with the tubing passed through a wave guide. Finally, intermittent intravenous anesthetic bolus injections from zone III or zone IV can be administered.

3. Easy access to hospital information systems should be available.
4. Access to emergency communication (phone or code button) should be readily available.
5. An evacuation plan should be in place in the event of a quench or medical emergency, with a designated location outside zone IV with accessible monitors, oxygen, suction, and resuscitation equipment.
6. Complex airway management should be performed outside of zone IV in a controlled environment.
7. Alternative airway devices should be available in the MRI suite.
8. Suction should be immediately available.
9. A recovery area should be available for patients who received anesthesia services.

When planning and designing an MRI suite, the anesthesiologist should confer with the facility biomedical engineer to determine the best location of anesthesia equipment in terms of safety and accessibility in relation to gauss lines within the MRI suite.[12] Locations of gauss lines indicating the magnitude of the magnetic field in zone IV that are clearly marked throughout the room are an extra visual safety cue for personnel (Figure 2-1). These lines aid in safely positioning essential patient equipment when in use and also can help early in the design process in planning where to place medical gas, vacuum, and WAGD outlets.[12]

The MRI suite should be organized into four zones with each zone designed for different functions: patient interviews, physical examinations and changing areas, ferromagnetic detection systems, access control, and site-specific clinical

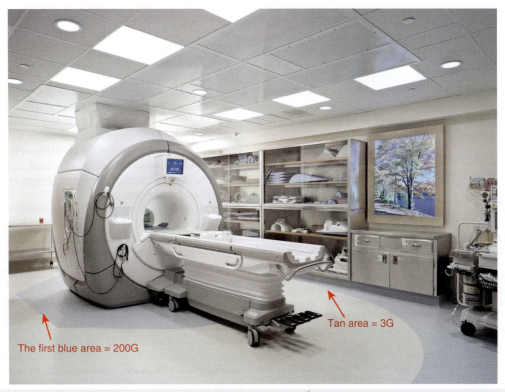

Figure 2-1 The magnetic resonance imaging (MRI) scanner area of an intraoperative MRI suite. Colored floor markings are used to indicate gauss lines in an intraoperative MRI. (Photograph courtesy of Mike Rebholz; caption courtesy of eppstein uhen architects, Milwaukee, WI.)

and operational needs.[2] As the zones increase in number, the potential hazards increase (Table 2-3).[13]

The Guidelines state that the MRI suite needs to be designed to ensure that unscreened individuals are unable to freely enter the area within 5 gauss around the MRI scanner.[2] An anteroom, visible from the control room, is an area for people to pass through before actually entering the scanning or control room.[2] A separate self-contained air-conditioning unit and other specialty support equipment may be required depending on the manufacturer requirements.[2] When anesthesia services are used in the MRI suite, induction and recovery areas should have medical gases and be monitored.[2] This area may be in the patient holding area for convenience. An area where emergency care can be provided outside of the MRI room (zone IV) should be available.[2]

The MRI suite is generally on the bottom floor of the hospital because of the weight of the magnet, but this location is not absolute as a result of the current lower weight of magnets. The floor needs to be able to support the weight of the scanner equipment and prevent environmental vibrations.[2] A knock-out panel in the ceiling should be installed to easily access and change the magnet when needed.[2] A lay-in ceiling is recommended by The Guidelines because of its easy installation, service, and remodeling.[2] Other design considerations for the MRI suite include installation of radiofrequency shielding; a lighted sign and a red light to indicate when the magnet is on; finishes, fixtures, and equipment that decrease the need for maintenance because the magnetic fields in the area can be hazardous; a cryogen quench exhaust pipe and room exhaust with pressure equalization in case a cryogen breach should occur; and various finishes or markings to easily identify the critical field strength zones surrounding the MRI scanner.[2]

HYBRID OPERATING ROOMS

As technology increases and radiographic services are increasingly being used during surgical procedures, hybrid spaces are becoming more common. Examples of these include, but are not limited to, a cardiac catheterization laboratory or cardiac operating room where cardiac valves can be replaced minimally invasively, an MRI or neurosurgical operating suite where intracranial tumor resections or deep brain stimulator insertions can be performed, an intraoperative angiography room where embolectomies and abdominal aortic aneurysm repairs can be done, and an intraoperative radiotherapy room where tumor isolation and radiation can be performed. When combining radiographic technology with an operating room, these components each supply their own set of challenges and concerns that need to be considered. The logistics of two hybrid spaces, an intraoperative MRI suite and an intraoperative angiography suite, will be addressed here.

Intraoperative Magnetic Resonance Imaging

The advantages of an intraoperative MRI (IMRI) suite are especially evident for delicate intracranial neurosurgical procedures because the neurosurgeon can have timely feedback of progress or confirmation of completeness of tumor resections. In the design of an IMRI suite, all operating room personnel need to be especially aware of gauss lines, ferromagnetic objects, and fixed and mobile anesthesia equipment, all of which can be overlooked during critical moments intraoperatively. A complete operating room is adjacent to a fully functional MRI scanner with its strong magnetic field; thus the operating area needs to be far enough away for safe operating conditions using ferromagnetic items and the ability to adequately maintain a sterile environment, yet close enough to limit unnecessary distance for personnel to have to move within the area to accomplish tasks.[5]

To maximize the use of the expensive MRI scanner from a business standpoint, consideration could be given to position the MRI scanner in a location in which both ambulatory patients and intraoperative patients can access it.[5] Either way, the scanner itself should be separated from the operative suite by large shielded partition doors. See Figure 2-2 for a suggested design and rendition of an IMRI suite.

In one IMRI design the patient is moved from the operating area to the MRI scanner on a MRI-compatible transport table with a fixed anesthesia monitor. The other design is to have the MRI scanner itself move to and around the patient.[5] Because of technical challenges with both of these designs, all parties need to be involved in design planning from the start. Note that the latter design costs significantly more than the former.

Because of the advanced physics challenges that exist in constructing an IMRI room, medical physicists should be involved in the design of the area from its beginning stages. Outside radiofrequency can interfere with images, so a Faraday cage, made of aluminum or copper, needs to be built around the entire IMRI to block outside electric fields from interfering with MRI scans.[5] Additionally, because of the close vicinity of the strong magnetic field, bars attached to the walls to anchor moveable items with cords should be considered.[5] Color-coded lines on the floor indicating gauss lines are even more important to have in an IMRI suite than in a normal MRI suite, especially if a movable MRI magnet design is chosen.

Anesthesia equipment should be MRI-safe if using the same equipment in the IMRI operating area and the

Table 2-3	Magnetic Resonance Imaging Suite Zones
Zone	**Activity**
Zone I	This area is freely accessible to the public.
Zone II	This area is where patients are interviewed and screened. They should be supervised by MRI personnel and should not have free movement throughout this zone.
Zone III*	This area is where the MRI scanner's magnetic fields are strong enough that ferromagnetic objects can cause serious injury or death. Anesthesia personnel can monitor the patient from here if needed.
Zone IV*	This area is where the MRI scanner itself is located.

Modified from American Society of Anesthesiologists Task Force on Anesthetic Care for Magnetic Resonance Imaging. Practice advisory on anesthetic care for magnetic resonance imaging. *Anesthesiology.* 2009;110:459-479.

*All access to zones III and IV is to be strictly restricted and controlled by MRI personnel.

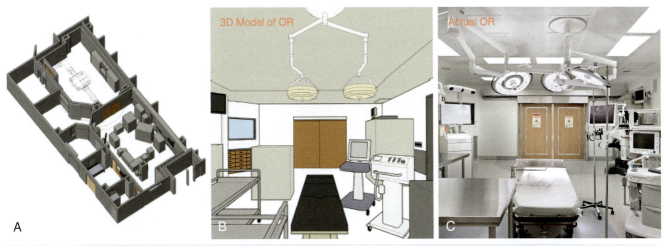

Figure 2-2 A three-dimensional rendition **(A)** and sketch **(B)** of an intraoperative magnetic resonance imaging (IMRI) suite done by architects. **C,** The actual intraoperative MRI suite. Photo is taken from the operative area looking toward shielded partition doors that open to the MRI scanner area. (Photograph, three-dimensional rendition, and sketch courtesy of eppstein uhen architects, Milwaukee, WI; intraoperative MRI photograph courtesy of Mike Rebholz.)

MRI scanner. Alternatively, if the design setup is that in which the patient is moved to the scanner, portable MRI-safe equipment can be used during the scanning phase and standard equipment can be used in the operating area; however, because of the numerous lines, tubes, and wires, this option can be time-consuming when transporting the patient back and forth. Anesthesia personnel should be responsible for ensuring that all anesthesia equipment is nonferromagnetic, including overlooked items such as flashlights, stethoscopes, intravenous poles, laryngoscopes and blades, scissors, clamps, timers, and vaporizers.

A final inspection and examination should be made to check for ferromagnetic items before a scan.[5] This inspection could be similar to the preoperative time-out adapted for the MRI scan. A defined protocol indicating which team member is responsible for what can be helpful.

Because communication with the outside world is imperative, especially during a medical emergency, yet the high magnetic field prohibits the use of pagers, telephones, and computers. IMRI team members should develop a detailed protocol defining what is to be done in a medical emergency, including how and where to call for a medical code, where the patient is to be taken for resuscitation, and location of emergency equipment.[12]

Intraoperative Angiography

Intraoperative angiography (IA) is becoming increasingly prevalent because it allows the surgeon to see vascular structures in real time during procedures. Designers and users of IA face the task of combining the separate challenges of radiation exposure from radiography and a traditional operating room environment. IA requires lead lining of all walls, floors, ceiling, windows, and doors.[5] The minimum required lead thickness is determined by medical physicists based on the NORA site's weekly workload, occupancy of the NORA site and adjacent areas, and the distance from the source of radiation to the nearest occupied area on the opposite side of the radiation barrier.[14] The Guidelines states that a certified physicist or other expert should recommend the type, location, and

amount of radiation protection that needs to be installed according to the final room layout and imaging equipment selected.[2]

In a traditional operating room, anesthesia machines are generally located to the right of the head of the operating room table, with the breathing circuits to the left side of the machine,[4] but this arrangement may have to be altered to accommodate large x-ray machines. Anesthesia equipment and personnel should be as close to the head of the interventional table as possible to maintain vigilance, and x-ray machines can be stationed at the other end of the table. Because the x-ray machine needs to be able to spiral 360 degrees around the patient, all anesthesia equipment must have extra length to avoid tangling in the imaging equipment (Figure 2-3). Careful planning must be done because the imposing x-ray equipment will also compete for ceiling and air space with surgical lights, booms, intravenous poles, and viewing screens.[5]

Angiography and fluoroscopy emit an immense amount of radiation through scatter; thus anesthesia personnel are at great risk because they are very close to the patient.[5] Portable lead screens are helpful but do not protect well against scatter. To maximally protect themselves, personnel should wear front and back lead aprons and a lead thyroid shield, be greater than 36 inches from the ionizing source, and stay behind a portable lead screen when possible.[5]

Conclusion

When designing a NORA site, all personnel who will actually be working in the area, such as interventionalists, anesthesiologists, nursing staff, and technicians, should be involved in the design process. Whether building in a new location or retrofitting into an existing area, each NORA site has unique challenges. To save time and money, it is worth the time and effort to research needs and then seek information from others who have designed a similar NORA site on what works and what does not work for each phase of the design process. An architect, specifically a medical architect, should be chosen who is familiar with the

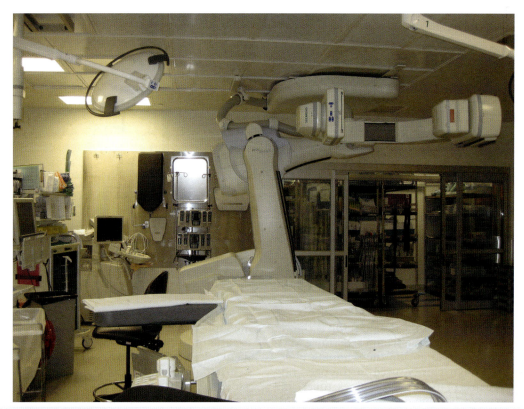

Figure 2-3 Intraoperative angiography.

location of the space. The American College of Healthcare Architects is a good place to begin when searching for medical architects. Additionally, local contractors are generally recommended, particularly ones with experience working in the existing facility, because they are most familiar with local standards and the building infrastructure. The AIA, TJC, and individual state departments of health should be consulted on specific building requirements.

When planning the actual layout of a room, NORA supply cabinets should not be located in the anesthesia work area if possible. If this is unavoidable, gas lines should not obstruct access to cabinets.[3] If anesthesiology requires storage space in the NORA site, it should be immediately adjacent to the anesthesia work area. Because visualization of the actual working space is difficult for many, even when looking at detailed design development documents, the medical architect can aid by showing a computer-generated three-dimensional model with the design and layout of the area, including actual locations of gas outlets, electrical outlets, door swing radii, and imaging equipment rotation radii. Also helpful is a mock-up of the NORA site in which actual equipment is brought into the NORA space to easily visualize workflow and locations of outlets and lights.[3]

Practice runs simulating as much as possible the time a patient arrives at the front door until the patient leaves again, with all personnel and equipment, should be done before the go-live date, to identify potential areas for improvement. This practice can be done at various intervals throughout the design process to aid progress[4], such as after the first design development is completed by the medical architect and then again after construction.

The number of radiographic and surgical procedures is increasing. Imaging equipment is getting smaller, but its capabilities are growing. Technology that was new 10 years ago is now obsolete; a "normal" MRI scanner was 1.5 tesla 10 years ago, and now the "normal" scanner is 3 tesla. This increase in imaging strength is also associated with a need for more generators, cooling systems, and related equipment. To grow with technology, it is most convenient to start with a room with the largest square footage possible. Because budgets are often limited, the best way to plan for current and future NORA sites is to have soft spaces around the NORA locations. This means having nursing lounges, locker rooms, and storage closets nearby that can be easily renovated into areas to accommodate an expanding NORA site and its associated needs. The biggest concerns and costs when expanding an existing area are those associated with medical gases and electricity; careful planning with consideration for future needs of these two systems is required. The only way to plan now is to budget for construction in the future.

Implementing a NORA design can be an arduous process whether building new or retrofitting into an existing area. See Table 2-4 for an approximate timeline. Note that many variables contribute to deviations from this estimate, including departmental personnel availability, contractor availability, hospital rules and regulations, and, often, unforeseen factors.

Providing anesthesia services outside the traditional operating room is very challenging for multiple reasons, not the least of which is a cramped or illogical room design from the point of view of the anesthesiologist. Anesthesiology should work closely with room design teams from the very beginning to create a safe and efficient NORA site for patients.

Table 2-4 Timeline for Design and Implementation of a Non–Operating Room Anesthesia Site

Activity	Time (wk)
Choose equipment and vendor, schematic room design and design development by medical architect (locations of gas outlets, lighting, etc.)	6-8
Prepare construction documents (i.e., guides for the contractors on how to build the area)	6
Design approval by the state	6
Construction	10 (including ~2 wk at the end for the equipment vendors to guide installation)
Medical personnel training	2
"Go live": area open to patients	Total time: 32 wk

Acknowledgments

The authors would like to thank Kurt Smith and eppstein uhen architects in Madison and Milwaukee, Wisconsin, for their generous donation of time and expertise to the composition of this chapter.

References

1. Committee of Origin. Standards and Practice Parameters: statement on nonoperating room anesthetizing locations. Approved by the ASA House of Delegates on October 15, 2003, and amended on October 22, 2008. http://www.asahq.org/For-Members/Standards-Guidelines-and-Statements.aspx.
2. Facility Guidelines Institute. *Guidelines for design and construction of health care facilities: 2010.* Chicago: American Society for Healthcare Engineering of the American Hospital Association; 2010.
3. Ehrenwerth J. The anesthesiologist's overview of the operating room. In: *2012 operating room design manual.* Park Ridge, IL: American Society of Anesthesiologists; 2012. https://www.asahq.org/for-members/practice-management/asa-practice-management-resources/operating-room-design-manual.aspx.
4. Loeb R. Ergonomics and workflow. In: *2012 operating room design manual.* Park Ridge, IL: American Society of Anesthesiologists; 2012. https://www.asahq.org/for-members/practice-management/asa-practice-management-resources/operating-room-design-manual.aspx.
5. Rogoski J. Hybrid operating rooms. In: *2012 operating room design manual.* Park Ridge, IL: American Society of Anesthesiologists; 2012. https://www.asahq.org/for-members/practice-management/asa-practice-management-resources/operating-room-design-manual.aspx.
6. Maheshwari K. Room ventilation systems. https://www.asahq.org/for-members/practice-management/asa-practice-management-resources/operating-room-design-manual.aspx
7. Functional testing and design guides: from the fundamentals to the field. Portland, OR, peci. http://www.peci.org/ftguide/ftg/System-Modules/AirHandlers/AHU_ReferenceGuide/FTG_Chapters/Chapter_8_Reheat.
8. Helfman S. Gas and vacuum supplies. In: *2012 operating room design manual.* Park Ridge, IL: American Society of Anesthesiologists; 2012. https://www.asahq.org/for-members/practice-management/asa-practice-management-resources/operating-room-design-manual.aspx.
9. Helfman S. Electrical service. In: *2012 operating room design manual.* Park Ridge, IL: American Society of Anesthesiologists; 2012. https://www.asahq.org/for-members/practice-management/asa-practice-management-resources/operating-room-design-manual.aspx.
10. Moss E, Nagle T. Medical air. Indianapolis, IN: Anesthesia Patient Safety Foundation.http://www.apsf.org/newsletters/html/1996/summer/apsfmedair.html.
11. Centers for Disease Control and Prevention. Waste anesthetic gases: occupational hazards in hospitals. Department of Health and Human Services, Centers for Disease Control and Prevention, National Institute for Occupational Safety and Health. Publication number 2007-151. September 2007. http://www.cdc.gov/niosh/docs/2007-151/pdfs/2007-151.pdf.
12. Rogoski J. Remote and hazardous locations. In: *2012 operating room design manual.* Park Ridge, IL: American Society of Anesthesiologists; 2012. https://www.asahq.org/for-members/practice-management/asa-practice-management-resources/operating-room-design-manual.aspx.
13. American Society of Anesthesiologists Task Force on Anesthetic Care for Magnetic Resonance Imaging. Practice advisory on anesthetic care for magnetic resonance imaging. *Anesthesiology.* 2009;110(3):459–479.
14. National Council on Radiation Protection and Measurements. *Structural shielding design for medical x-ray imaging facilities,* report 147. Washington, DC: National Council on Radiation Protection and Measurements; 2005.
15. United States Department of Energy. *DOE technical standard: specification for HEPA filters.* DOE-STD-3020-2005. Washington, DC; 2005.
16. U.S. Department of Labor. Anesthetic gases: guidelines for workplace exposures. Occupational Safety & Health Administration. 2000. https://www.osha.gov/dts/osta/anestheticgases/index.html.

3 Room Setup, Critical Supplies, and Medications

MARK C. PHILLIPS

An increasingly large number of anesthetic cases are performed outside the traditional operating room environment. Procedures performed in areas such as the electrophysiology laboratory and interventional radiology department are becoming more complicated and often take longer. Patients are presenting with more complicated histories and comorbidities. Because of the complexity of the procedures and patients' conditions, anesthesiologists are requested to provide services in these remote locations with increasing frequency. Non–operating room anesthesia (NORA) sites pose challenges. This chapter will address room setup, supply, and medication issues in these off-site locations. Unlike in the main operating room, each NORA site has equipment unique to that area that can pose challenges for the anesthesia care team.

Room Setup

NORA procedures occur in a wide array of locations (Box 3-1). These sites range from a designated area in the postanesthesia care unit (PACU) where electroconvulsive therapy is performed to specially designed multiroom suites for gastrointestinal endoscopy. The equipment, supplies, and medications needed in each area will depend on the planned anesthetics and the frequency of their occurrence. The American Society of Anesthesiologists (ASA) issued a Statement on Nonoperating Room Anesthetizing Locations (Figure 3-1)[1] that provides minimal guidelines applicable to all anesthesia care in locations outside the operating room.

One challenge for anesthesia practitioners in remote locations is space. Procedural areas are often planned and built without considering that anesthesia care might be needed in that area. As a result, the anesthesia team is often given inadequate space and not always near the patient. The anesthesia team often works around C-arms in

interventional radiology and an endless array of monitors and C-arms in the cardiac electrophysiology laboratory. These spaces become very crowded areas with the introduction of anesthesia equipment and monitors (Figure 3-2).

Before providing anesthesia services in a NORA location, it is important to evaluate the area to ensure that the guidelines as put forth in the ASA Statement on Non–Operating Room Anesthetizing Locations are followed, along with institutional policies. If the proper equipment and systems are not in place to ensure patient safety, the area should not be used to provide anesthesia services until such changes are made.

The anesthesia department sometimes sends older equipment to the remote anesthesia areas. Remote areas are perceived as not needing the newest equipment because these areas are often not used to the same extent as rooms in the main operating room. It is an unwise practice to send older equipment to remote areas. Using older equipment in a remote area raises the possibility of unfamiliarity with the equipment and machine malfunction. If a problem arises with the equipment, the practitioner may not be able to troubleshoot the problem. Assistance may take much longer to arrive than it would in the main operating room. The ASA Committee on Equipment and Facilities published Guidelines for Determining Anesthesia Machine Obsolescence.[2] This document has not been approved as a practice parameter or policy statement by the ASA House of Delegates, but it does provide practical advice regarding essential features needed in an anesthesia machine to provide a safe anesthetic for patients. Equipment and supplies should match as closely as possible the equipment in the main operating room. Having uniformity of equipment and supplies in all locations provides familiarity for the anesthesia providers who rotate through these areas.

Anesthesia machine check in NORA locations is just as important as in the main operating room. Anesthesia machines in remote locations may not be used every day, so it is important to do a complete machine check at the start of the day. It is important to ensure that the soda lime is fresh in an anesthesia machine that might not have been used recently. In NORA procedure areas, the anesthesia team shares the space with the procedure team. Anesthesia care may not be provided for each case in the room during the day. During nonanesthetic procedures, the procedure nurses may use monitors on the anesthesia workstation. This raises the possibility, for example, that the anesthesia machine may be moved, connections unplugged, or breathing circuits dislodged. If nonanesthesia cases were performed between anesthesia cases, the machine needs to be thoroughly checked before the next anesthesia procedure. Anesthesia machines and equipment in NORA

Box 3-1   Non–Operating Room Locations Commonly Requiring Anesthesia Services

Gastrointestinal endoscopy suite
Cardiac catheterization laboratory
Cardiac electrophysiology laboratory
Pulmonary bronchoscopy laboratory
Interventional radiology department
Interventional neuroangiography department
Computed tomography suite
Magnetic resonance imaging suite
Radiation therapy suite
Electroconvulsive therapy suite

STATEMENT ON NONOPERATING ROOM ANESTHETIZING LOCATIONS

Committee of Origin: Standards and Practice Parameters

(Approved by the ASA House of Delegates on October 15, 2003 and amended on October 22, 2008)

These guidelines apply to all anesthesia care involving anesthesiology personnel for procedures intended to be performed in locations outside an operating room. These are minimal guidelines which may be exceeded at any time based on the judgment of the involved anesthesia personnel. These guidelines encourage quality patient care but observing them cannot guarantee any specific patient outcome. These guidelines are subject to revision from time to time, as warranted by the evolution of technology and practice. ASA Standards, Guidelines and Policies should be adhered to in all nonoperating room settings except where they are not applicable to the individual patient or care setting.

1. There should be in each location a reliable source of oxygen adequate for the length of the procedure. There should also be a backup supply. Prior to administering any anesthetic, the anesthesiologist should consider the capabilities, limitations and accessibility of both the primary and backup oxygen sources. Oxygen piped from a central source, meeting applicable codes, is strongly encouraged. The backup system should include the equivalent of at least a full E cylinder.

2. There should be in each location an adequate and reliable source of suction. Suction apparatus that meets operating room standards is strongly encouraged.

3. In any location in which inhalation anesthetics are administered, there should be an adequate and reliable system for scavenging waste anesthetic gases.

4. There should be in each location: (a) a self-inflating hand resuscitator bag capable of administering at least 90 percent oxygen as a means to deliver positive pressure ventilation; (b) adequate anesthesia drugs, supplies and equipment for the intended anesthesia care; and (c) adequate monitoring equipment to allow adherence to the "Standards for Basic Anesthetic Monitoring." In any location in which inhalation anesthesia is to be administered, there should be an anesthesia machine equivalent in function to that employed in operating rooms and maintained to current operating room standards.

5. There should be in each location, sufficient electrical outlets to satisfy anesthesia machine and monitoring equipment requirements, including clearly labeled outlets connected to an emergency power supply. In any anesthetizing location determined by the health care facility to be a "wet location" (e.g., for cystoscopy or arthroscopy or a birthing room in labor and delivery), either isolated electric power or electric circuits with ground fault circuit interrupters should be provided.*

6. There should be in each location, provision for adequate illumination of the patient, anesthesia machine (when present) and monitoring equipment. In addition, a form of battery-powered illumination other than a laryngoscope should be immediately available.

7. There should be in each location, sufficient space to accommodate necessary equipment and personnel and to allow expeditious access to the patient, anesthesia machine (when present) and monitoring equipment.

8. There should be immediately available in each location, an emergency cart with a defibrillator, emergency drugs and other equipment adequate to provide cardiopulmonary resuscitation.

9. There should be in each location adequate staff trained to support the anesthesiologist. There should be immediately available in each location, a reliable means of two-way communication to request assistance.

10. For each location, all applicable building and safety codes and facility standards, where they exist, should be observed.

11. Appropriate postanesthesia management should be provided (see Standards for Postanesthesia Care). In addition to the anesthesiologist, adequate numbers of trained staff and appropriate equipment should be available to safely transport the patient to a postanesthesia care unit.

*See National Fire Protection Association. Health Care Facilities Code 99; Quincy, MA: NFPA, 1993.

With permission American Society of Anesthesiologists

Figure 3-1 American Society of Anesthesiologists Statement on Nonoperating Room Anesthetizing Locations.

locations need to have regular preventive maintenance, as do machines in the main operating room.[3]

At times an anesthesia machine is transported to a location where anesthesia service is infrequently provided. In these situations, the machine needs to be checked very carefully because transportation of the machine can potentially damage the machine or loosen connections. It is essential to ensure that the anesthesia machine, monitors, and equipment are all in good working order before beginning anesthetic care.

In certain locations where sedation is the only planned action, a compact monitor with the capability of monitoring electrocardiography, blood pressure, oxygen saturation, and end-tidal carbon dioxide ($ETCO_2$) is very useful and does not take up much space (Figure 3-3). $ETCO_2$ monitoring should be included in the monitoring for procedural sedation or general anesthesia in any NORA location.

In areas where anesthesia care is provided, even if sedation is the only planned action, the anesthesia provider

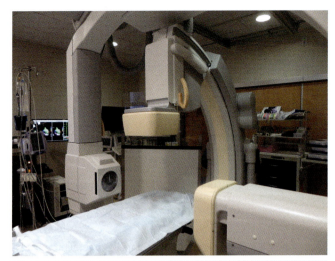

Figure 3-2 Crowded environment in the cardiac electrophysiology laboratory. Anesthesia workstation is behind the lead glass shield.

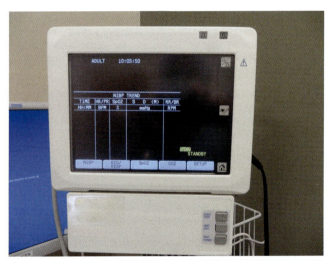

Figure 3-3 Compact monitor with end-tidal carbon dioxide monitoring capability.

should be able to administer general anesthesia and manage the airway. A defibrillator and emergency resuscitation cart should be immediately available to the anesthetist.

The NORA location ideally should have oxygen, air, and nitrous oxide available via a central supply. It is essential to ensure an adequate supply of oxygen is available for the duration of the case. If central supply oxygen is available, a full E-type tank of oxygen should be present as a backup. If oxygen tanks are to be used for the case, it is important to ensure adequate supplies for the case are available, as well as a backup tank. The tank key must be present before beginning anesthetic care.

Central suction may not be available in NORA locations. It is important to ensure suction is available via a suction machine if central suction is not available.

The procedure tables in NORA locations often do not move into the variety of positions available with the main operating room tables. It may be advisable to induce and emerge from anesthesia on the stretcher on which the patient is brought to the procedure room. Using the stretcher will allow heads-up, Trendelenburg, and reverse

Trendelenburg positioning if needed. Certain procedures, such as endoscopic retrograde cholangiopancreatography, are commonly done in the prone position. The procedure staff must keep the stretcher next to the procedure room in case the patient needs to be immediately turned to the supine position.

Monitoring standards in NORA locations should be the same as in the main operating room. Electrocardiography, pulse oximetry, blood pressure, and $ETCO_2$ are minimal requirements. Gas analysis is also advised if use of volatile anesthetics is planned.

Postprocedure recovery should be the same standard as that of the main operating room. Ideally, the patient should recover in a monitored environment close to the procedural area. If this is not possible, the patient should be transported to the main PACU for recovery from anesthesia. The patient should be transported with supplemental oxygen, a transport monitor, an Ambu bag, and emergency medications in case of an emergency during transport.

Other pieces of equipment are needed in NORA locations. Many procedures done in NORA locations are done under sedation or with total intravenous anesthesia (TIVA). Using an intravenous infusion pump for medications such as propofol is very helpful in achieving an adequate level of sedation or anesthesia. A forced-air warming system is needed to ensure patients do not develop hypothermia. Certain NORA locations such as magnetic resonance imaging (MRI) and computed tomography (CT) suites are kept cool to help protect equipment, thus placing patients at risk for hypothermia. An intravenous fluid warmer is needed if there is the possibility of blood transfusion or the need for large amounts of intravenous fluids. Transducers to measure arterial blood pressure and central venous pressure should be readily available. A bispectral index monitor or other depth of anesthesia monitor is also a useful device to have available.

It is beneficial to have point-of-care laboratory testing available in NORA locations. NORA locations may be far from the operating room or main hospital laboratories; having point-of-care testing will improve efficiency. This availability will allow laboratory tests such as blood glucose, potassium level, and hematocrit to be quickly checked.

In any area where anesthesia care is to be provided, the anesthesia provider should know the location of oxygen shutoff valves and fire extinguishers. Safety and emergency evacuation procedures in NORA spaces should be reviewed with the personnel in those areas. The anesthesia provider should also ensure the presence of a defibrillator and resuscitation cart in any location where anesthesia care is to be provided.

In the main operating room, personnel are accustomed to assisting and being attentive during the movement of the patient into the room, during anesthetic induction, and during emergence from anesthesia. This is not the case in many NORA locations. Personnel in these locations are used to their routines and are unaware of the concerns of the anesthesia team. Time spent familiarizing these personnel with the issues and concerns of the anesthesia team regarding care of the patient before service is begun will be very helpful to the anesthesia team.

The anesthesia and procedural teams should collaborate to create a quiet environment during anesthetic induction and emergence. This hushed setting benefits the patient and allows the anesthesia care team to effectively communicate. The importance of safety straps on the patient needs to be stressed, especially during emergence from anesthesia. The procedural team should be instructed on the importance of being attentive and nearby during emergence from anesthesia. Spending time familiarizing the team with the anesthesia machine and airway devices such as Eschmann stylets is very helpful. If assistance is needed with bag-mask ventilation or with airway supplies, prior familiarity is much better than trying to instruct in the middle of a stressful event. Anticipation of and planning for problems that might arise in these locations is important, because help from the main operating room may take an extended time to arrive.

In many NORA locations, the setup is similar to that of the main operating room once space issues are negotiated. Setup differs significantly in two locations—radiation therapy and MRI suites.

ROOM SETUP IN RADIATION THERAPY

Providing anesthesia care for patients undergoing radiation therapy poses challenges for the anesthesia provider. Radiation therapy can consist of traditional external beam radiation therapy or can be delivered in a targeted fashion via a Gamma Knife or CyberKnife. The CyberKnife delivers gamma-ray beams via a robot arm that moves around the patient and delivers radiation from different directions. In this situation, the anesthesia provider must make sure all hoses and tubing, the anesthesia machine, and the cart are away from the area traveled by the robot arm. Because of the high levels of scatter radiation during radiation therapy treatment, the anesthesia provider cannot remain in the room during treatment. The anesthesia monitors and patient must be viewed via video surveillance. It takes 20 to 30 seconds to stop treatment and open the heavy lead door if immediate access to the patient is required.

ROOM SETUP IN MAGNETIC RESONANCE IMAGING

Providing anesthesia services in the MRI suite poses problems not encountered in other anesthetizing locations. If proper precautions are not taken, the MRI suite can be a hazardous environment for both the anesthesia provider and the patient. Descriptions of the science and technical aspects of MRI have been published elsewhere and are beyond the scope of this chapter.[4,5] MRI has advantages in that this imaging modality does not expose the patient to ionizing radiation and thus does not have cumulative effects when serial examinations are required. The number of MRI scans done each year continues to grow, and the need for anesthesia services in the MRI suite continues to grow as well.

In 2007 the American College of Radiology published a Guidance Document for Safe MR Practices.[6] In 2009 the ASA Task Force on Anesthetic Care for Magnetic Resonance Imaging published a practice advisory on anesthetic care for MRI.[7] These documents provide detailed information about safe practices within the MRI environment.

The major concern in providing anesthesia care in the MRI suite is the strong magnetic field present around the

Table 3-1   Magnetic Resonance Suite Zones

Zone	Activity
Zone I	All areas freely accessible to the general public. This is the area through which personnel and patients access the MRI area.
Zone II	The area between the uncontrolled zone I and the strictly controlled zone III. This is the area where patients are greeted, histories obtained, and questions answered. Movement by non-MRI personnel and patients is under the supervision of MRI personnel.
Zone III	This is a restricted area. Movement in this area is strictly controlled by MRI personnel. Access to this area is only after screening for the presence of ferromagnetic material. Ferromagnetic objects may produce a serious hazard if brought into this area.
Zone IV	This is the MRI scanner room itself. By definition it is within zone III.

MRI, Magnetic resonance imaging.

scanner at all times. It takes several days to generate the magnetic field used in MRI. Therefore the magnetic field is always on, even when there is not a patient in the scanner. The magnetic field is measured in tesla units (T); 1 T equals 10,000 gauss. The earth's magnetic field is approximately 0.5 gauss. MRI scanners used for clinical purposes are generally 1- to 3-T machines. Thus the MRI scanner generates a magnetic field thousands of times stronger than the earth's magnetic field. Any item of equipment that contains ferromagnetic material will be attracted to the magnet. In addition to the static magnetic field that is always present, during image acquisition, radiofrequency pulses are applied. Both the static magnetic field and the intermittent radiofrequency pulses create the safety issues associated with MRI.

Four zones have been identified in the MRI environment, with increasing danger from the magnetic field with each increase in zone (Table 3-1).[6] Signs should be posted to indicate each zone in the MRI suite.

In an area in the MRI suite known as the 5-gauss exclusion zone, ferromagnetic items become very significant risks because of abnormal operation and being drawn to the magnet. This area is generally demarcated by a red line. The distance of the 5-gauss line from the scanner bore varies depending on the strength of the MRI and the shielding of each device.

Multiple incidents have been reported of ferrous-containing objects, hospital beds, anesthesia carts, intravenous poles, oxygen tanks, and other items being drawn to the magnet (Figures 3-4 and 3-5). Serious injury or death can occur in these situations. A paper clip has a terminal velocity of 40 miles per hour in a 1.5-T magnetic field.[8] Larger objects have greater velocity and force. These items can become high-speed projectiles when they enter the magnetic field of the scanner It is imperative that all personnel, patients, and objects be screened for the presence of ferrous-containing materials before being allowed in zone III or zone IV areas.

If an employee or patient is trapped by an object drawn to the magnet, such as an anesthesia cart, the MRI has to be shut down emergently. This very expensive and potentially hazardous procedure is called a quench. The MRI scanner is super-cooled with inert gases such as liquid helium. In a quench, these gases are suddenly released to shut down the magnetic field. They usually escape by a pressure valve to the outside. If these gases do not exit outside but rather empty into the scanner room, hypoxia may occur as hundreds of thousands of liters of helium is released into the scanner room, displacing oxygen. This gas can also pressurize the room, making it impossible to open doors. The room can then become a fire hazard because flammable liquid oxygen can form as a result of the rapid drop in room temperature.[6]

A quench is very expensive in terms of the cost of getting the scanner back on line. An emergency quench can damage the coils of the magnet as a result of the rapid change in temperature as the cryogenic material is released. The scanner has to be checked very carefully to ensure it is not damaged. Refilling the cryogen materials is also very

expensive. A significant economic impact occurs from lost revenue during the time the scanner is down. An emergency quench should be initiated by MRI personnel only in life-threatening emergencies.

The MRI does not need to be quenched if a piece of equipment is attached to the magnet but no life is in jeopardy. The MRI and engineering personnel can lessen the magnetic field so that the object can be safely removed from the magnet.

The best way to avoid an emergency quench is to ensure that proper MRI procedures are followed at all times and to follow the instructions of the MRI personnel. Some institutions require personnel going into the MRI environment to complete an educational program and training before being allowed in the MRI area. It is also important to ensure that anesthesia personnel are screened for the presence of foreign bodies or implanted devices containing ferromagnetic material before being allowed to work in the MRI environment.[7]

The American Society of Testing and Materials developed terminology regarding equipment and devices in the MRI environment. Equipment and devices are given the designations MRI safe, MRI conditional, and MRI unsafe. MRI safe equipment is identified as having no ferromagnetic parts or radiofrequency interference. MRI unsafe equipment is identified as having ferromagnetic parts or being affected by radiofrequency interference. MRI conditional equipment may be safe in certain areas of the MRI suite but cannot be identified as having no ferromagnetic parts.[7]

Many manufacturers make MRI safe and MRI conditional anesthesia machines. It is preferable to have these machines in the MRI suite (Figure 3-6). If an MRI safe or MRI conditional anesthesia machine is not available, it is important that the anesthesia machine be kept at a safe distance and that a long anesthesia circuit be used.

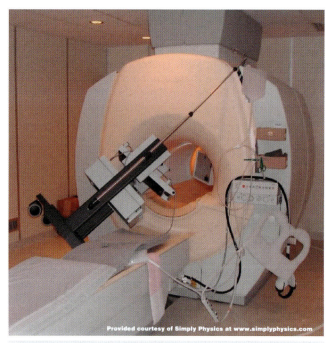

Figure 3-4 Intravenous pole attached to magnetic resonance imaging magnet bore. (Courtesy Simply Physics. http://www.simplyphysics.com.)

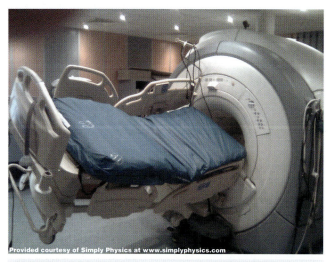

Figure 3-5 Hospital bed drawn to magnetic resonance imaging magnet bore. (Courtesy Simply Physics. http://www.simplyphysics.com.)

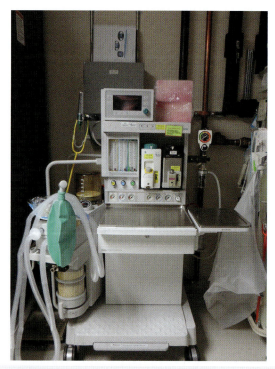

Figure 3-6 Anesthesia machine for use in magnetic resonance imaging environment.

If an infusion pump is going to be used, it should be MRI safe or MRI conditional (Figure 3-7). If it is not, it should be kept outside the scanning room and the tubing threaded through a waveguide to the patient in the scanner.

As mentioned earlier, radiofrequency pulses are emitted during MRI scanning. The radiofrequency pulses can interfere with monitors and equipment because they can heat up monitor wires and leads. The risk for patient burn exists if these leads are looped or coiled. To lessen the risk for burns, monitoring wires should be examined to ensure that insulation is intact. Leads and cables should be straight and in line with the body. Leads and cables should not be in direct contact with the skin. It is now common to have specially shielded pulse oximeters for use in MRI with wireless communication to the monitor. MRI safe electrocardiography electrodes are available. The electrocardiogram (ECG) can be transmitted via telemetry and eliminate a wire to the monitor.

In addition to the risk for patient burns related to radiofrequency pulses, risk to the hearing of patients and personnel is also an issue. The radiofrequency pulses make noise up to 90 decibels. The 3-T machines are much louder than 1.5-T machines. The patient as well as any personnel or visitors present in the scanner room should wear hearing protection provided during the procedure.

In the event of cardiac or respiratory arrest while the patient is in the scanner, basic life support measures should be started while the patient is emergently removed from the magnet room to a magnetically safe location for full resuscitation measures to take place. If resuscitation is done in the magnet room, it raises the possibility of danger from ferromagnetic objects used in the resuscitation. If the hospital resuscitation team is called to the MRI room,

team members must follow MRI safety protocols. In responding to the emergency, the hospital resuscitation team may not realize the significant hazards associated with the magnetic field and thus inadvertently take a ferrous object into the magnet room, creating a serious hazard. This underscores the importance of removing the patient to a magnetically safe place for resuscitation. In addition, it is often difficult to interpret ECG data while in the magnet room, which could hamper resuscitation efforts.

In many institutions, the patient is anesthetized in an area outside the scanner room, then moved onto the MRI gantry and taken into the scanner room (Figure 3-8). This process allows the anesthesia provider to use any equipment needed during the anesthetic induction. If induction is to take place in the scanner room, care must be taken to ensure that nonferrous equipment and supplies are used. It is important to ensure that the anesthesia circuit and intravenous lines are long enough to allow for movement of the MRI gantry during scanning.

Before being brought into the scanner, the patient is questioned carefully regarding the presence of any ferromagnetic devices such as pacemakers, implantable cardioverter-defibrillators, prosthetic heart valves, aneurysm clips, bullets, or shrapnel. If the patient is unable to answer, family members are questioned. Other means such as looking for scars or using plain films can be employed to determine if the patient has a device. If it cannot be determined the patient is safe to have the procedure, it should not be done.

The anesthesia provider will in most circumstances not be in the scanner room during the scan. The anesthesia provider needs to have visualization of the patient through a window and also by video cameras. The anesthesia

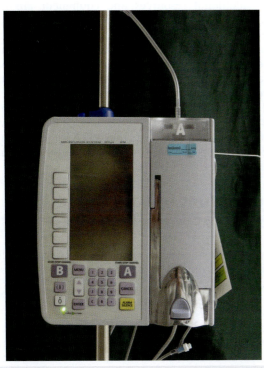

Figure 3-7 Infusion pump for use in magnetic resonance imaging environment.

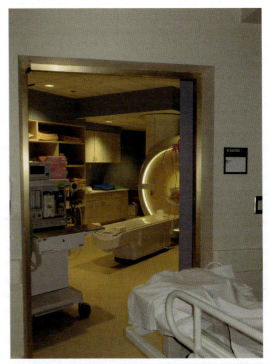

Figure 3-8 Anesthesia induction for magnetic resonance imaging can take place outside the scanner room, with the patient then moved to the scanner.

monitors also must be visible. This can be achieved using a video camera focused on the monitors. Ideally this should be by means of a slave display at the MRI control desk.

Pregnant personnel can work throughout their pregnancies in the MRI environment. However, it is recommended that they move away from the magnet bore during actual scanning.

Cooperation and consultation between the MRI personnel and anesthesia staff are very important in the MRI environment. A good working relationship and understanding of the concerns of both the MRI personnel and the anesthesia staff will ensure a safe experience for the patient.

Critical Supplies

NORA locations need to be supplied even better than the main operating rooms. Because of the remoteness of some locations, supply support from the main operating room is often infrequent. It is important to make sure that adequate supplies are present before beginning anesthetic care. If additional supplies are needed in the middle of a procedure, it may take some time for them to arrive.

NORA locations where services are provided multiple times per week should have well-supplied anesthesia carts. These carts should remain in place. In locations where service is very infrequent, an anesthesia cart with supplies can be taken to that location on the day of a procedure. In an area where service is provided daily it is recommended to have an anesthesia supply storage area nearby, just as in the case of the main operating room. This will allow for easy stocking of anesthesia carts between cases. It is sometimes difficult to obtain space for an anesthesia supply storage area; however, the argument that efficiency will be improved and room turnaround faster will go a long way toward acquiring space. Having a dedicated anesthesia technician assist with room turnover in busy multiroom areas such as the gastrointestinal endoscopy or cardiac electrophysiology suites also improves efficiency.

The supplies needed in NORA locations are often the same as those in the main operating room, with a few exceptions. Because of the distance from the anesthesia machine to the patient in many of these locations, a longer anesthetic circuit is often needed than those used in the main operating room. Likewise, longer intravenous tubing is also necessary. A flashlight other than a laryngoscope provides illumination in darkened rooms, assisting in finding and drawing up medications and observing the patient.

A list of important phone numbers should be posted in a clearly visible place in the procedure room. This list of numbers should include the main operating room anesthesia board to request additional anesthesia assistance, the operating room pharmacy if additional medications or malignant hyperthermia supplies are needed, the number to call for anesthesia supplies, and the number to call for the difficult airway cart. Trying to remember phone numbers in the middle of an emergency is difficult. Having the team in the room make needed phone calls allows the anesthesia provider to concentrate on the emergency.

The ability to manage an airway is needed in any area where anesthesia care is provided. Sufficient airway supplies to manage an airway should be immediately available

Box 3-2	**Airway Supplies Checklist**

Ambu bag and various size face masks
Various sizes of endotracheal tubes
Endotracheal tube stylet
Tongue blades
Oral airways of various sizes
Nasal airways of various sizes
Lubricating gel
Laryngoscope (with extra batteries)
Miller and Macintosh laryngoscope blades
Laryngeal mask airways of various sizes
Eschmann intubating stylet
Cook airway exchange catheter
Magill forceps
Videolaryngoscope
Nasal cannula with carbon dioxide sampling capability
Syringe
Tape

(Box 3-2). It is helpful to have a video laryngoscope in NORA locations. An argument also can be made for having a difficult airway cart with a fiberoptic endoscope in NORA locations. Practical and economic concerns, however, would advocate having the cart permanently available only in busy NORA locations such as a multiroom gastrointestinal endoscopy suite. If it is necessary to call for the difficult airway cart, the personnel responsible for bringing it to the remote site need to be familiar with the remote location and the fastest route to deliver the equipment.

In circumstances in which the patient has a known difficult airway, the difficult airway cart can be called for and additional anesthesia personnel can be arranged to assist. An alternative for patients with a known difficult airway is to perform the intubation in the main operating room, where additional resources and equipment are readily available, and then transport the patient to the NORA location for the procedure. Transporting an intubated patient poses the risk for inadvertent extubation if the endotracheal tube or breathing circuit gets snagged during transport. If the patient has to be transported a considerable distance, it is recommended a transport ventilator be used rather than hand ventilating the patient with an Ambu bag. The decision to intubate a patient with a known difficult airway in the main operating room or in the NORA location should be made weighing patient and institutional factors and arriving at the best decision for the particular case.

Safety Issues in Non–Operating Room Anesthesia Locations

Safety issues for anesthesia personnel are often magnified in the NORA environment (Box 3-3).

RISK FOR TRIPS AND FALLS

NORA locations have various monitors, equipment, and cables not seen with such frequency in the main operating room. In areas not initially designed for the provision of anesthesia services, power outlets may be poorly positioned, thus leaving power cords across walking pathways. Cables

Box 3-3   **Safety Considerations in Non–Operating Room Anesthetizing Locations**

Trips and falls
Exposure to trace anesthetic gases
Radiation exposure
Magnetic resonance imaging safety

and infusion lines are often suspended across walking paths. The lights in the room are often dimmed to improve visualization of imaging for the proceduralist. These factors, coupled with the remote location in the room that the anesthesia team is often provided, are a recipe for a trip and a fall. Likewise, C-arm beams and video monitors often are positioned close overhead, posing a hazard for a head injury. Caution must be taken to avoid head injury. The risks for contaminating the field, pulling out intravenous infusion lines or catheters, and disrupting the procedure also exist. Situational awareness of the location of cords, cables, and equipment is necessary at all times.

EXPOSURE TO TRACE ANESTHETIC GASES

Studies have raised the issue of possible dangers involved in repeated exposure to trace concentrations of waste anesthetic gases.[9,10] Later analysis of these studies found flaws in the study design.[11,12] A later prospective study found no causal relationship between exposure to trace anesthetic gases and adverse health events.[13] The National Institute for Occupational Safety and Health has established standards for allowable trace gases, as follows[14]:

- *Volatile anesthetic alone:* 2 parts per million (PPM) over 1 hour
- *Nitrous oxide alone:* 25 PPM for an 8-hour time-weighted average
- *Volatile gas with 25 PPM nitrous oxide:* 0.5 PPM over 1 hour

One of the means of lowering trace gases in the OR is frequent air exchanges. The current requirement is 15 to 21 air exchanges per hour, of which 3 must be with fresh outside air. NORA locations adapted for the presence of anesthesia may not have as robust an air exchange system and thus have higher trace gas measurement. If volatile gases are to be used, a gas scavenging system should be in place. If no gas scavenging system is available, TIVA should be used for general anesthesia cases. Other means of minimizing trace gas levels include using low gas flows, being vigilant regarding circuit leaks and disconnects, and not turning on gases until the anesthesia circuit is connected to the patient.

RADIATION EXPOSURE

Exposure to ionizing radiation is another safety concern for anesthesia personnel providing anesthesia in NORA locations such as the cardiac electrophysiology laboratory, interventional radiology department, and gastrointestinal endoscopy suite. Radiological imaging, especially fluoroscopy, is used routinely in many of these procedures. It is important that anesthesia staff be educated about the hazards of radiation exposure, the importance of wearing personal protective equipment, and limiting exposure as much as possible.

Exposure to ionizing radiation is potentially harmful for several reasons, including development of leukemia and fetal abnormalities resulting from genetic injury.[15]

Radiation exposure is measured in terms of roentgen equivalent man (rem) units. The rem is a unit used to derive a quantity termed the equivalent dose. It relates the absorbed radiation dose in human tissue to the effective biological damage of the radiation. The rem is often expressed in terms of thousandths of a rem, or mrem. The unit of measurement for a biological radiation dose outside the United States is the Sievert (Sv); 1 Sv equals 100 rem. The maximum annual occupational exposure is to be no more than 5000 mrem per year or 50 mSv. For pregnant personnel, the total dose allowed during the pregnancy is 500 mrem. The exposure from a chest x-ray is approximately 25 mrem. The exposure from whole-body CT is 1100 mrem. The exposure from a C-arm fluoroscopy unit is 1200 to 1400 mrem/min. Exposure during fluoroscopy is much higher than from CT or regular x-rays.

In 2005 a study by Katz[16] demonstrated that the radiation exposure to an anesthesia department doubled after the department began providing anesthesia services in a cardiac electrophysiology laboratory. Although the annualized limits were still well below the occupational exposure limits, the study did show a significant increase when providing services in an area where fluoroscopy is heavily used.

Radiation exposure may occur from primary exposure from the source collimator, as leakage from the device, or from scatter radiation. Scatter radiation is radiation reflected from the patient or other surfaces. Scatter radiation is responsible for the majority of occupational exposure and is the largest danger for the anesthesia provider. Scatter radiation increases when the power output of the beam and the size of the imaged field increases. Fluoroscopy has more scatter radiation than a CT machine with a focused beam.

Anesthesia personnel should use the ALARA principle: always attempt to keep radiation exposure As Low As Reasonably Achievable. ALARA is founded on the following three concepts of limiting exposure to radiation:

1. Reducing radiation time
2. Increasing distance from the source of radiation
3. Barriers to radiation

Limiting radiation time is under the control of the proceduralist. Distance and barriers are under the control of the anesthesia provider.

Exposure to radiation decreases with the inverse square of the distance from the radiation source. Anesthesia team members should remain at least 3 to 6 feet from the radiation source if possible. Exposure is minimal beyond 3 feet. Six feet of air provides the equivalent protection of 9 inches of concrete or 2.5 mm of lead.[17] Being 6 feet away from the beam decreases scatter exposure to the same level as wearing five lead aprons. Lead aprons attenuate 97% to 98% of scatter.

Full wraparound lead vests and skirts are recommended. Full-wrap lead will lessen radiation exposure if the anesthesia practitioner has his or her back turned during imaging. Full-wrap lead is heavy, and it is important that it is

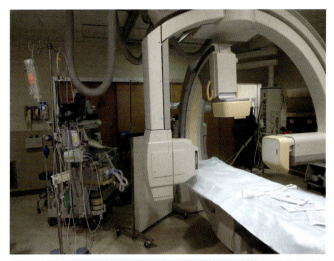

Figure 3-9 Lead glass shield between the anesthesia workstation and fluoroscopy unit makes access to the patient difficult.

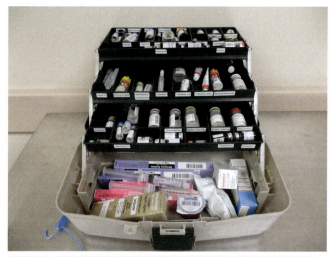

Figure 3-10 Tackle box containing medications

appropriately sized and fits correctly. Thyroid shields are also recommended. Lead skirts and vests are often removed from areas where needed and end up in a locker or lounge. The anesthesia service should have dedicated personal protective equipment identified as belonging to the anesthesia service to prevent its misappropriation. Lead glasses are recommended to protect the corneas from radiation exposure.

A movable lead glass shield between the anesthesia practitioner and the radiation source affords additional protection (Figure 3-9). The lead glass shields can be difficult to maneuver into position in an already crowded space and can make access to the patient difficult. Communication from the procedural team regarding the initiation of imaging allows the anesthesia team to take appropriate precautions, such as moving farther away during imaging if possible.

It is important that anesthesia team members wear appropriate lead protection when entering the room during a procedure. Entering the room without appropriate protection is distracting to the proceduralist and may interrupt the procedure if imaging has to be stopped to avoid exposing an unprotected person. If imaging is not stopped, the individual is exposed to an unnecessary risk.

It is recommended that dosimeters be worn by any anesthesia personnel working on a routine basis in an area where radiation exposure is a concern. Pregnant personnel should not work in areas where radiation exposure occurs.

Medications

Medications needed in NORA areas are the same as those used in the main operating room. Remote areas, however, pose special concerns regarding medications. Most operating rooms have a pharmacy located in the immediate vicinity; NORA rooms usually do not. It is thus important to have an adequate supply of all anticipated medications. It may take some time to obtain a medication if the anesthesia team has not brought it with them. The significant morbidities and coexisting diseases of patients undergoing procedures in NORA locations necessitate having a wide range of medications available.

Another concern in NORA areas is medication error resulting from the low lighting in the procedure rooms. Often the procedure rooms have the lights dimmed or turned off to improve visualization of images on the monitors. This low-light environment raises the possibility of the wrong medication being administered. A flashlight should be on the anesthesia cart in remote areas.

In areas where anesthesia is given infrequently and procedural sedation only is planned, drugs may be transported in a tackle box (Figure 3-10). More often, an anesthesia cart with anesthesia medications and supplies is used. Standardization of medication trays between NORA locations and the main operating room is recommended. This will provide familiarity with the location of medications on the drug tray, and anesthesia providers will know what drugs are available. It is important to check that medications and supplies are not expired. This is especially true in an area where anesthesia service is infrequently provided.

An emergency cart with a defibrillator, emergency drugs, and equipment needed to provide cardiopulmonary resuscitation should be in any NORA location. The anesthesia provider should know the location of this cart and how to operate the defibrillator.

Medications used in NORA locations run the spectrum from benzodiazepines and opioids used for sedation to agents used for general anesthesia. Sedation is used more frequently in NORA locations than in the main operating room. Sedation can range from minimal to moderate to deep sedation. Medications and supplies must be available to rescue a patient whose level of sedation becomes deeper than originally planned.

Several medications are of particular use in NORA locations where procedural sedation is commonly used. These medications include midazolam, propofol, dexmedetomidine, and ketamine.

MIDAZOLAM

Midazolam is a mainstay of therapy for procedural sedation as well as an adjunct for general anesthesia. Midazolam is a benzodiazepine. Benzodiazepines produce sedation, anxiolysis, and anterograde amnesia. Midazolam does not provide significant analgesia. Midazolam was the first benzodiazepine developed primarily for use in anesthesia.[18] After intravenous administration, onset of action is within 2 to 3 minutes. Termination of effect is from redistribution, and metabolism occurs in the liver.

In the cardiovascular system, midazolam causes mild systemic vasodilation and decrease in cardiac output. Heart rate is not usually affected. Cardiovascular effects may be pronounced in hemodynamically compromised individuals and the elderly, especially if given in a large dose or in conjunction with opioids.

Midazolam causes a mild decrease in respiratory rate and tidal volume. Respiratory depression may be significant if midazolam is given in conjunction with an opioid.[19] Respiratory effects may be magnified in the elderly and those with respiratory disease.

Midazolam has amnestic, anticonvulsant, muscle relaxant, and sedative hypnotic properties in the central nervous system. It causes a decrease in cerebral blood flow and cerebral metabolic rate.[20]

Midazolam 0.1 to 0.4 mg/kg can be given to induce general anesthesia. Sedation can be achieved with dosages of 0.01 to 0.1 mg/kg. Most commonly during procedural sedation, midazolam is used as part of a multidrug therapy in combination with opioids, propofol, or ketamine, depending on the patient's condition, procedure, and clinical goals.

Midazolam has an antagonist, unlike other intravenous agents such as propofol and ketamine, which do not. Flumazenil is a competitive antagonist at the benzodiazepine binding site on γ-aminobutyric acid receptors in the central nervous system. It acts within 2 minutes, with peak effect in 10 minutes. The half-life of flumazenil is short, and thus this agent may require repeat administration. Patients who have received flumazenil should be observed for signs of resedation.[21] Dosage of flumazenil begins with 0.2 mg/min intravenously. Total dose is usually 0.6 to 1 mg.

PROPOFOL

Propofol is an ultra–short-acting hypnotic agent that has sedative, amnestic, and hypnotic effects but no analgesic properties. Onset of action is within 30 to 60 seconds, and duration of effect is 4 to 8 minutes.[21]

Propofol is used for induction of general anesthesia, as an infusion during total intravenous anesthesia, and for procedural sedation. It is very useful in areas where inhaled anesthetic agents cannot be used because of the lack of a scavenging system.

Propofol is the most commonly used agent for induction of general anesthesia. The usual induction dose is 1 to 2.5 mg/kg. Patients of advanced age and those with significant comorbidities will need a reduced dose. Premedication with benzodiazepines or opioids will lessen the induction requirement.[21]

Propofol causes significant vasodilation and reductions in both preload and afterload.[20] Elderly patients and patients with reduced intravascular volume are at risk for significant hypotension when propofol is administered, especially if it is given rapidly. Titrated doses of propofol given slowly can help avoid this hypotension.

Propofol is a respiratory depressant. It often causes apnea after an induction dose. Propofol causes a significant reduction in upper airway reflexes, making it an excellent choice when a laryngeal mask airway is going to be placed.

Patients frequently report pain on injection of propofol. Administration of lidocaine 50 to 100 mg before or with the propofol often will attenuate this problem. Administering the propofol in a larger vein also lowers the incidence of pain on injection.

Propofol has a rapid onset and short duration of action. In addition to its usefulness to provide induction of general anesthesia, it can be used as an infusion as part of a total intravenous anesthesia regimen, often in combination with benzodiazepines and opioids. Propofol infusion also can be used as part of a balanced anesthetic technique with volatile agents, opioids, and nitrous oxide. Infusion rates between 100 and 200 mcg/kg/min are typically used in combination with opioids or nitrous oxide to provide general anesthesia. Propofol is often used in titrated boluses or as an infusion to provide procedural sedation. Infusion rates between 25 and 75 mcg/kg/min are typically used for procedural sedation. Because of the respiratory depressant effect of propofol, it is recommended that it be administered only by individuals trained in airway management.

Propofol has an antiemetic effect. This makes it a useful agent in patients prone to postoperative nausea and vomiting.

DEXMEDETOMIDINE

Dexmedetomidine is a highly selective α_2-adrenergic agonist approved for clinical use in 1999.[22] It has sedative and analgesic effects. Dexmedetomidine is similar to clonidine; however, it is much more selective and shorter acting than clonidine. After intravenous administration, it undergoes rapid redistribution and is extensively metabolized in the liver.

After administration, dexmedetomidine produces a sedated but arousable state that resembles a natural sleep state. It causes minimal respiratory depression. Ventilatory response to hypercarbia is maintained.[20] For these reasons, it may be particularly useful in certain patient populations such as the morbidly obese and patients with obstructive sleep apnea. These patients may be at risk for respiratory depression and obstructed airway if administered a benzodiazepine and opioid combination for procedural sedation.

Dexmedetomidine can cause bradycardia and hypotension. Agents such as glycopyrrolate and ephedrine should be readily available to treat bradycardia and hypotension should they occur.

For procedural sedation in adults a loading dose of 1 mcg/kg is infused over 10 minutes, followed by an infusion of 0.6 mcg/kg/hr. The rate of infusion should be titrated to achieve the targeted level of sedation. This will usually be at an infusion rate of 0.2 to 1 mcg/kg/hr.[21]

Dexmedetomidine can enhance the effects of sedatives, hypnotics, anesthetic gases, and opioids. If these agents are given in conjunction with dexmedetomidine, the amounts administered of these agents or the dexmedetomidine infusion may need to be adjusted.

KETAMINE

Ketamine is a phencyclidine derivative. It was first introduced into clinical practice in 1965. It has a rapid onset of action because of its high lipid solubility. After administration of ketamine, the patient's eyes remain open with a slow nystagmus. This cataleptic state is known as dissociative anesthesia.[20] Ketamine produces significant analgesia with minimal respiratory depression. Ketamine relaxes bronchial smooth muscle, making its use beneficial in patients with reactive airway disease. Salivation is often increased by ketamine. Premedication with an anticholinergic can be given to limit this effect.

From a cardiovascular standpoint, ketamine can cause increases in blood pressure, heart rate, and cardiac output from centrally mediated sympathetic stimulation. Ketamine, however, is a direct myocardial depressant. This effect can be seen when ketamine is administered to critically ill patients who have limited sympathetic reserve. Ketamine should be used with caution in patients with coronary artery disease or pulmonary hypertension.

In contrast to the other intravenous anesthetic agents, ketamine is a cerebral vasodilator and can cause increases in cerebral blood flow and cerebral metabolic rate. It is usually not used in patients with intracranial pathology or patients in whom increases in intracranial pressure would be detrimental.

One of the effects of ketamine that has limited its use over the years is unpleasant emergence reactions. Patients may experience bad dreams, hallucinations, and out-of-body experiences. When benzodiazepines are given along with the ketamine, emergence reactions are significantly reduced and amnesia is increased.

One advantage of ketamine is that it can be given by a variety of routes—intravenously, intramuscularly, and orally. Anesthesia can be induced with 1 to 2 mg/kg intravenously or 4 to 6 mg/kg intramuscularly. Ketamine is available in a variety of concentrations, from 10 mg/mL to 100 mg/mL. It is important to pay close attention to the concentration to avoid giving an inappropriate dose. Ketamine also can be administered as small bolus doses of 10 to 20 mg intravenously as part of a procedural sedation regimen.

Ketamine and propofol have been mixed together to produce ketofol for procedural sedation. One study mixed equal amounts propofol 10 mg/mL with ketamine 10 mg/mL. Bolus doses of 1 to 3 mL were titrated to effect.[23] It was felt the addition of ketamine to propofol counteracts the respiratory depression seen when propofol alone is used. Propofol blunts the adverse psychological effects of ketamine. Ketamine also provides an analgesic effect, which propofol does not have.

Allergic Reactions

The ability to manage and treat anaphylactic and anaphylactoid reactions should be available in remote anesthesia areas. Patients are at risk in the operating room for allergic reactions from latex and numerous medications, primarily muscle relaxants and antibiotics. In NORA locations, patients are at risk for adverse reactions from these agents and from intravenous contrast agents.

Intravenous contrast agents are used millions of times each year in radiological procedures to facilitate imaging. Older contrast agents were ionized, hyperosmolar, and fairly toxic. These agents have in large part been replaced by newer nonionized contrast agents. The incidence of adverse side effects has diminished since the introduction of the newer agents.[24]

Although the incidence of contrast reactions has decreased since the introduction of newer low-osmolarity agents, adverse reactions still occur. Patients with a history of asthma, a history of allergy, or prior contrast reaction and medically debilitated patients are more likely to develop a contrast reaction.[24] Symptoms can range from mild nausea and headache to severe life-threatening reactions with bronchospasm and cardiovascular collapse. Usually these reactions occur within the first 15 minutes after injection of the contrast agent. Should an adverse reaction occur, treatment should be symptomatic. Oxygen and inhaled bronchodilators should be administered to patients with bronchospasm. Patients with refractory bronchospasm or cardiovascular collapse should receive epinephrine. Steroids and antihistamines also should be administered (Box 3-4). If a patient experiences a severe reaction while under sedation, strong consideration should be given to proceeding to intubation. Patients can develop severe glottic edema, making intubation difficult. Intubation and mechanical ventilation may be needed to facilitate oxygenation and ventilation in a patient experiencing severe bronchospasm.

If patients have experienced a previous contrast reaction, they should be given prophylaxis before subsequent procedures. Prophylaxis should include steroids and histamine-1 and histamine-2 receptor antagonists.

Contrast-induced nephropathy is a complication of radiological procedures and is a leading cause of hospital-acquired acute renal failure.[15] Acetylcysteine and periprocedure hydration are used to lessen the incidence of contrast-induced nephropathy.

Benzocaine Spray and Methemoglobinemia

Benzocaine spray is often used to provide topical anesthesia for transesophageal echocardiography and gastrointestinal endoscopy cases. Application of topical benzocaine can lead to the development of methemoglobinemia. Methemoglobinemia can be a serious and potentially fatal adverse drug effect. Development of cyanosis in the presence of normal arterial oxygen saturation is an indication of the

---

Box 3-4   Treatment of Anaphylaxis and Anaphylactoid Reactions

Stop causative agent or medication
Administer 100% oxygen
Bolus intravenous fluids
Epinephrine 10-100 mcg IV: Increase if no response
Consider epinephrine infusion 1-10 mcg/min
Vasopressin 2-5 units
Histamine-1 blocker: Diphenhydramine 50 mg IV
Histamine-2 blocker: Famotidine 20 mg IV or ranitidine 50 mg IV
Steroid: Hydrocortisone 50-150 mg IV

IV, Intravenously.

development of methemoglobinemia. If a patient develops methemoglobinemia, the treatment is supplemental oxygen and methylene blue. Methylene blue 1% solution 1 to 2 mg/kg intravenously is given slowly over 5 minutes.[25] Methylene blue restores the iron in hemoglobin to its normal oxygen-carrying state.

Malignant Hyperthermia

It is not necessary to store a supply of dantrolene in each NORA location for treatment of malignant hyperthermia. However, a procedure should be in place to quickly obtain dantrolene and other malignant hyperthermia treatment supplies. Procedures should also be in place to quickly obtain the additional resources needed should a patient develop malignant hyperthermia. Nursing personnel in NORA locations should receive instruction regarding malignant hyperthermia and their role should an event occur. If the NORA location is more than 5 to 7 minutes from where the dantrolene is stored, then a malignant hyperthermia treatment kit should be stored in that NORA location.

Conclusion

Providing an anesthetic in a non–operating room setting presents a unique set of challenges to the anesthesiologist. Because of the longer distance to the operating rooms, the unique arrangements of the NORA suite, and the hazards involved, such as radiation, diligent planning is needed before the patient enters the suite. Careful attention must be given to ensure proper room setup to provide a safe and satisfying experience for the patient, staff, and practitioners.

References

1. American Society of Anesthesiologists. Statement on nonoperating room anesthetizing locations, amended in 2008. http://www.asahq.org/For-Members/Standards-Guidelines-and-Statements.
2. American Society of Anesthesiologists. Guidelines for determining anesthesia machine obsolescence. http://www.asahq.org/For-Members/Standards-Guidelines-and-Statements.
3. Souter KJ. Anesthesia provided at alternate sites. In: Barash PG, Cullen BF, Stoelting RK, et al, eds. *Clinical anesthesia*. New York, NY: Walters Kluwer/Lippincott Williams & Wilkins; 2009:861–875.
4. Currie S, Hoggard N, Craven I, et al. Understanding MRI: basic MR physics for physicians. *Postgrad Med J*. 2013;89(1050):209–223.
5. Berger A. Magnetic resonance imaging. *BMJ*. 2002;324(7328):35.
6. Kanal E, Barkovich A, Bell C, et al. ACR guidance document for safe MR practices: 2007. *Am J Roentgenol*. 2007;188(6):1447–1474.
7. American Society of Anesthesiologists. 2009. Practice advisory on anesthetic care for magnetic resonance imaging: a report by the American Society of Anesthesiologists Task force on Anesthetic Care for Magnetic Resonance Imaging. *Anesthesiology*. 2009;110(3):459–479.
8. ECRI Institute. The safe use of equipment in the magnetic resonance environment (guidance article). *Health Devices*. 2001;30(12):421–444.
9. Cohen E, Bellville J, Brown B. Anesthesia, pregnancy, and miscarriage: a study of operating room nurses and anesthetists. *Anesthesiology*. 1971;35(4):343–347.
10. Knill-Jones R, Rodriques L, Moir D, Spence A. Anaesthetic practice and pregnancy: controlled survey of women anaesthetists in the United Kingdom. *Lancet*. 1972;1(7764):1326–1328.
11. Buring J, Hennekens C, Mayrent SL, et al. Health experiences of operating room personnel. *Anesthesiology*. 1985;62(3):325–330.
12. Tannenbaum T, Goldberg R. Exposure to anesthetic gases and reproductive outcome: a review of the epidemiological literature. *J Occup Med*. 1985;27(9):659–668.
13. Spence A. Environmental pollution by inhalational anesthetics. *Br J Anaesth*. 1987;59(1):96–103.
14. Rothschild J, Winters B, Brenan-Rothschild K. Highway to the danger zone: hazmat. In: Gallagher C, Ginsberg SH, Lewis MC, et al, eds. *Anesthesia unplugged*. 2nd ed New York, NY: McGraw Hill Medical; 2012:541–549.
15. Stensrud P. Anesthesia at remote locations. In: Miller RD, Eriksson LI, Fleisher LA, et al, eds. *Miller's anesthesia*. 7th ed. New York, NY: Churchill Livingstone; 2009:2461–2484.
16. Katz J. Radiation exposure to anesthesia personnel: the impact of an electrophysiology laboratory. *Anesth Analg*. 2005;101:1725–1726.
17. Nicholau D, Arnold W. Environmental safety including chemical dependency. In: Miller RD, Eriksson LI, Fleisher LA, et al, eds. *Miller's anesthesia*. 7th ed. New York, NY: Churchill Livingstone; 2009:3053–3073.
18. Reves J, Fragen R, Vinik H, Greenblatt D. Midazolam: pharmacology and uses. *Anesthesiology*. 1985;62(3):310–324.
19. Bailey P, Pace N, Ashburn M, et al. Frequent hypoxemia and apnea after sedation with midazolam and fentanyl. *Anesthesiology*. 1990;73(5):826–830.
20. Eilers H. Intravenous anesthetics. In: Miller R, Pardo M, eds. *Basics of anesthesia*. Philadelphia, PA: Elsevier; 2011:99–114.
21. Reves J, Glass P. Intravenous anesthetics. In: Miller R, Eriksson LI, Fleisher LA, et al, eds. *Miller's anesthesia*. 7th ed. New York, NY: Churchill Livingstone; 2009:719–768.
22. Kamibayashi T, Maze M. Clinical uses of alpha$_2$ adrenergic agonists. *Anesthesiology*. 2000;93:1345–1349.
23. Willman E, Andolfatto G. A prospective evaluation of "ketofol" (ketamine/propofol combination) for procedural sedation and analgesia in the emergency department. *Ann Emerg Med*. 2007;49(1):23–30.
24. Morcos S, Thomsen H. Adverse reactions to iodinated contrast media. *Eur Radiol*. 2001;11(7):1267–1275.
25. Armstrong C, Burak K, Beck P. Benzocaine induced methemoglobinemia; a condition of which all endoscopists should be aware. *Can J Gastroenterol*. 2004;18(10):625–629.

4 The Role of the Non–Operating Room Anesthesiologist

E. HEIDI JEROME, MANON HACHE, and LENA S. SUN

In recent years, the number of non–operating room anesthesia (NORA) procedures has increased significantly. At our institution—Morgan Stanley Children's Hospital of New York-Presbyterian—40% of all anesthesia procedures (~4000/10,000 cases) were done outside of the operating room in 2011, in contrast to 20% in 2001 (~1400/7000 cases). A similar trend is occurring nationwide.[1]

Many reasons account for this change. First, many more procedures, such as bone marrow aspiration and lumbar puncture, require minimal supplies and can be performed in several locations outside the operating room. Some procedures, such as organ-selective chemotherapy, require specialized equipment that must be housed in specific locations outside the operating room—for example, an interventional radiology department.

Second, sophisticated diagnostic imaging methods are becoming increasingly available for medical investigation. These imaging procedures can be prolonged and require the patient to be completely still, often requiring anesthesia. Magnetic resonance imaging (MRI) and single-photon emission computed tomography (SPECT) scanning for seizure activity are two examples.

Third, for pediatric patients in particular, parents and referring physicians expect these young patients will have access to the same diagnostic and minimally invasive procedures that are offered to adults and that these patients will be taken care of safely, comfortably, and efficiently. These procedures often require anesthesia. These diagnostic and minimally invasive procedures, even those that do not require special equipment, are often best conducted in non–operating room venues. This has the additional benefit of being a cost-saving measure so that operating rooms are reserved for sterile procedures requiring a more invasive approach. As we see more procedures performed outside the operating room, the anesthesiologist will be asked to play several roles. Anesthesiologists will have oversight of sedation and anesthesia at all NORA sites. They will develop these programs to ensure that all procedures are conducted with a level of safety similar to that in procedures performed in the operating room. They will provide training for anesthesia residents and nonanesthesia personnel. Anesthesiologists will also be providing much of the hands-on care for patients undergoing these procedures.

Oversight of Non–Operating Room Anesthesia

As the number of procedures conducted outside the operating room has increased, so has the number of practitioners providing anesthesia and sedation services to these patients. Many of these patients seen in non–operating room locations are still cared for by anesthesiologists, but providers increasingly come from the departments of medicine, pediatrics, emergency medicine, dentistry, oral surgery, and radiology. Although many factors are driving this change, the involvement of multiple specialties has occurred because many non–operating room procedures do not require a surgical plane of anesthesia. For example, a claustrophobic patient undergoing MRI or an adolescent having a cardiac catheterization who will receive local anesthesia may require only anxiolysis. A toddler having MRI will require deep sedation, whereas an adult undergoing bronchoscopy may require a moderate level of sedation. Nonanesthesiologists have embraced these procedures, as evidenced by the increasing publication of studies of procedural sedation and analgesia in their respective specialty journals.[2] Published investigations by anesthesiologists often include sedation teams with nurse practitioners and pediatricians or radiologists as the personnel providing hands-on sedation.[3,4] Care by nonanesthesia personnel also may be driven by insurance companies that may not wish to pay for the additional cost of anesthesia services for some of these procedures.

As this transition to multispecialty providers occurs, anesthesiologists remain central to ensuring that all sedation care is as safe as possible. As the pioneers of operating room safety, anesthesiologists are recognized by The Joint Commission as key players in the oversight of non–operating room sedation and anesthesia services, as well as operating room anesthesia. The requirement recently issued by the Centers for Medicare and Medicaid Services (CMS)* that all deep sedation and anesthesia services be under the oversight of a single physician in any hospital caring for their patients has led most institutions to assign that role to anesthesiologists, although the CMS does not require this physician to be an anesthesiologist. Thus anesthesiologists will continue to play a major role in all NORA sites where sedation or anesthesia is provided, even when the providers of such care are not anesthesiologists.

The roles of credentialing, establishing practice guidelines, and providing quality assurance for sedation and analgesia services conducted by other specialties have brought significant challenges to anesthesia departments. Two of these challenges are establishing nil per os (NPO, or nothing by mouth) standards and credentialing practitioners

---

*Centers for Medicare and Medicaid Services: http://www.cms.gov/Regulations-and-Guidance/Guidance/Transmittals/downloads/R59SOMA.pdf.

for the use of propofol infusions. Anesthesiologists have long accepted NPO times of 2 hours for clear liquids and 6 hours for other liquids and food to diminish the risk for aspiration. Emergency medicine physicians often encounter patients who would benefit from sedation and analgesia but do not meet these NPO criteria. Several authors from this specialty have questioned the risk for aspiration in nonfasted patients and have attempted to demonstrate the safety of shorter NPO times. The American College of Emergency Physicians published a complex clinical advisory to determine what depth of anesthesia may be given to patients in the emergency room based on fasting from 0 to 3 hours, the urgency and duration of a procedure, and the health of a patient. This advisory uses the terms *dissociative sedation, non–extended moderate sedation,* and *brief deep sedation* to describe levels and duration of sedation.[5] These terms are not familiar to most anesthesiologists, nor are NPO times of less than 2 hours for clear liquids or 6 hours for solids acceptable to most anesthesiologists. The American Academy of Pediatrics also has published a guideline on sedation that allows the practitioner to balance the benefit of sedation for emergency procedures against the risk for aspiration for patients who are not on NPO status.[6] Changing attitudes toward NPO times by nonanesthesiologists will be important issues for anesthesiologists who have oversight of these practitioners.

The second controversial issue is credentialing nonanesthesiologists in propofol sedation. Gastroenterologists enthusiastically embraced the use of propofol for patients undergoing endoscopy, starting a debate on the safe use of this drug for deep sedation.[7-9] The American Society of Anesthesiologists' (ASA's) 2004 statement on the safe use of propofol limited use of propofol to "persons trained in the administration of general anesthesia." In 2009, however, the ASA acknowledged the use of propofol and other anesthetic drugs by other specialists when it published a Statement on Granting Privileges for Deep Sedation to Non-Anesthesiologist Sedation Practitioners. This document describes training, skills, monitoring, and quality assurance review of nonanesthesiologist practitioners to ensure safe delivery of sedation. It requires that a trained individual be solely responsible for sedation and monitoring during propofol administration. Anesthesiologists must continue to provide such guidance to nonanesthesiologists as non–operating room procedures evolve.

Although many articles have been published regarding the safety and efficacy of various sedation regimens and NPO status, caution must be exercised when establishing guidelines for sedation by nonanesthesiologists. Severe complications, including death, are rare, so any comparison of the relative safety of different regimens in hundreds of patients simply lacks the power to establish safety. In addition, moderately severe complications such as respiratory depression are often poorly measured in these studies.

One approach that has been extensively used in anesthesia is the ASA Closed Claims analysis. This method allows examination of adverse events and may help determine risk factors for these events. In 2009, non–operating room closed claims were compared to those in the operating room.[10] Adverse respiratory events, including inadequate oxygenation and ventilation, were the most common cause for NORA claims. Monitored anesthesia care (MAC) was the most common anesthetic, and oversedation and lack of end-tidal carbon dioxide monitoring was the most common scenario encountered. These events happened in older, sicker patients, most often in the gastroenterology suite, and more often resulted in death than events in the operating room. However, closed claims analysis provides only a retrospective look at adverse events, without the benefit of a control group or large number of patients. The Pediatric Sedation Research Consortium was created to improve the understanding of the nature and frequency of adverse events in patients undergoing anesthesia or sedation outside the operating room. The Consortium collects data from 37 different institutions and is thus able to look at sedation encounters in thousands of patients. It recently published articles comparing sedation by pediatricians to that by nonpediatricians, including anesthesiologists, intensive care physicians, emergency room physicians, advanced practice registered nurses, pediatric nurse practitioners, physician assistants, dentists, surgeons, certified registered nurse anesthetists, registered nurses, medical technologists, and radiologists.[11] The Consortium described monitoring modalities used during sedation, compared adverse events among various providers,[12] looked at adverse events during propofol sedation by emergency room physicians,[13] compared propofol to pentobarbital sedation for MRI imaging,[14] compared etomidate versus pentobarbital for CT scans,[15] looked at the incidence and nature of adverse events outside the operating room,[16] and looked at adverse events specifically with propofol sedation outside the operating room.[17] It confirmed that serious adverse events are rare and found no statistically significant difference in the rate of adverse events related to different providers of sedation. However, the Consortium concluded that the safety of pediatric sedation depends on the systems' ability to manage less serious adverse events.

Levels of Sedation and Anesthesia

The various procedures or diagnostic imaging conducted outside the operating room require different levels of sedation or anesthesia. Diagnostic imaging is usually painless and therefore requires minimal analgesia, whereas interventions may require intraoperative analgesics or postoperative pain management. The continuum of sedation and analgesia can be categorized in different ways. The ASA published a statement[18] defining different levels on the continuum of sedation that apply for any practitioner: Minimal sedation (anxiolysis) applies to the patient who is maintaining verbal contact with the practitioner administering sedation. Moderate (previously called conscious) sedation applies to patients who purposefully respond to verbal command or light touch. No airway support should be required, and spontaneous ventilation and hemodynamic stability are maintained. Moderate sedation is often used for short procedures or diagnostic imaging. Deep sedation and analgesia apply to patients who do not respond to light touch but will respond to painful or repeated stimuli. Spontaneous ventilation may not be maintained, and the patient may require intervention to maintain a patent airway. Deep sedation may be appropriate for pediatric patients who must be asleep to be immobile for imaging or for more invasive procedures in adult patients.

In contrast, MAC applies only to a patient who receives care from an anesthesiologist for non-painful or minimally painful procedures in which local or regional anesthesia is provided. MAC allows for administration of sedative and analgesic medicines in doses that exceed those used for moderate sedation and includes the possibility of having the patient go through all of the levels of sedation to general anesthesia, as needed. Even if no medications are used, the presence of the anesthesiologist is required to safely monitor patients who may become unstable.

For many diagnostic and minimally invasive non–operating room procedures, particularly in pediatric patients, the level of sedation required to obtain optimal conditions often is deep sedation. Because the nature of sedation is fluid, it is easy for the patient to go from one level of sedation to the next. All personnel administering sedation to patients outside the operating room must be properly credentialed and trained in rescuing patients from a sedation level deeper than was intended. A practitioner who is planning deep sedation must be able to manage a patient who becomes truly anesthetized. This skill is part of credentialing for anesthesia practice, but many nonanesthesiologist practitioners will need to acquire additional skills and training to gain this ability.

Organizing Safe Practice

The anesthesiologist's role as the administrator giving oversight to all NORA procedures and as the hands-on care provider for individual patients is to ensure the safety and comfort of all patients.

The first priority should always be safety. It is of paramount importance that patients undergoing procedures or diagnostic imaging have had a recent medical evaluation and that all preexisting conditions are optimized. This is no different from seeing patients before surgery in the operating room. A standard procedure is followed in the operating room for obtaining a history, undergoing a physical examination, signing consent forms, and providing insurance approval documentation. However, it is sometimes logistically difficult to organize all of the patient's information ahead of time in non–operating room settings. It can be helpful to designate a point person responsible for ensuring all NORA procedures are followed as smoothly as possible. That designated person should communicate with the referring physician and the team providing the procedural care so that all necessary documents are present and instructions are given before administering anesthesia. This point person or persons may be affiliated with the anesthesiology department or with the various non–operating room sites and services.

A gamma knife procedure is an excellent example of the complex interactions of several services. This treatment requires the presence of the anesthesiologist to sedate or intubate the patient, the neurosurgeon to place the head frame with pins, the MRI technologists to perform the scan, and the radiologists to make the radiation calculations based on the scan. The patient is transported by the anesthesiologists to the gamma knife, where the patient undergoes the radiation treatment with the help of gamma knife technologists and supervision of the radiologist. The procedure may take several hours. When the radiation is finished, the head frame is removed and the patient emerges from anesthesia or sedation and goes to the post-anesthesia care unit (PACU). Nurses and specially skilled nurse practitioners in preprocedure preparation, MRI and gamma knife setup, and PACU care are essential at each phase of the procedure. A single coordinating individual must be responsible to bring these 8 to 12 care providers in different settings together in proper sequence.

In addition to facilitating communication with all services to ensure patient safety, the anesthesiologist is responsible for ensuring proper documentation, including preanesthesia evaluation, intraprocedural monitoring of vital signs and all drugs given, and postprocedure evaluation confirming that the patient is back to baseline status. Anesthesiologists must be active participants in providing quality assurance for these patients.

For some NORA procedures, information unique to those settings is essential. Several examples follow. A careful screening for metal or device implants must be done before a patient enters the MRI scanner and is best done well ahead of time to prevent last-minute cancellation. For SPECT scanning, the patient must not receive intravenous glucose before the procedure. For cardiac catheterization, interventional radiology, and CT, a careful history for contrast dye must be obtained.

During the procedure, careful patient positioning must avoid any pressure injury while the patient is sedated or anesthetized. MRI beds can be hard, so pressure sites should be periodically relieved during long scans. Arm positioning during cardiac catheterization must be carefully done to avoid brachial plexus injury. Corneal abrasions are a particular risk for patients who are in several different planes of sedation. We may be reluctant to tape a patient's eyes closed with moderate sedation, but an abrasion may occur if this is not done when that patient becomes deeply sedated.

Another goal is efficiency in providing anesthesia care. This is easiest when well-established protocols for patient flow before, during, and after the procedure are in place. A well-staffed admitting area, procedure area, and PACU with good communication among administrative assistants, nurses, anesthesiologists, and procedural physicians is key to efficiency.

In addition to providing relief from pain and anxiety during the procedure, other aspects of patient comfort are also key to excellent patient care. Avoiding long waiting times, avoiding excessive NPO times, providing updates to waiting families, and providing postprocedural food and drink are some measures that can greatly improve a patient's experience. Although some of these are not under the direct control of the anesthesiologists, they should have a voice, both individually and administratively, in ensuring these types of comforts for their patients.

For emergency management of patients during regular hours or after hours, these non–operating room sites should have the same staffing, preprocedure evaluation, consent requirements and consideration of NPO status that occur during nonemergency care. A call system to bring in nurses, technologists, radiologists, other procedural physicians and the anesthesiologist should be in place. As increasing familiarity with NORA procedures is gained, it is recognized that some of them can be lifesaving or provide a diagnosis that leads to lifesaving surgery. Again, the anesthesiologist may not have direct control over all aspects of emergency care in NORA sites, but should have a role in planning for that care and surely have a role in making sure that any single emergency procedure goes as smoothly and safely as possible.

We are also responsible for the safety of hospital personnel and the public. It is important that medications, anesthesia machines, and equipment are secured while not in use to ensure that no one without proper training uses them. If anesthesia equipment and drugs are stored in off-site locations, they may be particularly vulnerable to such misuse. Ensuring the safety of co-workers also is essential. Education, appropriate screening, protective clothing, and lead glasses must be provided for anesthesia residents and nurse anesthetists who work with MRI scanners or in any site with x-rays or nuclear emissions. Anesthetic gases must be safely scavenged in NORA sites. When scavenging is not available, we should avoid the use of inhalational anesthetic agents.

When anesthesia is provided outside the operating room, unfamiliar surroundings and unfamiliar personnel may be a challenge. Considerable planning goes into providing anesthesia safely in these areas, and communication with all involved personnel is key. All practice guidelines must be followed, and all necessary equipment must be available before beginning the procedure.

Occasionally patients may come for a procedure or diagnostic test without having a primary physician within that institution. It is important to have guidelines in place to predetermine who will take ownership if the patient should require admission or further management of care.

Equipment

Several approaches are used to deliver NORA, but they broadly fall into two styles: mimicking the anesthesia equipment available in the operating room or bringing limited equipment and supplies for total intravenous anesthetic. Both styles have advantages and disadvantages. In mimicking operating room equipment, including anesthesia machines, monitors, and the supply cart, the anesthesiologist can provide a wide range of anesthetics, including general endotracheal anesthesia with inhaled anesthetic agents. This style also has the advantage of familiarity, which is particularly useful in residency training programs. The anesthesiology department maintains the equipment, and therefore it always should be in good condition.

Disadvantages of this complete anesthesia kit are that it is difficult to transport, so it is more suited to be permanently stationed in NORA sites. It occupies a fairly large space in these locations, which may be small; it requires maintenance at some distance from the operating room; it requires scavenging if inhaled anesthetics are to be used; and a source of gases must be available. Further, nonanesthesiologists, including laypersons, may have access to this specialized equipment if it remains in NORA sites after hours. If the equipment is to be moved back to the operating room, personnel must be assigned this task.

Advantages of bringing a light anesthesia kit are portability and the ability to provide care in smaller spaces. However, the anesthesiologist will likely depend on the unfamiliar monitoring equipment available at the NORA site. In addition, the anesthesiologist must remember all essential supplies or be forced to use unfamiliar ones. The type of anesthetic will be limited to use of intravenous medications, and the usual wide variety of airway support equipment in operating room settings will not be available. Endotracheal intubation equipment must always be immediately available, but, unless specifically planned, laryngeal mask airways and fiberoptic intubating equipment will not be available.

It may be convenient to induce anesthesia in an operating room setting or in another fully equipped site and then move the patient to a NORA site with only essential equipment. The transport must be carefully planned. The transport to the recovery area must be similarly well planned at the end of any anesthetic, with oxygen tanks and suction as necessary, regardless of whether the anesthesiologist used complete equipment or limited supplies.

In institutions where a computerized anesthesia record is used, a decision must be made a priori whether this capability will be present and maintained in NORA sites.

Personnel

Anesthesia coverage in NORA settings can be provided in several ways. Unlike operating rooms, NORA sites are rarely clustered in the same location, so the flexibility and efficiency of assigning anesthesia personnel based on type of procedure and ASA patient status often is not possible in outlying areas. A single anesthesiologist or anesthesia teams consisting of an attending and nurse anesthetist or resident will usually go to the NORA site. The best use of anesthesia personnel is to provide anesthesia care for several procedures in sequence at the outlying site. For example, a full day of interventional cardiac procedures or a full day of pediatric MRI scans is usually a more efficient schedule than single cardiac catheterizations requiring anesthesia a few days of the week or single pediatric MRI scans on a daily basis.

In some NORA settings, the physician requesting anesthesia care may ask for a subspecialty-trained anesthesiologist. For example, the neurointerventional radiologist may wish to have a neuroanesthesiologist care for a patient with an arteriovenous malformation in the radiology suite, or the cardiologist may wish to have a cardiac anesthesiologist care for a patient with congenital heart disease in the catheterization laboratory. For some patients with ASA physical status 4, this may be appropriate, but providing such coverage for all patients at these NORA sites will adversely affect anesthesia staffing for neurosurgical and cardiac surgery patients in the operating room. If many of the anesthesiologists in an institution become familiar with providing anesthesia at multiple NORA sites, flexibility for operating room cases can be maintained. The anesthesiologist's familiarity with NORA sites is important to maintaining their anesthesia safety. In our institution, we have found no difference in the complication rate during pediatric cardiac catheterization procedures attended by cardiac anesthesiologists and non–cardiac anesthesiologists.

In academic institutions, training of residents is an important role for attending anesthesiologists. As more procedures are done in NORA settings, teaching residents how to safely care for patients in many of these off-site facilities becomes an important goal of residency. It is often easier to assign a nurse anesthetist to a NORA site than train a resident who is unfamiliar with the unique challenges of these sites. However, the more familiar residents become with off-site anesthesia, the better they will be able to care for all patients in their future careers.

When off-site suites such as interventional radiology, cardiac catheterization, MRI, CT, or multiple gastroenterology procedure suites are clustered together, anesthesia care can be provided by an attending anesthesiologist simultaneously supervising two residents or four nurse anesthetists, if patient acuity permits. In these clustered off-site settings, preprocedural activities and PACU care can be run smoothly, similar to perioperative care.

When procedural sedation is provided by nonanesthesiologists, nurses and nurse practitioners may be supervised by trained medicine, pediatric, or emergency medicine specialists, or these trained specialists may directly provide care. Preprocedural evaluation and consent, physiologic monitoring during sedation, and postprocedural recovery must be conducted as it is when anesthesiologists provide care.

Conclusion

Despite the evolving nature of NORA, anesthesiologists must remain at the forefront to ensure patient safety and quality of care. The role of the anesthesiologist is not only to be present to provide anesthesia services but also to guide credentialing of all personnel administering moderate or deep sedation and ensure that proper quality assurance measures are being recorded. The choices of anesthesia equipment and monitoring devices for these procedures are crucial to providing safe care. Ensuring open communication among multiple services involved in these procedures and efficient scheduling of patients will allow a smooth encounter in NORA settings. Anesthesia practice needs to continue to evolve, along with new technologies and the modernization of our health care system.

References

1. Cravero JP, Blike GT. Pediatric anesthesia in the nonoperating room setting. *Curr Opin Anaesthesiol.* 2006;19(4):443–449.
2. Cravero JP, Havidich JE. Pediatric sedation: evolution and revolution. *Paediatr Anaesth.* 2011;21(7):800–809.
3. Mason KP, Lubisch N, Robinson F, Roskos R, Epstein MA. Intramuscular dexmedetomidine: an effective route of sedation preserves background activity for pediatric electroencephalograms. *J Pediatr.* 2012;161(5):927–932.
4. Sanborn PA, Michna E, Zurakowski D, et al. Adverse cardiovascular and respiratory events during sedation of pediatric patients for imaging examinations. *Radiology.* 2005;237(1):288–294.
5. Green SM, Roback MG, Miner JR, Burton JH, Krauss B. Fasting and emergency department procedural sedation and analgesia: a consensus-based clinical practice advisory. *Ann Emerg Med.* 2007;49(4):454–461.
6. American Academy of Pediatrics, American Academy of Pediatric Dentistry, Coté CJ, Wilson S, Work Group on Sedation. Guidelines for monitoring and management of pediatric patients during and after sedation for diagnostic and therapeutic procedures: an update. *Pediatrics.* 2006;118(6):2587–2602.
7. Rex DK, Deenadayalu VP, Eid E, et al. Endoscopist-directed administration of propofol: a worldwide safety experience. *Gastroenterology.* 2009;137(4):1229–1237 quiz 518–519.
8. Singh H, Poluha W, Cheung M, et al. Propofol for sedation during colonoscopy. *Cochrane Database Syst Rev.* 2008;4:CD006268.
9. Vargo JJ, Holub JL, Faigel DO, Lieberman DA, Eisen GM. Risk factors for cardiopulmonary events during propofol-mediated upper endoscopy and colonoscopy. *Aliment Pharmacol Ther.* 2006;24(6):955–963.
10. Metzner J, Posner KL, Domino KB. The risk and safety of anesthesia at remote locations: the US closed claims analysis. *Curr Opin Anaesthesiol.* 2009;22(4):502–508.
11. Monroe KK, Beach M, Reindel R, et al. Analysis of procedural sedation provided by pediatricians. *Pediatr Int.* 2013;55(1):17–23.
12. Langhan ML, Mallory M, Hertzog J, Lowrie L, Cravero J. Pediatric Sedation Research Consortium. Physiologic monitoring practices during pediatric procedural sedation: a report from the Pediatric Sedation Research Consortium. *Arch Pediatr Adolesc Med.* 2012;166(11):990–998.
13. Mallory MD, Baxter AL, Yanosky DJ, Cravero JP. Pediatric Sedation Research Consortium. Emergency physician-administered propofol sedation: a report on 25,433 sedations from the Pediatric Sedation Research Consortium. *Ann Emerg Med.* 2011;57(5):462–468.
14. Mallory MD, Baxter AL, Kost SI. Pediatric Sedation Research Consortium. Propofol vs pentobarbital for sedation of children undergoing magnetic resonance imaging: results from the Pediatric Sedation Research Consortium. *Paediatr Anaesth.* 2009;19(6):601–611.
15. Baxter AL, Mallory MD, Spandorfer PR, et al. Etomidate versus pentobarbital for computed tomography sedations: report from the Pediatric Sedation Research Consortium. *Pediatr Emerg Care.* 2007;23(10):690–695.
16. Cravero JP, Blike GT, Beach M, et al. Incidence and nature of adverse events during pediatric sedation/anesthesia for procedures outside the operating room: report from the Pediatric Sedation Research Consortium. *Pediatrics.* 2006;118(3):1087–1096.
17. Cravero JP, Beach ML, Blike GT, Gallagher SM, Hertzog JH. The incidence and nature of adverse events during pediatric sedation/anesthesia with propofol for procedures outside the operating room: a report from the Pediatric Sedation Research Consortium. *Anesth Analg.* 2009;108(3):795–804.
18. American Society of Anesthesiologists. *Continuum of depth of sedation: definition of general anesthesia and levels of sedation/analgesia.* 2009. https://www.asahq.org/coveo.aspx?q=continuum%20or%20depth%20of%20sedation.

General Management Principles

SECTION OUTLINE

5   *Continuous Quality Improvement for Non–Operating Room Anesthesia Locations*

6   *Critical Monitoring Issues for Non–Operating Room Anesthesia*

7   *Intravenous Anesthesia and Sedation Outside the Operating Room*

5 Continuous Quality Improvement for Non–Operating Room Anesthesia Locations

JULIA I. METZNER and KAREN B. DOMINO

As described throughout this book, non–operating room anesthesia (NORA) locations present a major challenge for safe anesthesia care. A vital quality improvement and risk management system is important to prevent patient harm and improve the quality of care. This chapter will discuss continuous quality improvement (CQI), selection of quality indicators, and methods to improve quality of care, including analysis of critical incidents and sentinel events using root cause analysis and systems analysis. Although these methods are typically employed in the operating room, they are also essential in NORA locations to improve patient safety. A checklist (Table 5-1) summarizes the steps necessary for establishing a CQI program in NORA settings.

Quality

Quality in health care means doing the right thing for every patient every time. The Institute of Medicine (IOM) defines quality as the "degree to which health services for individuals and populations increase the likelihood of desired health outcomes and are consistent with current professional knowledge."[1] To accomplish the desired goals, the IOM focuses on the following six principal areas of achievement:

1. *Safety:* Avoiding preventable injuries, reducing medical errors
2. *Effectiveness:* Providing services based on best clinical evidence
3. *Efficiency:* Using innovative strategies in allocation of limited resources; avoiding waiting time
4. *Patient-centered:* Individualizing care to the patient's unique needs
5. *Timely:* Reducing delays in delivery of care
6. *Equitable:* Providing consistent care regardless of patient characteristics and demographics

Quality improvement encompasses efforts to improve patient outcomes (health), system performance (care), and professional development (learning and teamwork).[2] CQI is a scientific approach to quality management that builds on traditional quality assurance methods by emphasizing the organization and systems of the health care system. CQI employs a systems approach to identifying and improving quality of care. CQI continually evaluates medical care to identify systematic problems and implements strategies to prevent their occurrence by a plan-do-study-act approach (Figure 5-1). By focusing on processes of care rather than individuals, latent system failures and errors are identified and corrected. Objective data are used to analyze and improve processes. Accurate and sensitive quality indicators, presented as a dashboard, are necessary to monitor performance according to benchmarks and improvements over time. When areas are identified for improvement, their current status is measured and documented. Changes are implemented, and the outcome is again measured after an appropriate time to determine whether improvement actually occurred.

Inspired by the Donabedian clinical indicators,[3] CQI programs are oriented toward defining the structure, process, and outcome of health care delivery. Following the Donabedian Quality-of-Care Framework, this model sees health care as a cyclic transformation mechanism. In this mechanism, patients are inputs entering a health care organization's structure. In this structure, these inputs undergo a process of care through which they will become outcomes or outputs. These outcomes/outputs will further inform the feedback loop back to inputs.[4]

Selecting Indicators

Structural indicators refer to the setting in which the care takes place. It describes the type and quantity of resources used by a health system or organization to deliver programs and services. Examples include organization, ownership, accreditation of facilities, ratio of practitioners to patients, qualifications of medical staff such as board certification, and technological complexity. Structural characteristics are considered necessary but insufficient elements in the delivery of health services. They are indirect measures of quality in that their presence enables but does not ensure the provision of quality health services, whereas the absence of these structural characteristics decreases the probability of quality outcomes.

Process indicators assess medical activities performed by the provider to ensure the "best" patient care and prevention, continuity of care, and physician–patient interaction. In the actual practice, process measures often imply compliance with standards of care such as the following:

- Was an adequate preanesthesia evaluation performed?
- Did the patient provide informed written consent before the procedure?
- Was the antibiotic administered in a timely manner?

Table 5-1 Quality Improvement Checklist for Locations Other Than the Operating Room

Steps	Description
Design a CQI infrastructure	Create a dedicated CQI committee with a designated chair and staff members
	Delineate responsibilities (data collection, metrics, outcome analysis, reporting)
	Provide resources (e.g., protected staff time, technical and IT support, electronic information system)
	Make the CQI program an integral part of the department's mission
	Ensure a nonpunitive culture
Create a list of quality indicators relevant for the practice and facility	Structure: Refers to hospital staff, facilities, material, and overall organization
	Process indicators: Coordination of patient care management activities (Was the antibiotic administered in a timely manner before incision? Was a preanesthetic evaluation performed and documented?)
	Outcomes: Measure patient-related end results of anesthesia care (e.g., mortality, morbidity, unplanned admission, patient satisfaction)
	See Table 5-2 for AQI quality indicators
Collect, analyze, and report data	Implement controlled and audited data collection (chart review, electronic anesthesia records) as well as self-reporting
	Use data element definitions that are clear, valid, and well defined
	Use tools to understand the process (e.g., flow charts, cause and effect diagrams, trend charts)
	Report data regularly to detect overall trends; calculate incidence rate (e.g., peripheral neurological deficit after regional anesthesia per total blocks performed)
	Compare data to national benchmarks
Detect problems and make improvements	Identify areas of recurring patterns; conduct a "focused review" of critical incidents and initiate root cause analysis
	Compare site-specific patterns with national trends
	Focus on systems, rather than on provider error
	Use a plan-do-study-act approach to make changes
Monitor for sustained improvement	Determine interval for reassessment (i.e., monthly, quarterly, yearly)
	Reassess indicators after change has been implemented
	Look for incremental performance improvement
	Communicate results to team, staff, and leadership
Submit QI data to a nationally endorsed anesthesiology registry, such as the Anesthesia Quality Institute	

CQI, Continuous quality improvement; *IT,* information technology; *QI,* quality improvement.

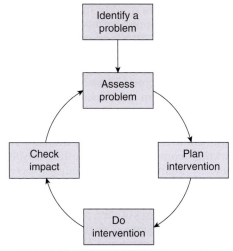

Figure 5-1 Continuous quality improvement (CQI) process uses a plan-do-study-act approach.

- Was central venous access obtained under strict sterile technique following established guidelines?
- Was hyperglycemia in a patient with diabetes treated according to an insulin protocol?

Although process indicators are considered more proximal indicators of quality than structural indicators, they cannot guarantee a quality outcome; they can only increase its probability.

Outcome indicators refer to the impact of treatments on patient well-being, including mortality, morbidity, disability, length of hospital stay, and patient functional status and satisfaction.

Validity of Continuous Quality Improvement Indicators in Anesthesiology

To confirm the validity of a quality indicator, the metrics must be connected to the accomplishment of a better outcome. Process indicators that evaluate care delivery paradigms, rather than patient outcomes, may be easier to measure and implement and can provide important insight into care.[5] Furthermore, process indicators might yield to positive or negative inputs concerning performance and consequently influence efficient improvement in patient care. Structural indicators are valuable only if they demonstrate an increase in either a good outcome or a process previously shown to yield better outcomes.

Because the outcomes of anesthesia care are so intertwined with surgery or procedural outcomes and patient comorbidities, choosing outcome measures sensitive to variations in quality of anesthesia care is difficult. Improvement in quality of anesthesia care was traditionally measured by a reduction in mortality and morbidity. However, mortality and serious morbidity attributable to anesthesia have decreased significantly over the last several decades to the point that they cannot currently be accepted as valid CQI measures.[6] In their review of

108 current anesthesia quality indicators, Haller et al[7] concluded that traditional perioperative morbidity and mortality data lacked criteria of sensitivity and specificity. Nearly half of the anesthesia quality indicators also measured surgical or postoperative care. Most indicators were either outcome (57%) or process (42%) indicators; only 1% of them were related to the structure of care. Patient safety (83%) and effectiveness (68%) were the two dimensions of quality of anesthetic care most often addressed, usually by outcome indicators. External benchmarking (comparison with other hospitals) and peer review by health care professionals were the primary methods used to identify possible quality issues.[7]

Despite these limitations, current quality-of-care indicators still measure processes of care, perianesthetic morbidity and mortality, and patient satisfaction for anesthesia care within both operating room and NORA settings. Because many severe adverse events in anesthesia are sufficiently rare, rates of more frequent outcomes such as nausea or vomiting, pain control, and critical incidents are often used as quality indicators. The Anesthesia Quality Institute (AQI) created a national clinical outcomes registry to capture data specific to anesthesia care, including quality of care.[8] Relevant quality indicators include rare outcomes (Table 5-2) (e.g., death), major adverse events (e.g., myocardial infarction and aspiration of gastric contents), minor adverse events (e.g., delirium and dental injury), administrative events (e.g., delays and documentation issues), and process events (e.g., difficult intubation and use of naloxone or flumazenil), as well as patient experience (Figure 5-2). These indicators are relevant to both operating room and NORA locations.

Methods to Improve Quality of Care: Quality Improvement Model Descriptions

Mishaps in anesthesia care are discovered through a variety of mechanisms. Historically, medical errors were revealed retrospectively through morbidity and mortality conferences and closed claims malpractice data.[9]

Review of a randomly selected or targeted sample of medical records has been used to identify problem areas and to collect data on adverse events.[10] Although collection of data in this manner may yield important epidemiologic information, it is costly and provides little insight into potential error reduction strategies. Moreover, chart review detects only documented adverse events and often does not capture information regarding their causes. Important errors that do not result in patient harm may go undetected by this method.

Critical Incidents

Critical incidents and adverse events reporting are innovations borrowed from the aircraft industry and adopted for anesthesiology quality improvement programs by Cooper[11] in the late 1970s. The goal is to report any unintended incident that could have jeopardized (if not corrected in a timely way) or did jeopardize patient safety. For example, a partial disconnect of the breathing circuit may be corrected before patient injury occurs, yet it has the potential to cause hypoxic brain damage or death.

Although learning from these incidents and "near-misses" might improve patient safety, the influence of well-recognized perception biases also will ultimately have an impact on the safety of care. These biases include under-reporting because of fear of punishment, inadequate documentation, unfamiliarity with the process, and lack of awareness of how the reported events will be analyzed.[12] Although most providers were aware of the existence of an incident reporting system in the United Kingdom, 25% did not know how to access the reporting form and over 40% of staff had never completed an accurate record of a reportable event.[13]

Incident reporting largely relies on the willingness of health care providers to voluntarily report them. The prevalence of underreported critical incidents has galvanized accrediting bodies such as The Joint Commission to promote mandatory reporting of select critical incidents and adverse outcomes as a requirement for institutional accreditation. The Joint Commission employs the term *sentinel event* in lieu of *critical incident* and defines it as "an unexpected occurrence involving death or serious physical or psychological injury, or the risk thereof."*

Sentinel Events

Sentinel events are single, isolated events that may indicate a systemic safety problem. A sentinel event may be an unexpected patient injury, such as an intraoperative death. Alternatively, a sentinel event may be a significant or alarming critical incident that did not result in patient injury, such as a syringe swap with administration of the wrong drug, noted and promptly treated.

The Joint Commission requires health care institutions to develop their own sentinel event policy. Such a policy would focus attention on underlying causes and risk reduction. The goal of the policy is to increase the general knowledge about medical errors, their causes, and prevention. This policy is seen as a way to have a positive impact on patient care and maintain public confidence in the accreditation process. The Joint Commission requires that this policy have a reporting, review, and planned feedback mechanism. Reportable events include, but are not limited to, incidents that involve wrong site or wrong patient surgery, incompatible blood transfusion reactions, awareness during general anesthesia, and, recently, preventing errors related to the use of common anticoagulants.*

The Joint Commission created a Sentinel Event Database as a component of its Sentinel Event Policy. This database accepts voluntary reports of sentinel events from member institutions, patients and families, and the press. The Joint Commission also mandates that accredited hospitals perform root cause analysis of critical sentinel events within 45 days.

---

*The Joint Commission: http://www.jointcommission.org/sentinel_event. aspx.

Table 5-2   Anesthesia Quality Institute Recommended Quality Indicators

Type of Indicator	Description	Type of Indicator	Description
Process	On-time starting percentages of first case		Surgical fire
	Cancellation rate		Skin or soft tissue injury
	On-time prophylactic antibiotic administration		Dental trauma
	Adherence to central line insertion protocol		Perioperative aspiration of gastric contents
	Temperature regulation		Vascular access complication
	Beta-blockade administration if preoperative beta-blocker		Pneumothorax
	Documentation compliance		Infection after regional anesthesia
	Patient complaints		Epidural hematoma
	Patient fall		High spinal
	Use of naloxone or flumazenil		Postdural puncture headache
	Regional block failure		Local anesthetic toxicity
	Unplanned dural puncture	Patient experience (see Figure 5-2)	Overall patient satisfaction
	Equipment malfunction		Rate of PONV
	Medication error		Adequacy of pain management
	Difficult intubation	Anesthesia Quality Institute recommended data collection	To assemble the indicators listed above, an anesthesia practice quality improvement program will need to electronically capture the following list of raw data for each case:
	Unplanned reintubation		
	Transfusion error		
	Prolonged emergence		Location (facility and location other than the operating room)
	Desaturation <90%, lasting >5 minutes		
	Bradycardia or tachycardia requiring treatment		CPT code(s)
	Hypotension requiring treatment		Surgeon
Clinical outcomes (major and minor adverse outcomes)	Death		Anesthesia provider(s)
	Cardiac arrest		Date
	Perioperative myocardial infarction		Time (or duration)
	Anaphylaxis or allergic reaction		Anesthesia type (e.g., general, regional, sedation, monitored anesthesia care)
	Malignant hyperthermia		
	Transfusion reaction		ASA class
	New stroke or brain damage		PQRS compliance (yes/no/not applicable for each of three variables)
	Visual loss		
	Eye injury		Occurrence of a listed complication (yes/no, and which one)
	Nerve damage		
	Incorrect patient, site, or procedure		Patient survey data (satisfaction, PONV, pain questions)
	Unplanned admission		
	Unplanned intensive care unit admission		Documentation completed, including QM form (yes/no)
	Intraoperative awareness		

From Dutton RP, DuKatz A. Quality improvement using automated data sources: the Anesthesia Quality Institute. *Anesthesiol Clin.* 2011; 29(3):439-454; and http://www.aqihq.org/qualitymeasurementtools.aspx.
ASA, American Society of Anesthesiologists; *CPT,* Current Procedural Terminology; *PONV,* postoperative nausea and vomiting; *PQRS,* Physician Quality Reporting System; *QM,* quality management.

Root Cause Analysis

Root cause analysis (RCA) is a system-based approach to investigate the underlying or contributing factors that lead to adverse events or critical incidents. The RCA was developed to analyze aviation and industrial accidents and is now widely implemented as an error analysis tool in health care. The goal of RCA is to determine what happened, why it happened, and what can be done to prevent it from happening again. This goal is accomplished by identifying the underlying problems and sequence of events in which the incident was rooted, not to "name and blame" individuals for the mistake. A typical RCA process follows a structured approach, which begins with data collection and reconstruction of the event through record review and participant interviews. A multidisciplinary team analyzes the sequence of events with the goal to spot why and how the incident occurred. Although identification of "active" errors is important, the major goal of the RCA is to uncover "latent" errors, such as system weaknesses hidden in a faulty operating system. To be thorough, an RCA must determine human and other factors, evaluate related processes and systems, analyze underlying cause and effect systems through a series of "why" questions, identify risks and their potential contributions, and suggest potential improvements in processes or systems.

Date		Provider ID	
MR #		CRNA ID	
ASA Class		Additional provider	

	QUALITY RATING					
	Strongly Positive	Somewhat	Neutral	Somewhat Negative	Strongly Negative	Don't Know
How satisfied were you with your anesthetic care?						
How likely are you to recommend the facility, personnel and anesthetic technique that you just underwent?						
After you left the recovery room or returned home…						
Did you experience nausea?	Yes	No				
Did you vomit at any time?	Yes	No				
How would you rate your pain on a scale of 1–10? (1 – no pain at all, 10 – worst pain ever)						
Has your pain medicine been effective	Yes	No				
Did you experience any unexpected events related to your procedure or the anesthetic?	Yes	No				

If so, please explain…	

This is a template. Please modify for local conditions.
The definitions for each measure can be found on the AQI website.   Not Part of Patient's Chart

Used with permission from the Anesthesia Quality Institute. Available at
http://www.aqihq.org/qualitymeasurementtools.aspx

Figure 5-2 Postanesthesia care patient satisfaction survey. (Used with permission from the Anesthesia Quality Institute. http://www.aqihq.org/qualitymeasurementtools.aspx.)

The knowledge gained from an RCA is used to make system changes that will prevent the sentinel event from occurring in the future. It is important for staff members to be engaged in discussions and participate in the development and implementation of practices or policies to reduce the risk for a similar event in the future. A plan for monitoring the effectiveness of new systems or procedures should be included as part of the plan.[14]*

*The Joint Commission: http://www.jointcommission.org/Framework_for_Conducting_a_Root_Cause_Analysis_and_Action_Plan.

Human Factors Analysis

Human factors analysis involves the study of human characteristics that may have an impact on patient safety. Examples of human factors include fatigue, stress, training, job environment, equipment, task, and environmental design. The science of human factors analysis is a multidisciplinary field with contributions from psychology, engineering, industrial design, graphic design, statistics, operations research, and anthropometry. The technology of examining human factors has been historically employed to improve aviation safety, and it is beginning to be used in health care in team training and in methods to reduce medication errors. It is also being incorporated into RCA.

Quality and Safety Improvement Efforts Outside the Operating Room

Surveillance of CQI processes at NORA locations must be as rigorous as in traditional operating room settings. Several of The Joint Commission's national patient safety goals give special attention to ambulatory and office-based practices. The goals are formulated based on the information provided by the Sentinel Event Advisory Group and thus are a synthesis of the reported sentinel events. The Joint Commission recommends program-specific patient safety goals for adoption; if the surveys show improvement in a specific area, the goals will be included in the accreditation standards. The Joint Commission revises, updates, and removes some goals each year while identifying new goals and requirements. These safety goals are found on The Joint Commission website.*

The Joint Commission's 2013 goals relevant to ambulatory and office-based anesthesia care are focused on prevention of infections and wrong patient and wrong site procedures. In an effort to reduce health care–associated infections, The Joint Commission set priorities for hand hygiene and catheter-associated urinary tract infection. Anesthesiologists have a crucial role in promoting hand and anesthetic apparatus hygiene and consequently preventing the transmission of intraoperative bacterial infections. Loftus et al[15] studied intraoperative bacterial transmission associated with anesthesia providers and equipment in a tertiary care center. Overall, 66% of provider hands were contaminated with one or more major pathogens, such as methicillin-resistant *Staphylococcus aureus,* methicillin-sensitive *S. aureus,* vancomycin-resistant enterococcus, *Enterococcus* spp, and Enterobacteriaceae. Bacterial organisms found on the hands of providers in a snapshot in time immediately before patient contact accounted for a fairly large proportion of the subsequent overall environmental and patient intravenous line stopcock set contamination. Furthermore, negligence for hand-transmitted bacterial contamination was shown by an observational study that monitored hand hygiene behavior of 226 nonscrubbed staff for a period of 60 hours and found that hand hygiene was applied no more than 0.14 times per individual per hour. Hand hygiene on entering or leaving the operating room was rare (2% and 8%, respectively). The team used a total of six or seven pairs of nonsterile gloves per surgical procedure.[16]

The Joint Commission also continues to stress its policy for preventing wrong person and wrong site procedures and wrong procedures. The Universal Protocol must be applied to all surgical and nonsurgical invasive procedures. Procedures that place the patient at the most risk include those that involve general anesthesia or deep sedation, although other procedures also may affect patient safety. The protocol is based on three intertwined elements: conducting a preprocedure verification process, marking the procedure site by directly involving the patient if possible, and performing a timeout before the procedure. The timeout is standardized, initiated by a designated member of the procedure team (usually the surgeon), and involves the immediate members of the procedure team. Team members agree about the patient identity, correct site, and procedure to be performed, and the timeout is documented. The surgical timeout has been recently expanded to improve team communication concerning equipment readiness, patient conditions, and anticipated intraoperative or postoperative concerns, with demonstrated reductions in surgical morbidity and mortality.[17] The American Society of Anesthesiologists' Committee on Ambulatory Surgical Care and the Society for Ambulatory Anesthesia's Committee on Office Based Anesthesia also have developed recommendations for safe anesthesia in NORA settings.* They recommend careful pre–site selection review, initiating thorough CQI and risk management programs, comparison of quality indicators with national benchmarks, a minimum of an annual check of anesthesia and emergency equipment, and regular CQI review by stakeholders.

THE FUTURE OF CONTINUOUS QUALITY IMPROVEMENT OUTSIDE THE OPERATING ROOM

Health care policy makers and national patient safety programs consider health information technologies (HIT) to be crucial to make the infrastructure of health care delivery safer, more efficient, and economical.[18,19]

Anesthesiology was one of the first medical specialties to champion HIT, known in the anesthesia literature as anesthesia information management systems (AIMS). The Anesthesia Patient Safety Foundation took a lead role in encouraging the use of AIMS to collect data, standardize anesthesia terminology, and stipulate major projects of outcome research and quality improvement.[20]

By definition, AIMS are a specific form of electronic medical record (EMR) systems that automatically capture, collect, and store patient data from the wide variety of monitors used perioperatively. In addition to providing basic recordkeeping functions, most AIMS also allow end users to access information for patient management, quality improvement, and research purposes. AIMS typically consist of a combination of hardware and software that interface with intraoperative monitors and in many cases hospital clinical data repositories or EMRs. All of this information is typically stored in a robust relational database that can be accessed simultaneously by multiple users through either a vendor's commercial application or standard database tools such as structured query language.[21]

CONTINUOUS QUALITY IMPROVEMENT AND ANESTHESIA INFORMATION MANAGEMENT SYSTEMS

Quality improvement may be supported by AIMS in several ways. First, these systems enable rapid collection of an enormous quantity of clinical data that can detect specific patterns and reveal deficiencies in the process of care. By gaining

*The Joint Commission: http://www.jointcommission.org.

*Becker's Hospital Review: http://www.beckershospitalreview.com/ anesthesia/15-quality-improvement-activities-for-office-based-anesthesia-recommended-by-asasamba.html.

insight into practices through uniform data collection, AIMS can smooth the progress of process improvement.

AIMS also facilitate reporting the continuously increasing number of quality metrics, such as timely administration of prophylactic antibiotics, preservation of normothermia, or indication for beta-blocker administration, as a condition of participation in pay-for-performance programs.

Clinical decision support systems also remind the provider about these care decisions and enhance the quality of care. For example, they can provide drug dosage guidance based on the patient's weight, alert the provider about changing clinical conditions such as low blood pressure or rhythm other than sinus, notify about drug allergies and drug interactions, send reminders regarding the need to re-dose antibiotics, or check blood sugar level in patients with diabetes. A recent report by Nair et al[22] showed that with the use of real-time reminders and feedback via clinical decision support, appropriate delivery of antibiotics was completed close to 100% of the time, and the compliance level remained stable over a period of 8 months despite staff turnover every month.

Finally, use of bar codes and automated alerts reduced medication errors in patients undergoing anesthesia. A recent, prospective randomized trial using a multimodal AIMS with bar code reading capabilities combined with decision support systems showed a reduction in the rate of drug errors by 21%.[23]

Conclusion

In summary, a robust CQI system is as important, if not more important, in the NORA setting as in the operating room. Dashboard analysis of quality indicators with benchmarking comparison to national standards is essential. Identification of safety concerns and critical incidents, thorough review of sentinel events using RCA to identify systems failures, initiation of systems changes, human factors analysis, and continuing assessment in a PDSA approach is vital to the success of a CQI program.

References

1. Institute of Medicine. *Crossing the quality chasm: a new health system for the 21st century.* Washington DC: National Academies Press; 2001.
2. Atkinson S, Ingham J, Cheshire M, Went S. Defining quality and quality improvement. *Clin Med.* 2010;10(6):537–539.
3. Donabedian A. The quality of care: how can it be assessed? *JAMA.* 1988;260(12):1743–1748.
4. Donabedian A. *An introduction to quality assurance in health care.* 44th ed. New York: Oxford University Press; 2003. 200.
5. Pronovost PJ, Miller MR, Dorman T, Berenholtz SM, Rubin H. Developing and implementing measures of quality of care in the intensive care unit. *Curr Opin Crit Care.* 2001;7(4):297–303.
6. Benn J, Arnold G, Wei I, et al. Using quality indicators in anaesthesia: feeding back data to improve care. *Br J Anaesth.* 2012;109(1):80–91.
7. Haller G, Stoelwinder J, Myles P, McNeil J. Quality and safety indicators in anesthesia: a systematic review. *Anesthesiology.* 2009;110(5):1158–1175.
8. Dutton RP, DuKatz A. Quality improvement using automated data sources: the Anesthesia Quality Institute. *Anesthesiol Clin.* 2011;29(3):439–454.
9. Higginson J, Walters R, Fulop N. Mortality and morbidity meetings: an untapped resource for improving the governance of patient safety? *BMJ Qual Saf.* 2012;21(7):576–585.
10. Shojania KG, Duncan BW, McDonald KM, Wachter RM, Markowitz AJ. Making health care safer: a critical analysis of patient safety practices. *Evid Rep Technol Assess (Summ).* 2001;43:1–668. i-x.
11. Cooper JB, Newbower RS, Long CD, McPeek B. Preventable anesthesia mishaps: a study of human factors. *Anesthesiology.* 1978;49(6):399–406.
12. Staender S. Incident reporting in anaesthesiology. *Best Pract Res Clin Anaesthesiol.* 2011;25(2):207–214.
13. Evans SM, Berry JG, Smith BJ, et al. Attitudes and barriers to incident reporting: a collaborative hospital study. *Qual Saf Health Care.* 2006;15(1):39–43.
14. Mahajan RP. Critical incident reporting and learning. *Br J Anaesth.* 2010;105(1):69–75.
15. Loftus RW, Muffly MK, Brown JR, et al. Hand contamination of anesthesia providers is an important risk factor for intraoperative bacterial transmission. *Anesth Analg.* 2011;112(1):98–105.
16. Krediet AC, Kalkman CJ, Bonten MJ, Gigengack AC, Barach P. Hand-hygiene practices in the operating theatre: an observational study. *Br J Anaesth.* 2011;107(4):553–558.
17. Haynes AB, Weiser TG, Berry WR, et al. Safe Surgery Saves Lives Study Group. A surgical safety checklist to reduce morbidity and mortality in a global population. *N Engl J Med.* 2009;360(5):491–499.
18. Bates DW, Gawande AA. Improving safety with information technology. *N Engl J Med.* 2003;348(25):2526–2534.
19. U.S. Department of Health and Human Services. Health Information Privacy. HITECH Act Enforcement Interim Final Rule. Washington, DC. http://www.hhs.gov/ocr/privacy/hipaa/administrative/enforcementrule/hitechenforcementifr.html.
20. Monk TG, Hurrell M, Norton A. Toward standardization of terminology in anesthesia information management systems. Anesthesia Patient Safety Foundation. http://www.apsf.org/initiatives.php?id=2.
21. Muravchick S, Caldwell JE, Epstein RH, et al. Anesthesia information management system implementation: a practical guide. *Anesth Analg.* 2008;107(5):1598–1608.
22. Nair BG, Newman SF, Peterson GN, Wu WY, Schwid HA. Feedback mechanisms including real-time electronic alerts to achieve near 100% timely prophylactic antibiotic administration in surgical cases. *Anesth Analg.* 2010;111(5):1293–1300.
23. Merry AF, Webster CS, Hannam J, et al. Multimodal system designed to reduce error in recording and administration of drugs in anaesthesia: prospective randomized clinical evaluation. *BMJ.* 2011;343. d5543.

6

Critical Monitoring Issues for Non–Operating Room Anesthesia

JOHN P. SCOTT

The rise in the number of nonsurgical diagnostic and therapeutic interventions is driving the surge in volume of remote anesthesia and sedation services.[1] These procedures have simultaneously become increasingly complex as a result of technological advances and sicker patient cohorts. Complicating matters further, although these patients remain at high risk for anesthesia-related complications, they may be scheduled for such procedures precisely because they are poor surgical candidates. Settings requiring non–operating room anesthesia (NORA) include the interventional radiology department, cardiac catheterization laboratory, endoscopy suite, emergency room, magnetic resonance imaging (MRI) suite, and hyperbaric oxygen chamber. The primary logistical challenges that abound in NORA include issues related to location, personnel, equipment, power supply, patient accessibility, and preprocedural screening.[2]

One critical consequence of NORA expansion is a shortage of qualified anesthesiologist providers. This resource limitation has resulted in increased numbers of nonanesthesiologists providing sedation.[3] The American Society of Anesthesiologists (ASA) categorizes sedation into four distinct categories: minimal sedation, moderate sedation, deep sedation, and general anesthesia (Table 6-1).[4] Monitored anesthesia care (MAC) is another term commonly encountered during sedation. MAC does not describe a particular level of sedation but rather the delivery of anesthesia care during a procedure. This may involve the administration of sedation, local anesthesia, or no anesthesia at all, but the provider remains responsible for the monitoring and medical care of the patient.[5]

According to ASA mandate, general anesthesia is provided only by anesthesia professionals such as anesthesiologists, certified nurse anesthetists, and anesthesia assistants.[6] However, the Centers for Medicare and Medicaid Services permits nonanesthesiologists to provide minimal, moderate, or deep sedation. This group of providers includes physicians, dentists, oral surgeons, and podiatrists. Great variation exists in these heterogeneous groups in their training, basic skills, and practice patterns, resulting in inconsistent care delivery.

In an effort to reduce anesthesia-related complications and improve outcomes, the ASA performed multiple closed claims analyses seeking to identify the root causes of adverse events during anesthesia. Initial analyses were focused on operating room–based general anesthetics.[7] These sentinel studies revealed that the most adverse events were respiratory and frequently preventable with improved monitoring, specifically with the use of continuous pulse oximetry and capnography.[7] Consequently, these monitors are now considered standard for operrating room–based anesthetics and are nearly universally employed.

Subsequent analyses focusing on NORA have yielded similar results.[8-10] The majority of complications in these studies were respiratory events. However, morbidity related to hypoventilation, hypoxemia, and hypothermia occurred at increased rates during NORA. Severity of injury and overall mortality also increased during remote location procedures.[9,10] The endoscopy suite and cardiac catheterization laboratory were the most commonly identified locations. MAC was the most frequently documented anesthetic technique. Risk factors for complications during NORA included extremes of age, ASA III and IV physical health status (Table 6-2), obesity, and emergency procedures. The quality of anesthesia care was more likely to be substandard in NORA claims in contrast to operating room–based claims, thus resulting in a call for improved monitoring and standardization of minimum monitoring requirements.[8,9] The ASA now recommends adherence to the same basic monitoring standards for anesthesia used in both operating room and non–operating room procedures.[11]

Nonanesthesiologist investigations by emergency room physicians, radiologists, and gastroenterologists similarly underscore the importance of minimum standard monitoring.[12-19] Improved monitoring of respiratory function, specifically pulse oximetry and capnography, facilitates the detection of respiratory insufficiency. For providers lacking formal anesthesia training, standard monitoring is essential to mitigate delays in the recognition of respiratory or cardiovascular insufficiency and ensure safe care delivery.

Despite the development of monitoring guidelines and overwhelming evidence of the benefits of basic monitors, uniform implementation of monitoring standards for NORA has not occurred. Surveys of sedation providers demonstrate inconsistent application of basic monitors.[15] To effectively improve patient safety during NORA, it is imperative that all providers understand and consistently adhere to basic monitoring standards.

Basic Monitors

The ASA recommends that minimum standard monitors employed for anesthesia should enable an assessment of oxygenation, ventilation, and circulation.[11] No distinction is made for type of anesthesia or location of anesthetic delivery. For healthy patients (ASA I to II physical health status) undergoing uncomplicated procedures, this should include continuous monitoring of oxygenation with pulse oximetry,

Table 6-1 Continuum of Depth of Sedation: Definition of General Anesthesia and Levels of Sedation/Analgesia

	Minimal Sedation (Anxiolysis)	**Moderate Sedation/Analgesia ("Conscious Sedation")**	**Deep Sedation/Analgesia**	**General Anesthesia**
Responsiveness	Normal response to verbal stimulation	Purposeful response to verbal or tactile stimulation	Purposeful response following repeated or painful stimulation	Unarousable even with painful stimulation
Airway	Unaffected	No intervention required	Intervention may be required	Intervention often required
Spontaneous ventilation	Unaffected	Adequate	May be inadequate	Frequently inadequate
Cardiovascular function	Unaffected	Usually maintained	Usually maintained	May be impaired

From American Society of Anesthesiologists. *Continuum of depth of sedation: definition of general anesthesia and levels of sedation/analgesia—standards, guidelines and statements.* Park Ridge, Ill: American Society of Anesthesiologists; 2009.

Table 6-2 American Society of Anesthesiologists Physical Status Classification System

ASA 1	Healthy
ASA 2	Mild systemic disease
ASA 3	Severe systemic disease
ASA 4	Severe systemic disease that is a constant threat to life
ASA 5	Moribund and not expected to survive
ASA 6	Brain dead; organ donor

Modified from American Society of Anesthesiologists. *Physical Status Classification System.* Park Ridge, Ill: American Society of Anesthesiologists.
ASA, American Society of Anesthesiologists.

respiratory rate and ventilation with capnography, and cardiac monitoring with electrocardiography. Noninvasive blood pressure measurements should be performed at least every 5 minutes. Measurement of patient body temperature is also recommended. Decisions regarding advanced invasive and noninvasive monitoring should be made on a case-to-case basis depending on patient health status and procedural complexity. Monitor alarm limits must be adjusted to age-appropriate vital sign thresholds and be clearly audible.

PULSE OXIMETRY

The introduction of continuous pulse oximetry during the 1980s has greatly improved provider recognition of peri-procedural hypoxemia. The ASA now mandates continuous pulse oximetry during all anesthetics.[11] Modern pulse oximeters calculate the arterial oxygen saturation based on the Beer-Lambert law. The measured arterial oxygen saturation is derived from the absorption of probe-emitted red and infrared light by hemoglobin within arterial (pulsatile) blood. The four main hemoglobin species within adult blood are oxyhemoglobin (HbO_2), deoxyhemoglobin (HbR), met-hemoglobin (metHb), and carboxyhemoglobin (COHb).[20] Fetal hemoglobin (HbF) is present in neonatal blood. HbO_2 and HbR, the predominant species in normal individuals, absorb light at different wavelengths. HbO_2 absorbs near infrared light at a wavelength of 940 nm, and HbR absorbs red light at a wavelength of 660 nm. The pulse oximeter calculates arterial oxygen saturation according to the relative ratio of red and infrared light absorption.[20]

Continuous pulse oximetry during anesthesia reduces the incidence and severity of periprocedural hypoxemia, although it is unclear whether this has resulted in reduced morbidity.[21] Prospective studies have not shown improved outcomes resulting from pulse oximetry,[21] but as Eichhorn[22] pointed out in his 1993 editorial, the rate of hypoxia-related adverse events during anesthesia is relatively low, making it impractical if not impossible to perform a study powered to detect statistically improved outcomes related the use of pulse oximetry.[22] Nonetheless, it is reasonable to conclude that enhanced detection of hypoxemia through routine continuous pulse oximetry has led to clinically significant improvements in care delivery.

Pulse oximetry has limitations. It does not provide information regarding ventilation. Also, because pulse oximeters rely on pulsatile blood flow to determine oxygen saturations, physiological states associated with decreased pulsatility, such as shock, severe vasoconstriction, and low cardiac output, may result in spurious pulse oximetry readings.[23] The pulse oximeter probe is typically attached to fingertips. Nail polish on fingernails decreases tissue penetrance of probe-emitted light and obscures pulse oximetry readings.[20] Finally, increased levels of abnormal hemoglobin variants such as methemoglobin and carboxyhemoglobin are associated with inaccurate pulse oximetry values and require alternative methods such as co-oximetry to measure arterial oxygen saturation.

CAPNOGRAPHY

Capnography is the continuous measurement of the partial pressure of carbon dioxide over the respiratory cycle (Figure 6-1). Capnography quantifies the amount of infrared radiation absorbed by molecules of carbon dioxide. The amount of infrared radiation absorbed has an exponential relationship to the partial pressure of carbon dioxide.[14] The measured partial pressure of carbon dioxide at the end of exhalation is called the end-tidal carbon dioxide ($ETCO_2$). Classically, capnography has been used to assess ventilation in intubated patients. However, this technology may be used in nonintubated patients using nasal cannulas equipped with sidestream ports for sampling exhaled carbon dioxide.[14] Before the introduction of capnography, visual inspection and impedance plethysmography were used to measure respiratory rate and to detect hypoventilation and apnea during sedation. These methods largely have been replaced by capnography, which also allows for the continuous quantification of respiratory rate.

Capnography provides essential quantitative and qualitative information regarding the adequacy of ventilation.[14]

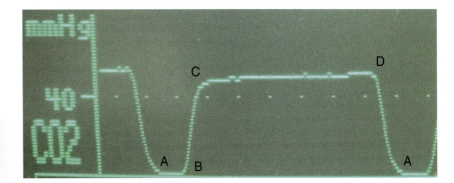

Figure 6-1 Normal capnogram. **A** and **B,** Dead space ventilation. **B** and **C,** Ascending expiratory phase (mixing of alveolar and dead space ventilation). **C** and **D,** Alveolar phase. **D,** End-tidal carbon dioxide. **D** to **A,** Inspiratory phase.

During procedural sedation complicated by hypoventilation, capnographic waveforms typically exhibit two types of changes. Bradypneic hypoventilation, a common side effect of opioids, is hypoventilation caused by a decrease in respiratory rate. The capnographic tracing in bradypneic hypoventilation displays increased $ETCO_2$ and decreased rate. Conversely, hypopneic hypoventilation, as commonly occurs with hypnotics such as propofol, is associated with decreased tidal volume and respiratory rate. A greater proportion of each exhaled breath is dead space ventilation, and $ETCO_2$ is consequently reduced with a widened arterial carbon dioxide level to $ETCO_2$ gradient.[14]

Studies evaluating capnography in nonintubated patients during NORA suggest that respiratory insufficiency may be detected by capnography well before hypoxemia is detected with pulse oximetry. In pediatric studies of remote procedural sedation in the emergency room and in MRI, capnography detected hypopneic hypoventilation 2 to 3 minutes before hypoxemia was detected with pulse oximetry.[17,18] Similarly, in adult patients undergoing propofol sedation in the emergency room or in the endoscopy suite, capnography was shown not only to provide earlier detection of hypoventilation but to also decrease the incidence of hypoxemia.[16,19] In patients undergoing procedural sedation receiving supplemental oxygen, capnography is crucial to the early detection of abnormal ventilation because hyperoxia delays the onset of hypoxemia.[13] The utility of capnography is not limited to monitoring ventilation; it is also useful in assessing circulation, perfusion, and total body metabolism. Capnographic waveforms exhibit quantitative changes in many pathophysiological states. Causes of increased exhaled carbon dioxide include hypoventilation, rebreathing of exhaled carbon dioxide, and hypermetabolic states such as malignant hyperthermia and hyperthyroidism. Causes of decreased exhaled carbon dioxide include unplanned airway disconnection (i.e., circuit disconnection or extubation), hyperventilation, increased dead space ventilation, and pulmonary hypoperfusion (i.e., profound shock, low cardiac output, pulmonary embolism, or venous air embolism).[24]

ELECTROCARDIOGRAM

Continuous electrocardiogram (ECG) monitoring is the simplest form of noninvasive cardiac monitoring. The ECG provides a graphic representation of the electrical activity of the heart, including its heart rate and rhythm. During anesthesia, continuous ECG monitoring is critical in the detection of myocardial ischemia, arrhythmias, or important electrolyte disturbances such as hyperkalemia.[24] However, the ECG provides little information regarding myocardial contractility or function.

Both three-lead and five-lead ECGs are employed for standard monitoring purposes. The three-lead ECG incorporates the I, II, and III limb leads first described by Einthoven. This provides basic ECG information, and only one lead may be viewed at a time. For more complex cases in at-risk patients, five-lead monitoring is recommended. This requires the placement of an additional limb lead and a fifth (V) intercostal lead, allowing for a more comprehensive examination. During five-lead monitoring, valuable information may be gathered by viewing leads II and V simultaneously. Lead II is useful in the detection of arrhythmias and inferior wall ischemia, and lead V is helpful in the detection of anterior and lateral wall ischemia.[24]

NONINVASIVE BLOOD PRESSURE

Noninvasive arterial blood pressure measurements should be performed at least every 5 minutes during NORA using either manual or automated methods.[11] These measurements are classically performed by placing an appropriate-size blood pressure cuff around the upper arm. Cuff inflation above the systolic blood pressure results in brachial arterial compression interrupting blood flow. Blood flow resumes with cuff deflation, allowing for an estimation of arterial blood pressures. Manual blood pressure monitoring requires a sphygmomanometer and a stethoscope placed over the brachial artery. This method relies on auscultation of the Korotkoff sounds to determine the systolic and diastolic blood pressure. The mean arterial blood pressure (MAP) may be calculated based on these pressures.

Automated blood pressure monitoring uses the principles of oscillometry described by Von Recklinghausen.[25,26] This method is based on the detection of oscillations transmitted as blood flow resumes in the previously compressed artery. Oscillometric blood pressure monitoring most accurately predicts the MAP, which occurs at the point of maximal oscillations. Systolic and diastolic blood pressure are calculated based on specific algorithms, but the systolic blood pressure normally corresponds to the beginning of oscillations and the diastolic blood pressure to when the oscillations cease.

Temperature

According to the ASA, "every patient receiving anesthesia shall have temperature monitored when clinically significant changes in body temperature are intended, anticipated or suspected."[11] Acceptable temperature monitoring sites include the axilla, nasopharynx, esophagus, rectum, and bladder.[27] Malignant hyperthermia is the most urgent temperature-related complication of general anesthesia with volatile gases. However, hypothermia is far more common, because most anesthetics induce a state of poikilothermia.

Temperature monitoring is equally important during NORA. Hypothermia is prevalent in remote locations, because many areas are not equipped with effective heating systems. Furthermore, some locations require active cooling to prevent equipment from overheating.[28] Hypothermia during anesthesia has been linked to multisystem morbidity, including myocardial ischemia, surgical site infections, and coagulation disorders.[27,29-31] Ultimately, undetected and untreated hypothermia is associated with prolonged length of hospital stay and increased costs.[28]

Advanced Monitors

INVASIVE INTRAVASCULAR MONITORING

All invasive intravascular monitoring systems require percutaneous placement of a vascular (i.e., arterial, central venous, or pulmonary artery) catheter and a pressure transduction system. Continuously transduced arterial or venous waveforms are displayed on monitors, allowing for the beat-to-beat assessment of arterial or venous pressures.[24]

Intraarterial blood pressure (IABP) monitoring is considered the most accurate method of blood pressure measurement. Decisions regarding arterial line placement for NORA should be based on patient health status and procedural complexity. Complex endovascular procedures in interventional radiology and the cardiac catheterization laboratory are likely to require IABP monitoring to assist with the maintenance of tight blood pressure control and vital end-organ perfusion pressure. In the mechanically ventilated patient, analysis of arterial pulse pressure waveforms and measurement of arterial pulse pressure variation during the respiratory cycle is predictive of preload responsiveness and may be used to guide fluid replacement therapy in hypovolemic patients.[32]

Common indications for central venous line placement include central venous pressure (CVP) monitoring and the need to deliver vasoactive or inotropic medications. Historically, the CVP was thought to accurately reflect the right ventricular end-diastolic pressure, pulmonary capillary wedge pressure, and left ventricular end-diastolic pressure. Based on these presumptions, the CVP was used as an indicator of ventricular preload responsiveness. Emerging evidence, however, suggests that CVP is not a reliable measure of intravascular volume status and should not be used in isolation to guide fluid resuscitation.[33]

The utility of pulmonary artery catheter (PAC) monitoring remains a source of great controversy within the anesthesia and critical care communities. PAC insertion allows for the measurement of right and left heart pressures and calculation of important hemodynamic variables, including cardiac output and vascular resistances. To date, no studies have linked PAC monitoring to improved patient outcomes. Instead, multiple observational studies suggest increased PAC-related morbidity and mortality.[34] Recognized complications of PAC insertion include arrhythmias, pulmonary artery rupture, and pulmonary hemorrhage.[35] Subsequently, PAC use for complex cardiac procedures and in the intensive care unit has declined in recent years. PAC monitoring during NORA should be reserved for experienced providers in select subsets of patients, such as those with left ventricular failure or liver transplants.

NEAR INFRARED SPECTROSCOPY

Near infrared spectroscopy (NIRS) is a completely noninvasive methodology used to assess regional tissue oxygenation and perfusion. NIRS also is based on the Beer-Lambert law and the absorption of near infrared light by hemoglobin species. NIRS probes contain a near infrared light source and two receivers. The light source emits near infrared light at 730- and 810-nm wavelengths to generate a tissue saturation.[36] The regional oxygen saturation (RSO_2) measured via NIRS is a mean tissue oxyhemoglobin saturation, which tends to reflect tissue venous saturation.[37] This RSO_2 value provides valuable information regarding regional oxygen delivery and consumption.[37] This is clinically important because reduced regional perfusion may be clinically silent until organ dysfunction occurs, resulting in increased morbidity and mortality.

NIRS is typically used in adults to monitor cerebral perfusion and blood flow. In terms of adult NORA procedures, bilateral cerebral RSO_2 monitoring has been used in interventional neuroradiology to detect critical changes in cerebral blood flow and oxygen delivery during endovascular procedures.[38] RSO_2 monitoring has been used in children to measure tissue saturations in the brain, kidney, and mesentery. For children with congenital heart disease, cerebral and renal or somatic, NIRS has become a widely accepted standard monitor of regional perfusion in the operating room and intensive care unit after open heart surgery. Many of these same children require future cardiac catheterizations, and NIRS monitoring may be helpful during these procedures. Similarly, critically ill children requiring NORA may benefit from NIRS monitoring to assess vital organ oxygen delivery.[39]

NIRS does have limitations. The probe emits near infrared light that penetrates a tissue depth of only 2 to 6 cm, which limits the utility of noncerebral RSO_2 monitoring in obese patients.[37] Additionally, because bilirubin also absorbs near infrared light, the device is not accurate in patients with hyperbilirubinemia, but it may still be used as a trend monitor.

BISPECTRAL INDEX MONITORING

Bispectral index (BIS) monitoring was developed to assess the levels of sedation and awareness during surgery. The BIS index, 0 to 100, is derived from continuous electroencephalographic and electromyographic data and corresponds to the patient's level of consciousness. A BIS of 0 equates to an isoelectric electrocardiogram (EEG) with no brain activity, and 100 to an awake and alert state.[40] BIS values less than 60 are associated with a state of general anesthesia and reduced incidence of patient recall.[41] BIS monitoring has been used during procedural sedation in remote locations to help providers titrate hypnotic and analgesic medications and avoid oversedation. Studies evaluating BIS monitoring for NORA confirm that patients under sedation frequently transition to a state of general anesthesia, which may be otherwise unnoticed by providers.[40] The Cochrane database reviewed BIS monitoring for anesthesia and procedural sedation and concluded that BIS monitoring was associated with reduced anesthetic requirements and shortened recovery times. The incidence of patient recall during painful procedures was also decreased, with shortened time to extubation during procedures requiring general anesthesia.[41] Other monitors of the EEG are not reviewed here but may be useful.

Site-Specific Monitoring Considerations

MAGNETIC RESONANCE IMAGING

MRI requires a motionless patient to generate optimal images without artifact. Radiologists request sedation or general anesthesia for patients who are unable to lie still. Many standard monitoring devices are not MRI compatible because of monitor interference or burn risks associated with ferromagnetic heating of wires and cables. Standard ECG monitoring is distorted by electromagnetic interference. Modern MRI-compatible ECG devices produce gated ECG waveforms that subtract electromagnetic interference. The measurement of pulse oximetry, capnography, and oscillometric blood pressure monitoring is largely unaffected by electromagnetic fields, but fiberoptic cables or wireless devices are required, as are MRI-compatible pulse oximeter probes and blood pressure cuffs.[42] Transducers for invasive arterial pressure lines and CVP lines contain copper, which is nonferrous and thus MRI compatible, but transducers should be kept off the MRI bed to reduce artifact and limit interference.[43] The use of NIRS and BIS monitors during MRI is contraindicated because of the risk for probe-related burns. Temperature should be routinely monitored because hypothermia is common as a result of the lengthy nature of these scans, especially in children or when general anesthesia is required.[28]

Modern MRI-compatible monitors are designed with wireless technology (e.g., Invivo, Gainesville, Fla.). These devices are equipped to measure noninvasive and invasive parameters. MRI-compatible monitors must be positioned an appropriate distance from the magnet and secured safely. MRI scanning is also very loud, and it is imperative that alarms on physiological monitoring equipment are set to appropriate volume levels.[44]

ENDOSCOPY SUITE

The ASA closed claims analysis for remote locations highlighted an increased complication rate of endoscopy suite procedures, including endoscopic retrograde cholangiopancreatography (ERCP), upper endoscopy, and colonoscopy.

Patients most likely to encounter complications were older (>70 years) and sicker (ASA status 3-5). Respiratory insufficiency was common during these cases. More than half of these claims were thought to be preventable with improved monitoring. Capnography was not employed in the majority of the claims.[8,10]

Endoscopic procedures requiring sedation are associated with various complications. The required sedation may diminish airway reflexes and increase aspiration risk. Endoscope placement frequently creates external airway compression and may worsen upper airway obstruction. Also, prone positioning required during ERCP is associated with worsened respiratory mechanics and limits provider access to the patient's airway. Early detection of respiratory insufficiency with continuous capnography and pulse oximetry is thus essential because the cases frequently involve shared airways and repositioning may be necessary to safely secure the patient's airway. Patients also may be at increased risk for hemodynamic lability after bowel preparation regimens or in the case of active gastrointestinal bleeding; thus continuous ECG and intermittent NIBP measurements also are indicated.[8]

CARDIAC CATHETERIZATION LABORATORY

The number of indications for cardiac catheterization in adults and children with heart disease is increasing. Historically, cardiac catheterization in adults was limited to percutaneous coronary interventions for coronary artery disease and electrophysiology studies for dysrhythmias. With the advent of percutaneous transcatheter valve replacement (TVR), patients with valvular heart disease who are poor surgical candidates may avoid the risks associated with surgical valve replacement and cardiopulmonary bypass.[45] These patients remain at high risk for anesthetic-related morbidity and mortality.

Cardiac catheterization may be performed under sedation with local anesthesia or general anesthesia. Irrespective of the choice of sedation, these individuals are at high risk because of cardiac disease and other comorbidities. Minimum standard monitoring for adult cardiac catheterization should include pulse oximetry, capnography, ECG, NIBP, and temperature. Invasive monitoring (i.e., IABP, CVP) should be based on patient health status and procedural complexity. For TVR procedures, both advanced noninvasive (NIRS) and invasive (IABP, CVP) monitoring modalities are recommended. Transesophageal echocardiography is frequently used as well.

Children with congenital heart disease may require multiple cardiac catheterizations during infancy and childhood. The spectrum of congenital heart disease is vast, encompassing cyanotic and acyanotic lesions. Given the degree of physiological complexity, advanced invasive and noninvasive monitoring is frequently required. NIRS has proved to be an extremely useful monitor in the assessment of oxygen delivery and consumption for children with heart disease.[39] Two-site cerebral and somatic regional oximetry provides vital information regarding the distribution of blood flow, oxygen delivery, and cardiac output. Invasive arterial pressure and CVP monitoring also may be necessary, depending on the type of lesion, patient health status, and procedural complexity.

HYPERBARIC OXYGEN CHAMBER

Hyperbaric oxygen therapy is prescribed for many conditions, the most common of which is for the treatment of nonhealing wounds in diabetic patients. However, critically ill patients with carbon monoxide poisoning secondary to smoke inhalation or necrotizing soft tissue infections may also require hyperbaric oxygen therapy. Invasive monitoring is often required for these patients. Hyperbaric oxygen chambers may be configured for single or multiple patients, and access to the patient and ease of monitoring differ accordingly.[46] In multipatient hyperbaric oxygen chambers, the monitoring devices are located within the chamber. In single-patient chambers, monitors are located outside the hyperbaric oxygen tank, and leads and cables must pass through pressure-sealed port holes to attach to the patient.[46] Continuous pulse oximetry is not universally indicated because of the high partial pressure of oxygen delivered. Dangers associated with monitoring during hyperbaric oxygen therapy relate to the inherent fire risks of high oxygen tensions. Thus all monitors used in hyperbaric oxygen chambers must be electrically safe and in compliance with National Fire Protection Association guidelines.[46] The development of wireless monitoring technology may help reduce fire risks and improve safety.[47]

OFFICE-BASED ANESTHESIA

Office-based anesthesia represents a rapidly growing segment of NORA. According to the American Hospital Association, the number of office-based anesthetics doubled from 1995 to 2005.[48,49] Dental, cosmetic, and maxillofacial procedures are commonly performed in office-based settings. These locations are not subject to the same governmental regulations as their hospital and ambulatory surgery center counterparts. Office-based anesthesia practices have minimal accreditation requirements.[50] Anesthetic techniques practiced in an office setting include local anesthesia, regional anesthesia, sedation, and general anesthesia.

Office-based practices should be equipped with the same standard monitoring capabilities (i.e., pulse oximetry, capnography, ECG, NIBP, and temperature) as hospitals and ambulatory surgery centers. Monitors must be well maintained and functional.[50] The ASA recommends compliance with the same minimum monitoring standards as hospital and surgery center anesthetizing locations. Available monitoring capabilities also must be equipped to meet patient needs in the event of emergencies and transfers.

INTENSIVE CARE UNIT

Patients in the intensive care unit are critically ill by definition. Transportation of critically ill patients can be destabilizing, with significant morbidity and mortality. This has resulted in a growing number of surgical and nonsurgical procedures for patients of all ages in the intensive care unit (Table 6-3). These patients are at extremely high risk for sedation-related morbidity and should be monitored accordingly. In situ invasive monitoring lines should be continued. For patients without advanced monitoring, it is important to recognize that

Table 6-3   Common Intensive Care Unit Procedures

Site	Procedures
Neonatal ICU	Patent ductus arteriosus ligation, balloon atrial septostomy, exploratory laparotomy, PICC insertion
Pediatric ICU	Bronchoscopy, endoscopy, delayed sternal closures after cardiac surgery, PICC insertion
Adult medical and surgical ICU	Bronchoscopy, endoscopy, percutaneous tracheostomy, percutaneous gastrostomy, external ventricular drain and intracranial pressure monitor placement, PICC insertion

ICU, Intensive care unit; *PICC,* peripherally inserted central catheter.

both the procedure itself and the required sedation may be life threatening. Thus additional invasive (i.e., IABP and CVP) and noninvasive (i.e., BIS and NIRS) monitoring may be required. BIS monitoring may allow for more precise titration of sedative and analgesic medications, because excessive sedation may result in hemodynamic instability. However, BIS monitoring has not been linked to reduced days of mechanical ventilation or intensive care unit length of stay.[51]

Conclusion

The implementation of monitoring standards for all anesthetics regardless of location represents an essential quality initiative to improve care delivery and patient safety. Basic monitoring for NORA should include pulse oximetry, capnography, ECG, and NIBP. Body temperature also should be measured. Anesthetics associated with increased risk, because of procedural complexity or patient comorbidities, require advanced monitoring. Facilities where complex procedures are performed on sick patients in remote locations must be equipped with monitoring capabilities to match patient needs.

References

1. Pino RM. The nature of anesthesia and procedural sedation outside of the operating room. *Curr Opin Anaesthesiol.* 2007;20(4):347–351.
2. Van de Velde M, Kuypers M, Teunkens A, Devroe S. Risk and safety of anesthesia outside the operating room. *Minerva Anestesiol.* 2009;75(5):345–348.
3. Lalwani K, Michel M. Pediatric sedation in North American children's hospitals: a survey of aesthesia providers. *Pediatr Anesth.* 2005;15(3):209–213.
4. American Society of Anesthesiologists. *Continuum of depth of sedation: definition of general anesthesia and levels of sedation/analgesia–standards, guidelines and statements.* Park Ridge, Ill: American Society of Anesthesiologists; 2009.
5. American Society of Anesthesiologists. *Distinguishing monitored anesthesia care (MAC) from moderate sedation/analgesia (conscious sedation): standards, guidelines and statements.* Park Ridge, Ill: American Society of Anesthesiologists; 2009.
6. American Society of Anesthesiologists. *Advisory on granting privileges for deep sedation to non-anesthesiologist sedation practitioners: standards, guidelines and statements.* Park Ridge, Ill: American Society of Anesthesiologists; 2010.
7. Caplan RA, Posner KL, Ward RJ, Cheney FW. Adverse respiratory events in anesthesia: a closed claims analysis. *Anesthesiology.* 1990;72(5):828–833.
8. Robbertze R, Posner KL, Domino KB. Closed claims review of anesthesia for procedures outside the operating room. *Curr Opin Anaesthesiol.* 2006;19(4):436–442.

9. Bhananker SM, Posner KL, Cheney FW, et al. Injury and liability associated with monitored anesthesia care: a closed claims analysis. *Anesthesiology*. 2006;104:228–234.

10. Metzner J, Posner JL, Domino KB. The risk and safety of anesthesia at remote locations: the US closed claims analysis. *Curr Opin Anaesthesiol*. 2009;22(4):502–508.

11. American Society of Anesthesiologists. *Standards for basic anesthetic monitoring: standards, guidelines and statements*. Park Ridge, Ill: American Society of Anesthesiologists; 2011.

12. Tuite C, Rosenberg EJ. Sedation and analgesia in interventional radiology. *Semin Intervent Rad*. 2005;22(2):114–120.

13. Burton JH, Harrah JD, Germann CA, et al. Does end-tidal carbon dioxide monitoring detect respiratory events prior to current sedation monitoring practices? *Acad Emerg Med*. 2006;13(5):5040–5044.

14. Krauss B, Hess DR. Capnography for procedural sedation and analgesia in the emergency department. *Ann Emerg Med*. 2007;50(2):172–181.

15. Fanning RM. Monitoring during sedation given by non-anaesthetic doctors. *Anaesthesia*. 2008;63(4):370–374.

16. Deitch K, Miner J, Chudnofsky CR, et al. Does $ETCO_2$ monitoring during emergency department procedural sedation and analgesia with propofol decrease the incidence of hypoxic events? A randomized, controlled trial. *Ann Emerg Med*. 2010;55(3):265–267.

17. Kannikeswaran K, Chen X, Sethuraman U. Utility of endtidal carbon dioxide monitoring in detection of hypoxia during sedation for brain magnetic resonance imaging in children with developmental disabilities. *Pediatr Anesth*. 2011;21(12):1241–1246.

18. Langhan ML, Chen L, Marshall C, Santucci KA. Detection of hypoxia by capnography and its association with hypoxia in children undergoing sedation with ketamine. *Pediatr Emerg Care*. 2011;27(5):394–397.

19. Beitz A, Riphaus A, Meining A, et al. Capnographic monitoring reduces the incidence of arterial oxygen desaturation and hypoxemia during propofol sedation for colonoscopy: a randomized, controlled study (ColoCap Study). *Am J Gastroenterol*. 2012;107(8):1205–1212.

20. Tremper KK, Barker SJ. Pulse oximetry. *Anesthesiology*. 1989;70(1):98–108.

21. Pedersen T, Moller AM, Pedersen BD. Pulse oximetry for perioperative monitoring: systematic review of randomized, controlled trials. *Anesth Analg*. 2003;96(2):426–431.

22. Eichhorn JH. Pulse oximetry as a standard of practice in anesthesia. *Anesthesiology*. 1993;78(3):423–426.

23. Severinghaus J, Spellman M. Pulse oximeter failure thresholds in hypotension and vasoconstriction. *Anesthesiology*. 1990;73(3). 532–527.

24. Stoelting RK, Miller RD, eds. *Basics of anesthesia*. 7th ed. Philadelphia: Churchill Livingstone; 2002.

25. Von Recklinghausen H. *Neue Wege zur Blutdruckmessung*. Berlin: Springer-Verlag; 1931.

26. Mark JB, Slaughter TF, Reves JG. Cardiovascular monitoring. In: Miller RD, ed. *Anesthesia*. 5th ed. Philadelphia: Churchill Livingstone; 2000:1117–1206.

27. Torossian A. Thermal management during anaesthesia and thermoregulation standards for the prevention of inadvertent perioperative hypothermia. *Best Pract Res Clin Anaesthesiol*. 2008;22(4):659–668.

28. Missant C, Van de Velde M. Morbidity and mortality related to anaesthesia outside the operating room. *Curr Opin Anaesthesiol*. 2004;17(4):323–327.

29. Frank SM, Beattie C, Christopherson R, et al. Unintentional hypothermia is associated with postoperative myocardial ischemia: the perioperative ischemia randomized anesthesia trial study group. *Anesthesiology*. 1993;78(3):468–476.

30. Kurz A, Sessler DI, Lenhardt R. Perioperative normothermia to reduce the incidence of surgical wound infection and shorten hospitalization: study of wound infection and temperature group. *N Engl J Med*. 1996;334(19):1209–1215.

31. Putzu M, Casati A, Berti M, Pagliarini G, Fanelli G. Clinical complications, monitoring and management of mild perioperative hypothermia: anesthesiological features. *Acta Biomed*. 2007;78(3):163–169.

32. Marik PE, Cavallazzi R, Vasu T, Hirani A. Dynamic changes in arterial waveform derived variables and fluid responsiveness in mechanically ventilated patients: a systematic review of the literature. *Crit Care Med*. 2009;37(9):2642–2646.

33. Kumar A, Anel R, Bunnell E, et al. Pulmonary artery occlusion pressure and central venous pressure fail to predict ventricular filling volume, cardiac performance, or the response to volume infusion in normal subjects. *Crit Care Med*. 2004;32(3):691–699.

34. Cowie BS. Does the pulmonary artery catheter still have a role in the perioperative period? *Anaesth Intensive Care*. 2011;39(3):345–355.

35. Kearney TJ, Shabot MM. Pulmonary artery rupture associated with the Swan-Ganz catheter. *Chest*. 1995;108(5):1349–1352.

36. Denault A, Deschamps A, Murkin JM. A proposed algorithm for the intraoperative use of cerebral near-infrared spectroscopy. *Semin Cardiothorac Vasc Anesth*. 2007;11(4):274–281.

37. Boushel R, Langeberg H, Olesen J, Gonzales-Alonso J, Bulow J, Kjaer M. Monitoring tissue oxygen availability with near infrared spectroscopy in health and disease. *Scand J Med Sci Sports*. 2001;11(4):213–222.

38. Mazzeo AT, Di Pasquale R, Settineri N, et al. Usefulness and limits of near infrared spectroscopy monitoring during endovascular procedures. *Minerva Anestesiol*. 2012;78(1):31–45.

39. Chakravarti SB, Mittnacht AJ, Katz JC, Nguyen K, Joashi U, Srivastava S. Multisite near-infrared spectroscopy predicts elevated blood lactate level in children after cardiac surgery. *J Cardiothorac Vasc Anesth*. 2009;23(5):663–667.

40. Gamble C, Gamble J, Seal R, Wright RB, Ali S. Bispectral analysis during procedural sedation in the pediatric emergency department. *Pediatr Emerg Care*. 2012;28(10):1003–1008.

41. Punjasawadwong Y, Phongchiewboon A, Bunchungmongkol N. Bispectral index for improving anaesthetic delivery and postoperative recovery. *Cochrane Database Syst Rev*. 2007;17(4):CD003843.

42. Patterson S, Chesney J. Anesthetic management for magnetic resonance imaging: problems and solutions. *Anesth Analg*. 1992;74(1):121–128.

43. Taber KH, Thompson J, Coveler LA, Hayman LA. Invasive pressure monitoring of patients during magnetic resonance imaging. *Can J Anaesth*. 1993;40(11):1092–1095.

44. Melloni C. Morbidity and mortality related to anesthesia outside the operating room. *Minerva Anestesiol*. 2005;71:325–334.

45. Covello RD, Ruggeri L, Landoni G, et al. Transcatheter implantation of an aortic valve: anesthesiological management. *Minerva Anestesiol*. 2010;76(2):100–108.

46. Weaver LK. Hyperbaric oxygen in the critically ill. *Crit Care Med*. 2011;39(7):1784–1791.

47. Zheng JN, Wu BM, Wang Q. Development of physiological monitors based on the Zigbee technology for hyperbaric oxygen therapy. *Chin J Med Instrument*. 2008;32(3):193–197.

48. American Heart Association. *AHA trend-watch chartbook: trends affecting hospitals and health systems: May 2005*. Chicago: American Heart Association; 2005.

49. Evron S, Ezri T. Organizational prerequisites for anesthesia outside the operating room. *Curr Opin Anaesthesiol*. 2009;22(4):514–518.

50. American Society of Anesthesiologists. *Guidelines for office-based anesthesia*. Committee of Origin: Ambulatory Surgical Care (Approved by the ASA House of Delegates on October 13, 1999, and last affirmed on October 21, 2009). Park Ridge, Ill: American Society of Anesthesiologists; 2009.

51. Weatherburn C, Endacott R, Tynan P, Bailey M. The impact of bispectral index monitoring on sedation administration in mechanically ventilated patients. *Anaesth Intensive Care*. 2007;35(2):204–208.

7 Intravenous Anesthesia and Sedation Outside the Operating Room

ANIL GUPTA and JOHAN RAEDER

The operating room is considered to be the most expensive part of the hospital, and therefore only procedures that require specific surgical care of the patient or dedicated anesthesia resources and postoperative care should be performed in this environment. Business managers in particular are not keen on using expensive operating room resources when a procedure can be performed under local anesthesia or during sedation and analgesia without the need for anesthesiologists. Such procedures should, whenever possible, be performed outside the operating room environment. Over the years, a disparity has existed between resources available and production targets, and demands to increase theater efficiency have therefore increased. Patient demands to provide good sedation and analgesia have simultaneously increased. As doctors, we are forced to meet the requests made by patients while ensuring safety and providing high-quality care at lower costs. These factors have created the need for providing competent anesthesia care outside the operating room at virtually no increased total costs to the health care provider. Thus the environment is ripe for creating optimal patient management systems in a non–operating room anesthesia (NORA) environment at similar or reduced costs and providing safe care with increased patient satisfaction. No business environment within the health care sector has faced so many conflicting challenges, all at the same time, in the last decade.

Coupled with the issues around safe management at reduced costs outside the operating room is the challenge to provide satisfactory conditions for surgeons, physicians, and radiologists to be able to perform the procedure in a satisfactory way and subsequently discharge the patient home as soon as possible, preferably without using postanesthesia care unit (PACU) resources. Additionally, not only do patients want to be discharged home safely but they also want participate in decision-making, drive without being injured or injuring others, take care of their children at home, and often go back to work later the same day. Although many of these demands cannot always be fulfilled, careful planning and availability of short-acting intravenous drugs with minimal side effects has made the impossible now seem achievable. To contain costs, however, several facilities have resorted to using the services of non–anesthesia-trained personnel to achieve the goal of providing sedation or analgesia in a safe way. Under these circumstances, and with the added complexity of multiple comorbidities in an increasingly aged population, supervision by a trained anesthesiologist has become increasingly important when performing procedures outside the operating room environment. Clinical practices that best achieve the goals of safety, ease of management, and safe discharge after sedation and analgesia have become a hot topic for regular discussions in corridors and conference among doctors, nurses, and health care managers, as well as the subject of increasing scientific publications in peer-reviewed journals throughout the world.

From an anesthesiology perspective, it is essential that the care given to patients undergoing procedures outside the operating room under sedation is, above all, safe. Compromising safety above costs is not acceptable practice for doctors or nurses. A team of competent and trained staff is thus needed to offer safe care at affordable costs and with full patient satisfaction. In hospitals, most guidelines on sedation and analgesia outside the operating room are today made keeping in mind the availability of competent, informed, and educated personnel. However, it is impossible to extend the use the guidelines published in one country or hospital to other countries, because of differences in the availability of drugs, monitoring standards, staff education and competence, and restriction on administration of drugs, among other factors. Therefore local practices and personnel competence should be considered when making recommendations for safe practice in sedation or analgesia techniques within each country and hospital. For instance, whereas only anesthesiologists in Australia and New Zealand can administer propofol, in Scandinavia, anesthesia nurses may administer propofol under the supervision of anesthesiologists but not surgeons. Thus it is important to take into consideration local governance, practices, and recommendations pertaining to the use of drugs by competent persons trained in the safe use of these drugs.

This chapter aims to provide alternatives for the practice of safe sedation and anesthesia outside the operating room. The focus is on total intravenous anesthesia (TIVA) as the method of choice, the drugs commonly used, and their pharmacology and side effects, but brief summary of an inhalational anesthetic as an alternative has been mentioned. Furthermore, the monitoring standards that should be used during TIVA are discussed, as well as specific patient scenarios. Details on procedure-related issues are adequately and more extensively covered in other chapters. This chapter focuses on the essentials of TIVA instead of details in the management of patients with coexisting morbidities in complex environments. The reader is referred to further reading in other chapters in

Table 7-1   American Society of Anesthesiologists Definitions of General Anesthesia and Levels of Sedation and Analgesia

Evaluation Factors	Minimal Sedation (Anxiolysis)	Moderate Sedation/Analgesia ("Conscious Sedation")	Deep Sedation/Analgesia
Responsiveness	Normal response to verbal stimulation	Purposeful* response to verbal or tactile stimulation	Purposeful response* following repeated or painful stimulation
Airway	Unaffected	No intervention required	Intervention may be required
Spontaneous ventilation	Unaffected	Adequate	May be inadequate
Cardiovascular function	Unaffected	Usually maintained	Usually maintained

*Reflex withdrawal from a painful stimulus is *not* considered a purposeful response.
From American Society of Anesthesiologists. *ASA standards, guidelines and statements*, October 2007. http://www.asahq.org/publications/p-106-asa-standards-guidelines-and-statements.aspx.

this book and more specialized textbooks when dealing with patients with comorbidities.

Although anesthesia can probably be achieved equally well outside the operating room environment using inhalational anesthetics, this may not be appropriate for several reasons. For instance, procedural sedation has been described using nitrous oxide in children. However, the use of inhalational or gaseous anesthetics requires a dedicated anesthesia machine and scavenging systems, which not only add significantly to the hospital costs but may also be detrimental to the non–operating room environment. Additionally, to achieve adequate sedation using inhalation agents, personnel within the room would certainly be exposed to the potential harmful effect of these agents unless an endotracheal tube or laryngeal mask airway (LMA) device is used. These require a significantly deeper level of sedation anesthesia, with its attendant problems. A major feature and benefit of intravenous sedation and analgesia technique is the elegant and comfortable option (for both patient and anesthetist) in the smooth transition from being fully awake to anxiolysis through light sedation, deep sedation, and, if needed, general anesthesia. Another major feature with total intravenous techniques is the concept of separating the different components of sedation and anesthesia and analgesia in a tailored and independent manner. To handle such smooth transitions of the level of sedation and anesthesia while providing excellent quality for patients and with maximal safety, qualified anesthesia personnel are often needed. Compromised airway, apnea, or cardiovascular problems may occur unpredictably and must be dealt with immediately and adequately by competent personnel.

Sedation, Sedation and Analgesia, and Anesthesia

A clear difference needs to be made at the outset between the different levels of sedation (effect of drug dose) and the different quality of sedation (effect of drug choice) that should be achieved in the individual case and for a specific procedure. The level of sedation may be differentiated into light sedation, moderate sedation, and deep sedation (Table 7-1), and the quality of sedation may be differentiated into anxiolysis, hypnosis (from sleepy to unconscious), and amnesia. To each of these components, analgesia may be added during painful procedures. Several scores for the assessment of the level of sedation have been described,

Table 7-2   Ramsay Sedation Scale

Score	Response
1	Anxious, restless, or both
2	Cooperative, oriented, and tranquil
3	Responding to commands
4	Brisk response to light glabellar tap or loud auditory stimulus
5	Sluggish response to light glabellar tap or loud auditory stimulus
6	No response to stimulus

From Ramsay MA, Savege TM, Simpson BR, Goodwin R. Controlled sedation with alphaxalone-alphadolone. *Br Med J*. 1974;2(5920):656-659.

Table 7-3   Modified Observer's Assessment of Alertness/Sedation Scale

Responsiveness	Score
Agitated	6
Responds readily to name spoken in normal tone (alert)	5
Lethargic response to name spoken in normal tone	4
Responds only after name is called loudly and/or repeatedly	3
Responds only after mild prodding or shaking	2
Does not respond to mild prodding or shaking	1

From Cohen LB, DeLegge MH, Aisenberg J, et al. AGA Institute review of endoscopic sedation. *Gastroenterology*. 2007;133(2):675-701.

but the ones commonly used include the Ramsay Sedation Scale (Table 7-2) and the Modified Observer's Assessment of Alertness/Sedation Scale (Table 7-3). The choice of scale that should be used depends on local education, trends, and practices, but it is important to regularly and routinely register the level of sedation. It is usually helpful to make a plan together with the operator before starting the procedure as to what levels and qualities of sedation are needed and expected for a particular patient and the specific procedure. The plan may subsequently need to be adjusted during the procedure, depending on the patient's actual response, the course of the planned intervention, and the side effects of the drugs used. Many procedures require anxiolytic and/or hypnotic effect alone because no associated pain occurs, whereas others require predominantly analgesia, with the procedure being painful but not necessarily perceived as

include paracetamol, nonsteroidal antiinflammatory drugs (NSAIDs) or coxibs, and glucocorticoid, as well as local anesthetics injected into the wounds. For further discussion, the reader is referred to specialized textbooks for the management of postoperative pain.

Neuromuscular Blockers and Reversal Agents

The use of neuromuscular blockers has declined in modern anesthesia and ambulatory care. These should be used only with a specific indication, which could be during intubation or when the patient is not allowed to move, even minimally, during the procedure. Even in these situations, sufficient anesthesia depth usually ensures adequate relaxation.

Suxamethonium is a cheap, fast-acting and short-acting drug that does not need to be reversed after the end of the procedure. However, in addition to the common, known side effects, its use in ambulatory patients may result in troublesome muscular pains, sometimes lasting for up to 1 to 2 days. In many countries, among the drugs used in anesthetic practice, it is believed to be the most common drug associated with anaphylactic reactions.[9] Rarely (~1 in 4000 patients), a deficiency of the enzyme pseudocholinesterase occurs, which would prolong its metabolism and thus duration of action substantially.

Mivacurium is a fairly short-acting nondepolarizing muscle relaxant, not needing routine reversal because of breakdown by the pseudocholinesterase enzyme in the blood. Therefore enzyme deficiency, as with suxamethonium, may occur and prolong the effect of mivacurium. It is useful in ambulatory procedures of short to intermediate duration, but its slow onset of action has restricted its use in clinical practice.

Vecuronium and cisatracurium are well-established, safe alternatives for producing a nondepolarizing muscle block but also have a fairly slow onset and intermediate duration of action that requires monitoring and the frequent use of reversal at the end of the procedure.

Rocuronium has a much faster onset of action than other nondepolarizing agents, especially when used in high doses, which is almost comparable with suxamethonium. However, in these high doses, prolonged recovery from muscle relaxation will occur, unless the very rapid-acting, effective but expensive drug sugammadex is used (see later discussion).

Reversal of Neuromuscular Blockade. Although serious clinical problems with residual neuromuscular block in recovery are rare today, the increased incidence of pulmonary complications in the elderly has been demonstrated with inadequate reversal of neuromuscular block.[10] Today, it is believed that train-of-four ratios of less than 0.9 may also interfere with normal swallowing and thereby increase the risk for aspiration.[11]

For the combination of neostigmine and glycopyrrolate, the dose of neostigmine should be 50 to 70 mcg/kg to adequately reverse the effect of the muscle relaxant. However, when used in this dose, the risk for nausea and vomiting is increased[12] and sometimes other side effects may be seen, such as bronchial constriction or defecation. In addition, it can take up to 20 minutes for full reversal of the block in some patients.[13]

Sugammadex is a rapid-acting reversal agent for rocuronium and vecuronium. Complete reversal from muscle relaxation is achieved within 1 to 2 min (2 to 4 mg/kg) at any level of muscle relaxation but a much greater dose (16 mg/kg) is required when used immediately after muscle relaxation (as after intubation).[14] Therefore it may be useful during microsurgery when full muscle relaxation must be maintained until the end of the procedure or when the surgeon abruptly completes the procedure during full muscle relaxation. In this way, the operating room is effectively used without delay in patient turnover. Other indications for the use of sugammadex include poor pulmonary function and morbid obesity, in which a complete and rapid reversal of muscle relaxation may reduce the risk for postoperative complications. Sugammadex is still not available for use in the United States because of the risk for allergic reactions, and it is expensive in Europe.

Antiemetics

Even during sedation, the incidence of PONV may be fairly high, especially when opioids are used. The use of antiemetics in patients at risk, as suggested by Apfel et al,[15] may be advisable. No specific protocols exist for use of antiemetics during sedation or anesthesia outside the operating room. The well-evaluated protocols for ambulatory surgery probably also apply to these procedures. For details about the drugs that may be useful in this situation, the reader is referred to specialized textbooks and reviews on this subject.

Target-Controlled Infusion

Target-controlled infusion (TCI) devices allow intravenous infusion of anesthetic agents to ensure that sufficient drug is delivered by a preprogrammed computer to maintain adequate and stable levels of drug in plasma and at the effect site. The administration rate is determined by drug pharmacokinetics and pharmacodynamics, which have been extensively tested in computer-assisted models and subsequently in humans. The infusion pumps are programmed in consideration of one or more patient variables—for example, weight, age, and sex (Figure 7-1). The pumps may use different pharmacokinetic models, but the end points remain the same. The TCI system ensures

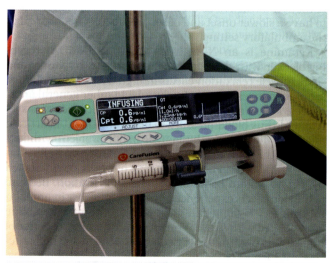

Figure 7-1 Target-controlled infusion (TCI) used during an endoscopic procedure.

rapid onset, stable effect, rapid offset or reduction in effect, and less work in mathematical calculations of doses of drugs to be administered.

The Target-Controlled Infusion Concept. With a manual scheme for administering propofol for rapid induction and subsequent maintenance of anesthesia in adults, the following general recipe can be used. Start with bolus of 2 mg/kg with an infusion of 10 mg/kg/hr for 10 minutes, then step-down infusion to 8 mg/kg/hr for another 10 minutes, then another step-down to 6 mg/kg/hr, which is maintained for the rest of the procedure. Subsequently, anesthesia depth can be regulated by stepping up or down by increments or decrements of 0.5 to 1 mg/kg/hr. This recipe may be put into a computerized pump and is based on the weight of the patient and simple mathematical calculations to administer a bolus dose and defined infusion rates. A computerized pump can be programmed to administer this automatically, and the resulting concentration, termed target concentration (or plasma concentration), and the concentration in the brain (effect site concentration) will correspond to approximately 2.5 to 3 mcg/mL. In other words, during maintenance of TIVA (after 15 to 20 minutes), a propofol infusion of 6 mg/kg/hr will correspond to a target (plasma or effect concentration) of about 2.5 mcg/mL.

With TCI the computer is programmed with the age and weight of the patient, and the computer then administers a bolus dose (based on body weight) and the infusion rate adjusts automatically depending on the plasma clearance and set target (plasma) concentration. Thus the only factor that is adjusted by the anesthesiologist is the target concentration of propofol, which, for maintenance of anesthesia, would correspond to a target concentration of approximately 2.5 mcg/mL. If a greater anesthetic depth is desired, the target concentration can be increased in small increments (e.g., to 3 mcg/mL), and the computer will automatically deliver a small bolus of drug to rapidly reach the set higher target concentration and subsequently adjust the infusion rate to maintain this greater anesthetic depth. If a shallower depth of anesthesia is desired and the target concentration reduced (e.g., to 2 mcg/mL), the computer automatically stops the infusion briefly and then starts it again at a lower target concentration.

The system is, however, not perfect, and one major limitation with using target concentration in plasma is that it does not take into account the delay in drug equilibration between plasma and brain (effect site) concentration. Because the anesthetic drug effect is not in the plasma but in the central nervous system, it would be better to have an infusion pump that could deliver a preset concentration of propofol into effect sites (in the brain) rather than plasma. Therefore the plasma TCI system can be reprogrammed into an effect site system. With these models, an overshoot in plasma concentration occurs initially (to account for the quicker equilibration to effect site in the brain) and with every increase in target concentration, to create a stronger drug gradient from plasma to brain, and thereby a more rapid effect can be achieved. One problem with effect site modeling is that the delay in effect may be variable among individuals and also depend on the rate of bolus dosing, state of the circulation, and other factors. However, the effect site modeling

gets closer to the clinical needs and has been proved to be very useful in clinical work. It should also be noted that some models compensate for weight-to-height ratio or age, whereas others only compensate for total weight. The common models do not compensate for differences in propofol sensitivity, which is lower in children and possibly in women. Multiple models are in use for propofol, the most common being the Schnider and the Marsh models; the latter is also available with some modifications. It is important for the anesthetist to become familiar with the clinical response to the targets of the model used in daily practice, because the Marsh model administers propofol in greater doses for a given target than the Schnider model.

In the case of remifentanil, only one TCI model is in common clinical use, the Minto model for both plasma and effect site concentration.[16,17] This model takes into consideration the patient's weight, height, and age for the plasma concentration modeling. When used in the effect site modus, it will deliver only a predetermined drug concentration in the brain and not adjust for patient pharmacodynamics or drug sensitivity, which is higher in elderly patients. For maintenance of analgesia during surgery, a remifentanil infusion of 0.1 mcg/kg/min will correspond to a target (plasma or effect) concentration of about 2.5 ng/mL. When remifentanil is used as an infusion in doses of less than 0.1 mcg/kg/min ($\approx$ effect concentration of 2.5 ng/mL), spontaneous respiration often can be retained, as during endoscopic procedures.[18] However, during surgery, usually a dose of 0.2 to 0.5 mcg/kg/min ($\approx$ effect concentration of 5 to 12 ng/mL) is needed. To tolerate a laryngeal mask insertion, a rule of thumb is to ensure a dose of 2 mcg/kg ($\approx$ effect concentration of 6 to 8 ng/mL) is administered over 2 to 3 minutes, whereas for intubation without muscle relaxant, a dose of 3 to 4 mcg/kg ($\approx$ effect concentration of 10 to 12 ng/mL) is needed. When using these doses, however, the ventilation needs to be controlled, because hypopnea and apnea are common. A general recommendation on doses of propofol and remifentanil during TIVA and TCI are presented in Table 7-4. The recommended doses are average based on body weight. These need to be adjusted for age and in individual patients depending on comorbidities. For more detailed discussion on pharmacokinetic modeling, the reader is referred to special literature.

Patient-Controlled Sedation

Some recent studies have looked at the administration of propofol using patient-controlled techniques, similar to the concept of patient-controlled analgesia. The natural advantage and in-built safety in the system is that oversedation is avoided and thereby the risk for respiratory obstruction prevented. In contrast to total intravenous anesthesia and analgesia using propofol, alfentanil, or both or nurse-administered sedation with midazolam, this technique was found to be associated with quicker recovery and greater patient satisfaction after endoscopic procedures[19] but not endoscopic retrograde cholangiopancreatography.[20] A method to close the loop by monitoring feedback from bispectral index–controlled sedation has been tested. More studies are needed on this important subject before definitive conclusions can be made.

Table 7-4   Propofol and/or Remifentanil Sedation Doses

Drug	TIVA (Propofol: mg/kg/hr; Remifentanil: mcg/kg/min)	TCI* (Propofol: mcg/mL; Remifentanil: ng/mL)
Spontaneous respiration		
Propofol (alone)	2-4	1-2
Remifentanil (alone)	0.1-0.15	2.5-3.5
Laryngeal mask		
Propofol (alone)	4-5	1.8-2.5
Remifentanil (assisted/controlled ventilation) (alone)	0.2-0.5	4-12
Spontaneous respiration (combination)		
Propofol	1-3	0.5-1.5
+ remifentanil	+0.05-0.1	+1-2.5
Controlled ventilation (combination)		
Propofol	4-5	1.8-2.5
+ remifentanil	+0.2-0.5	+4-12

TCI, Target-controlled infusion; *TIVA*, total intravenous anesthesia.
*The TCI propofol doses are for the modified (Struys) Marsh effect site model. For the Schnider model the targets should be approximately 25% higher, initially, then down to the levels in Table 7-4 after 10-15 minutes.

Monitoring During Total Intravenous Anesthesia and Analgesia

Poor monitoring should not compromise an otherwise perfect sedation or analgesia. In other words, not only is it adequate to provide satisfactory sedation and analgesia during the procedure outside the operating room but it is equally important to document that it has been performed safely. When things go wrong, and they sometimes do so, it is important to be able to go back to well-documented charts and be able to understand what went wrong, why it went wrong, when it went wrong, and what we can learn from the experience so that future patients receive the best clinical care. If not documented, it is considered "not done" by a lawyer if medicolegal problems arise from a case that does not go well.

When giving anesthesia to patients outside the operating room, the same monitoring standards are to be recommended as during anesthesia in the operating room. Just because a procedure is performed outside the operating room does not imply that safety standards should be reduced or compromised. Even when performing sedation or analgesia, monitoring standards should remain high and include, as the minimum, heart frequency, oxygen saturation, and blood pressure. In addition, it is important to measure certain respiratory variables, such as end-tidal carbon dioxide ($ETCO_2$) concentration and respiratory frequency. Although the former may not be completely accurate, depending on the breathing system being used, trends are important to register and a sudden drop in $ETCO_2$ or progressive increase in $ETCO_2$ and reduction in respiratory rate should alert the attending staff that all is not well with the patient. The former can result from respiratory obstruction, and the latter usually results from hypopnea. Constant observation of the

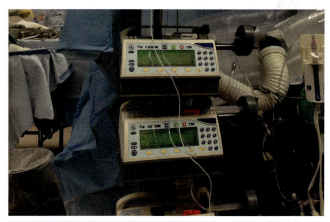

Figure 7-2 Total intravenous anesthesia used during a minor surgical procedure.

patient and the breathing pattern may alert the personnel of potential airway obstruction. A sudden drop in $ETCO_2$ with signs of paradoxical respiration is a sign of upper airway obstruction and often indicates a level of sedation that is too deep. Tidal volumes are difficult to measure under these circumstances, and excessive opiate use may go unnoticed until the $ETCO_2$ starts to increase, which could take up to 5 to 10 minutes in the healthy patient. Another important sign of opioid overdosing could be a progressive reduction in respiratory frequency below 8 to 10 breaths/min.

In patients undergoing the procedure under sedation, the level of sedation needs to be measured and documented. The most commonly used is the Ramsay scale (see Table 7-2), which is a 6-graded scale, but an alternative scale is also available—the Modified Observer's Assessment of Alertness/Sedation Scale (see Table 7-3). The main aim of anxiolysis or conscious sedation is to maintain continuous contact with the patient; therefore sedation scores should be maintained at 2 to 3 on the Ramsay scale. Any attempt at increasing to moderate or deep sedation risks compromising the airway, sometimes with disastrous consequences. Thus it is important that personnel caring for these patients should be well versed in using the Ramsay scale or the Modified Observer's Assessment of Alertness/Sedation Scale.

When TIVA is used for anesthesia or analgesia during certain surgical procedures (Figure 7-2), monitoring should follow the convention used in operating rooms, and no compromise on this principle should be accepted. In addition to routine monitoring, this may include monitoring of anesthesia depth, but the evidence for benefit in healthy patients who have not received muscle relaxation therapy remains controversial.

Side Effects and Complications

It is important to state at the outset that in untrained hands, sedation, analgesia, and TIVA are risky procedures and that deaths and serious complications occur, although these are not common. Therefore training and education should form a part of continuing medical education for personnel, and regular simulator training may help in avoiding very rare but potentially life-threatening complications.

One common complication seen during sedation and analgesia is airway obstruction, which usually results from too deep a level of sedation and lack of patient contact (Ramsay score ≥3) in relation to perceived patient stress. It sometimes takes time to detect oversedation because of the dark working environment in endoscopy rooms. Additionally, oxygen is often being supplemented by a catheter or mask during these procedures, and a delay in detecting hypoventilation or absence of ventilation may occur and not be detected by the SpO_2, thereby missing or misdiagnosing hypercarbia with resulting loss of consciousness. As mentioned earlier, the occurrence of paradoxical breathing should alert the personnel that the patient may not be maintaining a free airway. Depending on several patient factors, including age and comorbidities, some patients do not require much sedation before airway obstruction occurs. Thus, depending on several comorbid factors, airway obstruction can occur at surprisingly low doses of sedative drugs.

Respiratory depression is another common complication that might result from both excessive sedation and excessive use of opioid analgesics. Even apnea is known to occur in some patients given potent analgesics. This may manifest by a decrease in respiratory frequency or a progressive increase in $ETCO_2$. When respiratory depression occurs in the absence of deep sedation, the patient can be asked to breathe deeply and the problem is immediately corrected. However, when respiratory depression is accompanied by deep sedation or due to oversedation, it may require assisted ventilation, even in the absence of respiratory obstruction. It is important to be aware that deep sedation may occur without sedatives as a result of the progressive accumulation of carbon dioxide.

Hypotension is a well-known complication of sedation and analgesia, occurring during deep sedation or TIVA, more often in the presence of concomitant hypovolemia. Reducing the level of sedation usually reverses the problem, but management should otherwise follow conventional methods, such as initiating a Trendelenburg position, giving a bolus of intravenous crystalloids, and even administration of 5 to 10 mg intravenously of ephedrine or other vasopressors.

Hypertension may occur and may be a sign of either stress in a poorly sedated patient or pain. In all cases, the underlying causes must be determined and treated, but if not found, symptomatic treatment with a beta-blocker may be considered.

Bradycardia or tachycardia may sometimes occur. The former may be due to a combination of anesthetic and analgesic drugs, specifically the combination of propofol and fentanyl, both of which are known to independently cause bradycardia. Even vagal stimulation, as during insertion of the gastroscope into the pharynx and esophagus, may lead to bradycardia and may require prompt treatment with intravenous atropine 0.5 to 1 mg. During endoscopies, bradycardia may also occur due to vagal stimulation from dilated large intestines when air is injected to provide better visibility by the endoscopist.

With the increased use of remifentanil during TIVA over the last few years, muscle rigidity and postoperative hyperalgesia have been highlighted in several studies.[22] Although the latter is usually not an issue with most procedures performed outside the operating room because pain is not common after these procedures, muscle rigidity can be disturbing. Difficulty in ventilating an apneic patient should alert the physician to possible chest-wall rigidity. The dose of the analgesic used in a patient not receiving hypnotics simultaneously is often the key factor in muscle rigidity. As a rule of thumb, more than 1 to 2 mcg/kg of remifentanil is needed as a rapid bolus for the potential provocation of rigidity.

Rare and uncommon complications of endoscopy procedures could be bleeding and persistent abdominal pain after the procedure, which are always the result of surgical complications. Sore throat has been described frequently and may be the result of either gastroscopy or the use of an LMA or intubation. Spraying the pharynx with a local anesthetic may prevent the unpleasant sensation of a gastroscope going down the throat and may reduce postprocedural sore throat. Amnesia is not uncommon after benzodiazepine sedation and occasionally also with propofol sedation (although short-lasting); it is sometimes experienced as positive by patients, because memory of the unpleasant procedure is almost completely abolished. However, in some cases, amnesia is not beneficial, such as when the patient wants to communicate with the surgeon, watch the endoscopic procedure, or learn from the surgeon's instructions during the procedure.

Recovery and Discharge

Postprocedural recovery should follow well-established routines as during ambulatory surgery. Depending on the procedure performed and associated postoperative pain, patients need to be treated on an individual basis and according to common convention and established guidelines. In general, pain is usually not a common problem because many procedures are either painless or the patients have received local anesthetics and sometimes strong analgesics during the procedure. On the other hand, nausea and vomiting may occur, despite the use of TIVA. Therefore prophylactic antiemetics should be given to patients at risk.

Most patients recover quickly, specifically those who have had sedation or analgesia with propofol and with or without opiod analgesics. Those receiving midazolam may remain sedated and have amnesia for longer periods, depending on the total dose of midazolam administered. The discharge criteria for patients having sedation or analgesia are the same as after ambulatory surgical procedures. The score commonly used to assess recovery is the modified Aldrete score (Table 7-5) and to assess home discharge is the well-tested Post-Anesthetic Discharge Scoring System suggested by Chung et al[21] (Table 7-6). Home discharge requires that an adult person accompany the patient home in all cases, except when very low doses of propofol have been used to achieve sedation with or without the short-acting analgesics alfentanil or remifentanil. Even when fentanyl is used as an analgesic, recovery is usually rapid, but a small but significant risk for respiratory depression may remain at a later stage, depending on the doses used. It is rare that patients sedated or anesthetized outside the operating room need overnight admission to the hospital unless

Table 7-5 Modified Aldrete Scoring System

Activity	Score
Able to move four extremities voluntarily on command	2
Able to move two extremities voluntarily on command	1
Able to move no extremities voluntarily on command	0
RESPIRATION	
Able to breathe deeply and cough freely	2
Dyspnea or limited breathing	1
Apneic	0
CIRCULATION	
BP ± 20% of preanesthetic level	2
BP ± 20%-49% of preanesthetic level	1
BP ± 50% of preanesthetic level	0
PULSE RATE	
Pulse ± 20 beats of presedation rate	2
Pulse ± 50 to 21 beats of presedation rate	1
Pulse > ± 51 beats of presedation rate	0
CONSCIOUSNESS	
Fully awake	2
Arousable on calling	1
Not responding	0
OXYGEN SATURATION	
Maintains baseline saturation on room air	2
Needs O_2 to maintain >90% saturation	1
O_2 saturation <90% with O_2 supplement	0

Table 7-6 Post-Anesthetic Discharge Scoring System

Vital signs: Vital signs must be stable and consistent with age and preoperative baseline

BP and pulse within 20% of preoperative baseline	2
BP and pulse 20%-40% of preoperative baseline	1
BP and pulse >40% of preoperative baseline	0

Activity level: Patient must be able to ambulate at preoperative level

Steady gait, no dizziness, or meets preoperative level	2
Requires assistance	1
Unable to ambulate	0

Nausea and vomiting: The patient should have minimal nausea and vomiting before discharge

Minimal: Successfully treated with PO medication	2
Moderate: Successfully treated with IM medication	1
Severe: Continues after repeated treatment	0

Pain:

The patient should have minimal or no pain before discharge
The level of pain that the patient has should be acceptable to the patient
Pain should be controllable by oral analgesics
The location, type, and intensity of pain should be consistent with anticipated postoperative discomfort

Acceptability:

Yes	2
No	1

Surgical bleeding: Postoperative bleeding should be consistent with expected blood loss for the procedure

Minimal: Does not require dressing change	2
Moderate: Up to two dressing changes required	1
Severe: More than three dressing changes required	0

a complication has occurred during the procedure. An exception could be the aged patient with multiple comorbidities or a preterm baby, even after a minor procedure.

Total Intravenous Anesthesia for Specific Patients

In general, individual assessment of sedation is warranted for all patients during all procedures, and no cookbook recipe exists that can generalize doses and regimens, other than in broad terms, which have been outlined earlier. However, some specific patient factors should be considered because drug doses may need to be adjusted depending on several factors. Some of these situations are described in the following section, but it should be emphasized that the recommended doses should be taken with caution and individualized to each patient, depending on patient response.

OBESITY

In the obese, both remifentanil and propofol should be dosed by corrected ideal weight—that is, ideal weight plus 20% of the difference between ideal weight and actual weight. The obese are specifically prone to airway obstruction during sedation, and many of them may have sleep apnea syndrome. For these reasons, drugs should be titrated extra carefully in the obese, and patients should be monitored carefully during sedation. Recovery staff should be aware that the obese should be in recovery for a longer period and require careful monitoring. For further details, the reader is referred to specialized books on the care of the obese patients.

CHILDREN

Local anesthetic skin cream should be used in children before intravenous cannulation to make the venous puncture pain free. Propofol mixed with lidocaine may be used to reduce pain on injection of propofol, and sometimes an opioid may be needed. Younger children may not lie still during surgery under sedation; therefore a general anesthetic may be needed instead of sedation, and then an LMA may be more appropriate.

PREGNANCY

As with all types of surgery, the indication for doing the procedure under sedation should be carefully considered in the pregnant patient, specifically during the first trimester. With this said, most anesthetic drugs currently used are considered to be safe during pregnancy. Some exceptions may include NSAIDs, glucocorticoids, and nitrous oxide because their potential influence on DNA or cell growth in the fetus.

ALCOHOLICS AND DRUG ADDICTS

Patients who are unstable or under the influence of alcohol or narcotic medication should not be operated on except as emergencies. However, some of them may be stable and in a state of baseline sedative or opioid medication and others may be in a drug-free state, with or without accompanying restlessness. For these reasons the dose of the drugs used may need to be carefully titrated in these patients. If possible, opioids should be avoided for sedation. However, patients with a stable dose of opioid replacement therapy (e.g., methadone and buprenorphine) should have their baseline medication given before the procedure. Additionally, one should be generous in the use of depth of anesthesia monitoring in these patients.

Conclusion

The demands for better sedation and analgesia by patients combined with concerns expressed by the medical profession as to the safety of procedures being performed by non-anesthetic personnel has resulted in intense debate on the pros and cons of intravenous anesthetics administered by non–anesthesia-trained personnel for the safe management, earlier discharge, and greater satisfaction of patients after non–operating room procedures. Propofol has emerged as the agent of choice for sedation because of its better pharmacokinetic and pharmacodynamic profile that results in early recovery, quick discharge, and greater patient satisfaction. However, used incorrectly or in the wrong dosage, propofol may be associated with greater patient risks. Therefore anesthesiologists worldwide prefer to actively participate in the management of these patients when using propofol for sedation, and several publications have questioned its use by non–anesthesia-trained personnel. This debate is likely to continue. Midazolam is a safe alternative for sedation but results in longer discharge time and lower patient satisfaction. Additionally, the stronger amnesia from midazolam may be considered by many to be a negative attribute. When analgesics are needed during the procedure, alfentanil has the advantage of a quicker onset of action than fentanyl but a greater risk for respiratory depression. Remifentanil is a good alternative but should be given only by anesthesia-trained personnel. Dexmedetomidine and also the combination of ketamine and propofol are emerging as less respiratory-depressant alternatives to propofol or alfentanil for sedation and analgesia, but more studies are warranted, specifically on their safety profile and side effects. Finally, it is important to state that irrespective of who performs the sedation or analgesia, continuous monitoring of physiological parameters and depth of sedation by properly trained personnel are essential prerequisites for a safe practice of sedation and analgesia outside the operating room.

Acknowledgment

Anil Gupta would like to thank the Department of Anaesthetics, Gisborne Hospital, Gisborne, New Zealand, for the time he was given during the nonclinical sessions, which gave him the opportunity to complete this chapter.

References

1. De Baerdemaeker LE, Jacobs S, Den Blauwen NM, et al. Postoperative results after desflurane or sevoflurane combined with remifentanil in morbidly obese patients. *Obes Surg.* 2006;16(6):728–733.
2. Friedberg BL. Propofol-ketamine technique. *Aesthetic Plast Surg.* 1993;17(4):297–300.
3. Friedberg BL. Propofol ketamine anesthesia for cosmetic surgery in the office suite. *Int Anesthesiol Clin.* 2003;41(2):39–50.
4. Messenger DW, Murray HE, Dungey PE, et al. Subdissociative-dose ketamine versus fentanyl for analgesia during propofol procedural sedation: a randomized clinical trial. *Acad Emerg Med.* 2008;15(10):877–886.
5. Aouad MT, Moussa AR, Dagher CM, et al. Addition of ketamine to propofol for initiation of procedural anesthesia in children reduces propofol consumption and preserves hemodynamic stability. *Acta Anaesthesiol Scand.* 2008;52(4):561–565.
6. Goel S, Bhardwaj N, Jain K. Efficacy of ketamine and midazolam as co-induction agents with propofol for laryngeal mask insertion in children. *Paediatr Anaesth.* 2008;18(7):628–634.
7. Slavik VC, Zed PJ. Combination ketamine and propofol for procedural sedation and analgesia. *Pharmacotherapy.* 2007;27(11):1588–1598.
8. Lenz H, Sandvik L, Qvigstad E, et al. A comparison of intravenous oxycodone and intravenous morphine in patient-controlled postoperative analgesia after laparoscopic hysterectomy. *Anesth Analg.* 2009;109(4):1279–1283.
9. Mertes PM, Laxenaire MC. Anaphylactic and anaphylactoid reactions occurring during anaesthesia in France. Seventh epidemiologic survey (January 2001-December 2002). *Ann Fr Anesth Reanim.* 2004;23(12):1133–1143.
10. Berg H, Roed J, Viby-Mogensen J, et al. Residual neuromuscular block is a risk factor for postoperative pulmonary complications: a prospective, randomised, and blinded study of postoperative pulmonary complications after atracurium, vecuronium and pancuronium. *Acta Anaesthesiol Scand.* 1997;41(9):1095–1103.
11. Sundman E, Witt H, Olsson R, et al. The incidence and mechanisms of pharyngeal and upper esophageal dysfunction in partially paralyzed humans: pharyngeal videoradiography and simultaneous manometry after atracurium. *Anesthesiology.* 2000;92(40):977–984.
12. Hagemann E, Halvorsen A, Holgersen O, et al. Intramuscular ephedrine reduces emesis during the first three hours after abdominal hysterectomy. *Acta Anaesthesiol Scand.* 2000;44(1):107–111.
13. Kirkegaard H, Heier T, Caldwell JE. Efficacy of tactile-guided reversal from cisatracurium-induced neuromuscular block. *Anesthesiology.* 2002;96(1):45–50.
14. Dahl V, Pendeville PE, Hollmann MW, et al. Safety and efficacy of sugammadex for the reversal of rocuronium-induced neuromuscular blockade in cardiac patients undergoing noncardiac surgery. *Eur J Anaesthesiol.* 2009;26(10):874–884.
15. Apfel CC, Läärä E, Koivuranta M, et al. A simplified risk score for predicting postoperative nausea and vomiting: conclusions from cross-validations between two centers. *Anesthesiology.* 1999;91(3):693–700.
16. Minto CF, Schnider TW, Egan TD, et al. Influence of age and gender on the pharmacokinetics and pharmacodynamics of remifentanil. I. Model development. *Anesthesiology.* 1997;86(1):10–23.
17. Minto CF, Schnider TW, Shafer SL. Pharmacokinetics and pharmacodynamics of remifentanil. II. Model application. *Anesthesiology.* 1997;86(1):24–33.
18. Servin FS, Raeder JC, Merle JC, et al. Remifentanil sedation compared with propofol during regional anaesthesia. *Acta Anaesthesiol Scand.* 2002;46:309–315.
19. Kulling D, Bauerfeind P, Fried M, Biro P. Patient-controlled analgesia and sedation in gastrointestinal endoscopy. *Gastrointest Endosc Clin N Am.* 2004;14:353–368.
20. Gillham MJ, Hutchinson RC, Carter R, Kenny GN. Patient-maintained sedation for ERCP with a target-controlled infusion of propofol: a pilot study. *Gastrointest Endosc.* 2001;54(1):14–17.
21. Chung F, Chan V. A post-anesthetic discharge scoring system for home readiness afterambulatory surgery. *J Clin Anesth.* 1995;7:500-506.
22. Lenz H, Raeder J, Hoymork SC. Administration of fentanyl before remifentanil-based anaesthesia has no influence on post-operative pain or analgesic consumption. *Acta Anaesthesiol Scand.* 2008;52(1):149–154.

8 *Practice Procedure*

ERIC A. HARRIS

The provision of hospital-based, non–operating room anesthesia (NORA) has become a burgeoning part of almost every anesthesiology practice in the United States. Cost savings,[1] facilitated scheduling (as opposed to in the main operating rooms), and increased patient satisfaction are just a few of the reasons this branch of anesthesiology is expected to continue its exponential growth in the future. Medical device technology has advanced in tandem with NORA, allowing many surgical procedures once reserved for the operating room to be performed in a less invasive manner in an alternative site (e.g., intracranial coiling and stenting has obviated the need for many craniotomies).[2] In other procedures still performed in the operating room, anesthesia is administered at an alternative anesthetizing site before the main surgical procedure (e.g., a patient with placenta percreta may have uterine artery balloon occlusion catheters placed under anesthesia in the interventional radiology suite before a caesarean section in the operating room).[3] However, the provision of care in alternative sites has yet to garner the same level of academic scrutiny as the mainstream anesthesia subspecialties. Initial guidelines published almost 20 years ago[4] seem quaint considering the current diversity of alternative-site procedures requiring anesthesia and analgesia.[5]

Similar to the pediatric anesthesiologist who scoffs at the notion that an infant is merely a scaled-down adult, those who perform NORA testify that what they do is not simply a duplication of their operating room routines. Patients who require NORA are often elderly and quite ill[6] and may undergo procedures that are unfamiliar to the anesthesiologist. The NORA environment itself may at times appear dark, crowded, and cold. Anesthesiologists may have to rely on machines and monitors they are unaccustomed to using. Ancillary staff may be unfamiliar with the needs of the anesthesiologist, and assistance, when necessary, may not be available in a timely manner.

Patient Selection

The benefits of anesthesia for alternative-site procedures are recognized by both clinicians and patients, resulting in a vigorous demand for these services. Patients expect amnesia and analgesia for even the most pedestrian procedures. Clinicians appreciate the patient relaxation and immobility afforded by a deep or general anesthetic and the freedom from having to personally control the patient's sedation regimen. However, in the vast majority of cases, adequate patient comfort and cooperation can be ensured by a nurse familiar with sedation protocols who administers drugs under the direction of the physician performing the procedure. Although anesthesiologists may dictate and oversee the sedation policy in their institution, their direct involvement in these cases is often unwarranted. Which cases, then, typically require the services of an anesthesiologist during an alternative-site procedure?

PATIENTS WHO ARE UNABLE TO LIE STILL

This category encompasses a wide variety of patients, from those who are uncooperative because of mental or developmental disabilities, acute intoxication, or substance abuse, to those with movement disorders such as Parkinson's disease and Huntington's chorea. Both diagnostic imaging and interventional procedures often require the patient to remain motionless for prolonged periods. Other procedures require a cooperative patient to breath-hold at full inspiration or full expiration to target a lesion. As discussed earlier, many of these patients can be given a trial of nurse-administered sedation. If this fails, or if the situation is known to be challenging, an anesthesiology consult should be sought.

PATIENTS WHO CANNOT TOLERATE THE SUPINE POSITION

Patients in this classification have cardiopulmonary issues such as pulmonary edema or right heart failure or neuromuscular issues such as severe lower back pain and sciatica. In the latter cases, the amount of analgesia that the patient may require to complete the study might result in apnea.

PRACTITIONERS WHO ARE UNCOMFORTABLE PROVIDING THE NECESSARY LEVEL OF SEDATION

The American Society of Anesthesiologists (ASA) has delineated four levels of sedation that exist along a continuous scale—minimal sedation (anxiolysis), moderate sedation (previously referred to as conscious sedation), deep sedation, and general anesthesia.[7] Some have added a fifth level classified as dissociative sedation, produced by agents such as ketamine.[8] The importance of the fact that these levels exist along a continuum and are not discrete destinations cannot be overstated. Even experienced clinicians may find a patient easily slipping into a deeper level of sedation than expected. If adequate and brisk resuscitation methods are not instituted, a direct correlation can be found between unintended deep sedation and the likelihood of adverse events.[9] Given this facility to oversedate, The Joint Commission devised the sedation rescue philosophy, emphasizing that the clinician responsible for the sedation protocol must be able to rescue the patient from the next level of sedation beyond that intended.[10] Therefore if deep sedation is the target, the practitioner must be prepared for the unexpected descent into general anesthesia.

PATIENTS WHO ARE UNABLE TO CONTROL THEIR RESPIRATORY RATE

A small subset of patients undergoing invasive procedures within the radiology suite, most notably computed tomography (CT)-guided or ultrasound-guided ablations, will be required to perform voluntary breath-holds during certain phases of the procedure to allow precision targeting of a lesion. This is especially important for anatomic sites close to the diaphragm, including the kidneys, adrenal glands, liver, and basal lung segments.[11] Patients who are unable to cooperate because of developmental delays, language barriers, or immaturity may require paralysis and controlled ventilation under general anesthesia.

PATIENTS WITH SEVERE CLAUSTROPHOBIA

Although severe claustrophobia is typically more of a problem in magnetic resonance imaging (MRI) and CT, any procedure that requires the patient to be draped in a darkened room may be intolerable for a claustrophobic patient. Nurse-administered sedation may be adequate, but the most severe cases may require general anesthesia for even the most routine diagnostic tests.

INFANTS AND YOUNG CHILDREN

Pediatric patients typically account for the majority of patients requiring NORA. The presence of a parent in the room or techniques such as swaddling may be insufficient to keep the patient still and cooperative during the study or procedure.[12] Small vessels may make intravenous access difficult in the pediatric patient, precluding the option of intravenous sedation. Oral sedative agents such as chloral hydrate and midazolam have unpredictable effects and may cause a paradoxical hyperexcitable state in some children.[13-15] Finally, the lack of providers with Pediatric Advanced Life Support (PALS) certification may mandate (per institutional policy) the immediate availability of an anesthesiologist. However, in most institutions, the sheer volume of these cases would overwhelm almost any anesthesiology practice if each child required direct involvement. Therefore a selection protocol must be adopted that delineates which pediatric patients can be sedated in the absence of an anesthesiologist's uninterrupted supervision. Most children are given an initial trial of sedation provided by either a nurse under the direction of the clinician performing the procedure or staff from the pediatric intensive care unit. Chloral hydrate or midazolam, either oral or intravenous, is typically the first-line drug and is often successful. Some clinicians have reported success with regimens as simple as midazolam, and others have expanded their practice to include the use of propofol or dexmedetomidine.[16] If this regimen proves insufficient, the study or procedure is rescheduled for a time when it can be performed under the supervision of an anesthesiologist. Exclusions are made for children with a history of unsuccessful sedation, children with ASA class IV status or greater, and children with anatomic anomalies that may make airway management difficult; in these patients, anesthesia is administered immediately under the care of an anesthesiologist.

Pitfalls of Non–Operating Room Anesthesia

The sympathetic response before NORA can begin up to 1 hour before beginning the procedure. Tachycardia and tachypnea are often present, along with dry mouth and moist palms. Blood pressure may be mildly elevated, and gastrointestinal discomfort is almost universal. Surprisingly, these symptoms are present not in the patient but rather in the anesthesiologist assigned to the case. Most providers with stellar skills but limited NORA experience are loath to leave the security of the operating room. What is it about NORA that makes it seem so foreign?

DISTANCE FROM THE MAIN OPERATING ROOMS

Many anesthesiologists feel out of their element when asked to work outside the operating room. Their colleagues and the anesthesia technicians might not be familiar with the off-site anesthetizing locations, making it difficult and time-consuming to acquire extra drugs, equipment, or personnel to provide a break during the case.[17]

DISTANCE FROM THE PATIENT AND MONITORS

In some sites the patient is monitored from a different room through a window, by MRI or CT, or by closed-circuit television, such as in the radiation oncology suite (Figure 8-1). Changes in intravenous line flow rates, vaporizer settings, frequency of monitoring, or any other interventions that require direct contact ideally should be timed to occur during pauses in the diagnostic or therapeutic sequence.

ROOM CONFIGURATION

Anesthesiologists may find themselves positioned very close to the patient in a room that clearly was not designed to handle anesthetic equipment.[18] Standard operating rooms are built with space for the anesthesia machine and cart, ample lighting, gases and suction available from a wall or tower

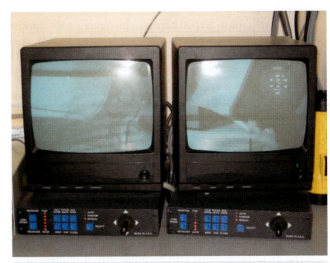

Figure 8-1 Closed-circuit televisions in the radiation oncology suite allow for remote monitoring of the patient.

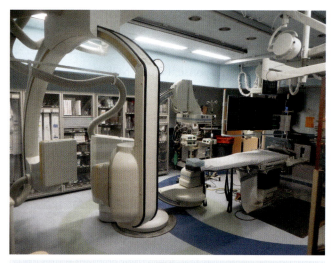

Figure 8-2 The various pieces of radiology equipment, in addition to the anesthesia machine and cart, often leave little room for the anesthesia provider.

source, and electrical outlets that will continue to provide power in the event of a generalized power loss. NORA sites may have none of these amenities, forcing the anesthesiologist to rely on items such as gas cylinders and portable suction devices. These extra pieces of equipment must compete for limited space with the bulky surgical equipment that is often used off-site, such as C-arm fluoroscopy units and endoscopy carts (Figure 8-2). Adequate lighting may be an issue, especially if the room is kept dark during fluoroscopic procedures. Loud, continuous noise may make alarms difficult to hear.[19] Positioning of the patient with an anticipated difficult airway may be problematic, because the tables in off-site locations typically are not as accommodating as tables in the operating room.[20]

LACK OF EMERGENCY EQUIPMENT

Most NORA sites are equipped with crash carts containing Advanced Cardiac Life Support (ACLS) drugs, intubation supplies, and a defibrillator. More specialized equipment, such as tools to access a difficult airway or supplies for treating malignant hyperthermia, however, will almost certainly be located near the main operating rooms at a remote location, thereby stripping another layer of comfort from the anesthesia provider.

SCARCITY OF SUPPORT STAFF

The personnel employed in the gastrointestinal suite, cardiac catheter laboratories, interventional radiology suites, and similar settings are well trained in their fields of expertise. Unfortunately, these fields have little to do with anesthesiology. Assistance with lines, difficult airways, or anesthetic emergencies may be delayed or completely unavailable.[21] A request for cricoid pressure that will be immediately fulfilled in the main operating room may be met with blank stares in a NORA site. Surgical airway assistance may likewise be delayed or unattainable. Furthermore, the staff present in these locations are typically not as well trained in ACLS as the personnel in the operating and recovery rooms.

RADIATION HAZARD

In addition to interventional radiology or neuroradiology areas that rely on a fixed source of radiation-based imaging, the anesthesiologist may be asked to work in the cardiac catheter laboratory or gastrointestinal suite, where the radiation source is portable or derived from the patient by nuclear medicine. Anesthesiologists must be familiar with the methods to reduce radiation exposure to both themselves and their patients and be willing to wear leaded aprons, wear glasses and shields, maintain a safe distance from the radiation source, or follow other institutional protocols to minimize this risk.

RENAL STATUS

Many cases performed with radiographic assistance require the use of contrast to identify fluid-filled structures. The contrast agent is often nephrotoxic above a certain dose; thus it is the shared responsibility of all the providers to ensure that this threshold is not exceeded. The use of contrast necessitates frequent flushing of the lines, so the anesthesiologist also must be mindful of the patient's volume status. Maintenance fluids should be reduced, and diuresis may be necessary.

ROOM TEMPERATURE

Pediatric and elderly patients may be especially sensitive to the temperature in many NORA sites, especially those in the radiology area. Patients with cold-sensitive conditions such as sickle cell anemia or cryoglobulinemia also may be at risk. Imaging machinery functions over a narrow (and often low) ambient temperature[22,23]; therefore the rooms are typically kept uncomfortably cold. To prevent temperature adjustment that might cause malfunction of the imaging equipment, no thermostats are located in the room. Instead, room temperature is controlled from a central, inaccessible location. Items such as forced-air warmers or fluid warmers may be difficult to obtain; challenging to fit in a limited space; and, in the case of MRI, impossible to use because of their ferrous components.

UNFAMILIAR EQUIPMENT

In some practices, NORA is still considered an inferior assignment within the department and thus older anesthesia machines and monitors may be relegated to NORA areas.[24] Many junior anesthesiologists may never have worked with or even seen some of the older equipment present at these sites.

Nowhere is the issue of unfamiliar equipment more salient than in the MRI suite,[25] where objects containing iron, cobalt, or nickel will be forcibly attracted to the magnet with a logarithmically increasing intensity. Depending on the volume of general anesthetics administered in the MRI scanner, the hospital may choose one of the following arrangements:

1. An anesthesia machine and monitoring equipment are stationed outside the room containing the magnet, and the door is left ajar to allow for the passage of cables and the breathing circuit. This is the least desirable configuration, because the open door can result in degradation of the MRI images.

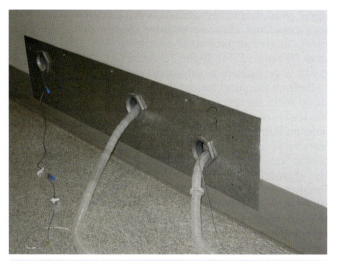

Figure 8-3 A reinforced floorboard in the magnetic resonance suite provides openings for intravenous tubing and circuit hoses.

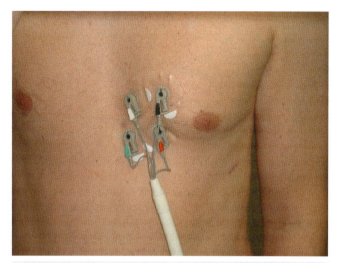

Figure 8-5 The cloverleaf pattern of electrocardiogram leads in the magnetic resonance imaging suite.

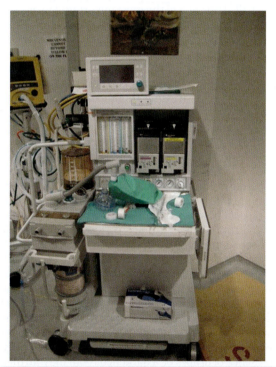

Figure 8-4 This magnetic resonance imaging–compatible anesthesia machine is similar to its standard operating room counterparts.

2. An anesthesia machine and monitoring equipment are stationed outside the room containing the magnet, but the door remains closed throughout the study. The cables and circuit are threaded through reinforced holes in the wall or floorboards (Figure 8-3).
3. An MRI-compatible anesthesia machine and monitoring panel are purchased that can safely remain in the MRI room at a certain distance—typically 6 feet—from the magnet bore. Most MRI-compatible machines are similar enough to their non-MRI counterparts to be familiar to most providers (Figure 8-4). Laryngoscopes are typically nonferromagnetic, although the batteries inside will be weakly attracted to the magnet unless they are MRI-compatible lithium batteries. Equipment

for vital sign monitoring is specific for the MRI suite, relying on distortion-free fiberoptic cables for the signal. The electrocardiogram may seem particularly foreign to the provider, because it will contain four graphite leads arranged in a cloverleaf pattern over the left sternal border (Figure 8-5). The short cable distance lessens the chance of a radiofrequency heating–induced burn.

4. An MRI-compatible infusion pump is used, which allows the practitioner to administer total intravenous anesthesia. If necessary, assisted ventilation is provided with an MRI-compatible ventilator. It is important that all infusion pumps used in the MRI area are MRI-compatible, because use of a standard pump may result in an infusion rate that differs from what is entered into and displayed on the device.

Risks and Safety of Non–Operating Room Anesthesia

As the volume of patients requiring alternative-site anesthesia continues to grow, so does the litany of anesthesia-related complications seen in this population. Examination of data from the ASA Closed Claims Project dispels the myth that patients who are too sick to undergo procedures in the operating room can be safely treated in a satellite location. The ASA Closed Claims Project is a collection of closed anesthesia-related malpractice claims from 1970 onward, representing 35 professional U.S. liability insurance companies.[26] The Closed Claims Analysis reflects only cases performed under the direct supervision of an anesthesiologist; cases done under the care of other health care providers, such as sedation in the gastrointestinal suite directed by the gastroenterologist, are not included in the results. Two recent analyses of these data[27,28] reveal a clearer picture of the risks associated with NORA. In total, 87 claims were filed for NORA cases, in contrast to 3287 claims for operating room anesthetics.

As the volume of NORA cases has risen over the decades, so has the number of reported complications. During the 1970s, NORA was cited in only 0.2% of the closed claims (n = 1) versus 1.2% (n = 24) from the period 1990 to 2001.[27] This rose to 2.8% (n = 62) from 2002 to 2009. Claims for patients who received NORA reveal that they are older, with 20% older than 70 years of age in contrast to 12% for operating room cases ($P < .01$). They are also sicker, with 69% of patients rated ASA class 3 to 5, in contrast to 44% in the operating room ($P < .001$). NORA procedures are more likely to be emergent, 36 percent versus 15 percent ($P < .001$).

Of these claims, 32% originated in the gastrointestinal suite. An earlier study found 50% of the claims were gastrointestinal-related, with one third of those occurring during endoscopic retrograde cholangiopancreatography.[27] More than half of the reported complications in the gastrointestinal area were the result of unintended oversedation. The cardiac catheterization and electrophysiological study laboratories accounted for another quarter of the claims, with the remainder occurring in the emergency room, the lithotripsy suite, and the radiology areas. Among all the radiology-related claims, 70% occurred during the administration of anesthesia in the MRI suite as a result of receiving burns from non–MRI-safe monitoring equipment, oversedation, and brachial plexopathy from patient positioning in the scanner. Oversedation is a noteworthy problem among children with developmental disabilities who receive anesthesia during an MRI examination; one study found the incidence among this population to be 11.9% versus 4.9% for children without these disabilities.[29] The authors speculated that the narrowness of the palate seen in these children, especially those with cerebral palsy, may make them susceptible to airway obstruction.

The majority of NORA claims involved monitored anesthesia care (MAC) (50% versus 6%, $P < .001$). General anesthesia cases represented only 26% of claims, whereas the percentage was three times as high among the operating room cohort. Of the NORA claims, 21% involved no anesthetic because they chiefly involved airway management provided by an anesthesiologist in the emergency room. Regional anesthesia, rarely performed in NORA sites, accounted for only 2% of claims versus 16% for the operating room.

The severity of injuries suffered by NORA patients was more substantial than their operating room counterparts, with a significantly larger number of operating room injuries rated as temporary or nondisabling. Although death was the most common complication in both groups, it occurred at almost twice the frequency among the NORA cohort (54% versus 29%, $P < .001$). Other complications, such as brain damage, myocardial infarction, and aspiration, occurred in roughly the same proportion. Only nerve damage was noted in a statistically significant higher percentage among the operating room group (19% versus 7%, $P < .01$.)

The primary mechanism of injury within both cohorts revolved around respiratory complications. However, the proportion of respiratory mishaps was double among the NORA group (44% versus 20%, $P < .001$) and the incidence of inadequate oxygenation or ventilation was seven times higher among the NORA patients (21% versus 3%, $P < .001$). Of the NORA claims, 30% (n = 26) involved respiratory depression as a result of drug overdose, with propofol (either alone or in combination with other drugs) the

agent most frequently cited as bearing responsibility. Factors associated with oversedation claims included obesity (56%), high-risk patients (ASA classes 3-5, 54%), and age over 70 years (27%). Of the 26 claims, 24 (92%) resulted in death or permanent neurological injury.

Perhaps the most salient figures to come from the study dealt with the preventability of injuries in NORA sites. Reviewers of the closed claims judged anesthesia care to be substandard in 54% of the remote location claims, in contrast to 37% in the operating room group ($P < .01$). Monitoring was cited as a key NORA deficiency, with 32% of the alternative site claims considered preventable by better monitoring, versus 8% in the operating room cohort ($P < .001$). The numbers were even higher in the gastrointestinal suite, where 86% of the cases were judged to have substandard care, including 62% of which were cited as having inadequate monitoring. The typical deficiency was the lack of end-tidal carbon dioxide ($ETCO_2$) monitoring; in the gastrointestinal cases, capnography was used in only 15% of the claim cases and another 15% relied on no respiratory monitoring at all. Thus one of the most important lessons learned from the NORA claims in the ASA Closed Claims Project is the vital importance of measuring $ETCO_2$ during the procedure. Although this is typically standard fare during a general anesthetic, analysis of the claims shows that it is often neglected during MAC cases. This occurs despite policy statements by the ASA stressing the importance of monitoring ventilation (as opposed to only oxygenation) during sedation.[31] Oversedation is common during NORA cases, during which the noxious stimuli may be intermittent. Introduction of the gastroscope, which aggravates the typical patient, may be followed by a protracted period of relative calm. The dose of sedatives, analgesics, or anesthetics to blunt the initial stimulus may result in oversedation and apnea afterward, especially when dealing with agents that display long elimination half-lives.[31] Apneic periods lasting 30 seconds or more are common, and in the absence of capnography or electrical impedance monitoring, apnea may be very difficult to recognize.[32] In one study, anesthesiologists blinded to capnography during MAC failed to identify a 20-second apnea period in every single cohort patient who displayed this lapse in breathing.[33] Another study among endoscopists showed that when blinded to capnography, they failed to diagnose a 30-second period of apnea in 63% of their sedated patients.[34] The presence of drapes or a darkened room may further hinder the ability to recognize apnea.

It is common for patients to be placed on supplemental oxygen while sedatives are being administered; paradoxically, this may delay the detection of apnea.[35] Pulse oximetry is not a sensitive monitor of apnea, especially if the patient is receiving supplemental oxygenation.[36-38] Patients who receive supplemental oxygen and then become apneic will maintain their saturation longer than patients maintained on room air[39]; by the time desaturation is noted, the patient may have developed significant hypercarbia and be well on the way to an adverse respiratory event. Capnography, on the other hand, is exquisitely sensitive; a recent study of patients in the gastrointestinal suite undergoing procedures under propofol sedation found no instances of apnea when $ETCO_2$ monitoring was added to pulse oximetry.[40] A similar study conducted among the pediatric population reported similar results when capnography was used with propofol MAC anesthesia.[41]

Studies confined to the pediatric population receiving sedation or anesthesia for procedures outside the operating room have echoed the findings cited earlier. A report from the Pediatric Sedation Research Consortium reviewed 35,000 pediatric alternative-site sedation cases.[42] The data revealed no deaths attributable to the sedation regimen and only a single cardiac arrest and a single case of aspiration (in a different patient), both attributed to the anesthesia care. However, the incidence of airway compromise was significant: 1 in 200 sedations required some type of unplanned airway assistance, and 1 in 400 patients progressed to develop stridor, laryngospasm, wheezing, or apnea. A subsequent, larger report from the same group reviewed the nature and rate of complications among 49,836 propofol-sedation episodes.[43] This report also claimed no deaths and only 2 episodes of cardiac arrest and 4 cases of aspiration related to the sedation. However, the incidence of airway compromise in these cases was much more significant. One in 10 patients required some type of unplanned airway intervention, with 31.6% of those patients requiring more advanced airway techniques, including bag-mask ventilation, oral airway insertion, and laryngeal mask airway or endotracheal tube placement. One in 65 patients progressed to develop stridor, laryngospasm, wheezing, or apnea. The authors concluded that although propofol sedation is undeniably safe in the NORA setting, it must be supervised by practitioners who are thoroughly skilled in the management of airway obstruction and respiratory embarrassment. Biannual PALS training using mannequins may not provide sufficient competency. Furthermore, $ETCO_2$ monitoring and the immediate availability of suction equipment should be standard.

Beyond propofol, ketamine continues to be a reliable agent for providing both anesthesia and analgesia during NORA cases. Concurrent use of a benzodiazepine and an antisialogogue may be necessary to moderate the side effects of ketamine. Dexmedetomidine is also a reliable choice for pediatric NORA cases,[44-47] but the manufacturers' recommended dose may provide insufficient anesthesia in this setting. Mason and associates[48] found that a dosing regimen of a 3-mcg/kg bolus over 10 minutes, followed by a 2-mcg/kg/hr infusion, improved the effectiveness of alternative-site sedation from 91.8% to 97.6% (versus a bolus of 2 mcg/kg and an infusion of 1-1.5 mcg/kg/hr[49]). Respiratory depression was not noted, yet bradycardia manifested in 16.1% of the patients in the sample, with 4% experiencing a heart rate drop of greater than 20%. Glycopyrrolate was successful in reversing the bradycardia, but was associated with an exaggerated hypertensive response,[48] likely as a result of the increased sympathetic vascular tone from the α_2 adrenoreceptor stimulation. These findings have been reported by other authors, thereby questioning the usefulness of dexmedetomidine in patients prone to developing bradycardia or heart block.[50]

The Future of Non–Operating Room Anesthesia

Advances in medical technology have allowed many procedures once reserved for the confines of the operating room to be performed in a variety of alternative locations. When cost savings, scheduling efficiency, and the decreasing willingness of patients to tolerate discomfort or anxiety are considered, little doubt should remain that NORA will continue to accelerate in the foreseeable future. Yet demand has begun to outstrip supply, because anesthesia departments must deal with staffing issues and limited reimbursement when trying to meet the requests for service. Some nonanesthesiologist physicians, frustrated by the lack of sufficient anesthesiologist coverage for their alternative-site cases, have begun to direct the delivery of sedation and anesthesia by themselves,[51] at times using drugs once reserved for use by anesthesia providers[52] (e.g., propofol,[53] alfentinil,[54] and remifentanil[55]). The danger of this practice is twofold: the gravest risk falls on the patients, who may receive drugs with unintended effects that cannot be adequately managed by the physician administering the medications. The secondary risk lies with anesthesiologists, who are often ultimately responsible for devising and overseeing sedation protocols for all health care providers at their hospital. The Centers for Medicare and Medicaid Services has echoed this, requiring that sedation and analgesia services be under the direction of the hospital's department of anesthesia.[56] The ASA strengthened this position in 2012, issuing a policy statement that any physician performing deep sedation must be qualified to recognize and rescue a patient from a state of general anesthesia.[57]

How will the medical specialty proceed beyond this crossroad? First, anesthesiologists must come to terms with the fact that in the future a proportionately larger percentage of NORA will be provided by nonanesthesiologists. Although some anesthesiologists may think this is ceding both control of the profession and income to others, it is merely acting in the patient's best interest by allowing a larger patient population to undergo necessary procedures free from anxiety and pain. However, it is necessary to continue to improve the safety of nonanesthesiologist-supervised NORA by providing education, direction, and consultation to colleagues.

The safety profile of nonanesthesiologist-directed NORA will improve with the introduction of new pharmacological agents that provide sedation and analgesia with a low risk for side effects. One such agent, fospropofol disodium (Lusedra), already has shown promise in the gastrointestinal suite.[58,59] Fospropofol is a water-soluble prodrug that releases free propofol after being hydrolyzed by alkaline phosphatase. The pharmacokinetic profile of fospropofol is thought to result in the avoidance of the high initial peak plasma concentration seen with the lipid emulsion formula of propofol. Unfortunately, several published reports of the pharmacokinetics and pharmacodynamics of this drug have been retracted because of an error in the assay procedure.[60-63] The dosing schedule begins with an initial bolus dose of 6.5 mg/kg. Redosing, when necessary, is given as a bolus of 1.6 mg/kg.

Another way to improve the safety of nonanesthesiologist-directed NORA is to place sedation management in the patients' hands. Similar to patient-controlled analgesia (PCA) pumps used to manage postoperative pain, patient-controlled sedation (PCS) devices allow the patient to self-administer a chosen sedative agent during the procedure. The patient presses a delivery button in response to pain or anxiety[64]; a certain level of consciousness is required to press the button, ensuring that the sedated patient will not receive an unnecessary dose. Similar to PCA pumps, PCS machines can be programmed with a lockout time to prevent the delivery of a rapid succession of doses. Target-controlled infusion systems may provide even more assurance against unintended oversedation. These delivery systems rely on a computer bench that accounts for both the pharmacokinetics of the drug and the physiological state of the patient to calculate and administer the ideal infusion rate.[65]

Ultimately, the best plan we have to minimize the risks of NORA is to hold it to the same rigorous patient preparation and intraoperative vigilance standards that apply to traditional operating room cases.[66] This preparation begins with the preprocedure evaluation of the patients, an exercise that is occasionally overlooked when preparing for a NORA case. In some instances, patients are scheduled for NORA procedures by an alternative scheduling practice and are not seen for an anesthesiology preoperative visit. Other patients are anticipated to require only sedation provided by a nonanesthesiologist, but the sedation proves to be inadequate to complete the procedure. The anesthesia team is then called to provide anesthesia care to a patient who has already been sedated, forcing a preoperative evaluation based more on chart review than physician–patient interaction. This situation also precludes the possibility of getting a proper informed consent from the patient to administer a more appropriate anesthetic. Excellent anesthetic care rests on the foundation of a thorough preprocedure assessment, and it is not always the case that this evaluation is completed with the same rigors and standards as for operating room cases.[67] It is because of this risk for inadequate preprocedure evaluation that the ASA has recommended that all NORA patients be channeled into the institutions' routine and customary preoperative assessment channels.[68]

The safety of operating room anesthesia can be duplicated in alternative sites only when the necessary equipment is present or readily available. These safety measures include properly functioning anesthesia machines, standard monitoring technology, and a pharmaceutical dispensing system that offers both routine and emergency drugs. Ancillary staff must be available to provide assistance when dealing with unexpected events. Many providers take these things for granted in the operating room, yet are permissive to perform NORA cases in their absence. This is a fundamental mistake and one that exposes the patient to harm and the provider to legal hazard; the ASA standards of care apply to all patients and do not vary with the location of the case.[4]

Postoperatively, patients who have received NORA should be directed toward the same postanesthesia care unit area into which patients from the operating room are channeled. Although many alternative sites have their own recovery areas, such as the cardiac catheter laboratory and gastrointestinal and interventional radiology suites, these are more suited for patients who have received only minimal sedation. The patient-to-nurse ratio may be too high, and the nurses themselves may be inexperienced in providing postanesthesia care.

The following chapters will delve more deeply into the intricacies of NORA in specific alternative sites. The common thread throughout will be the risks inherent to providing a safe anesthetic in each alternative location and ways to mitigate the hazard. Given the challenges of NORA, is it reasonable to wonder why a clinician would choose to practice under these difficult conditions? The answer from those who do a considerable amount of work in this field is that NORA is an enormously satisfying part of the specialty of anesthesiology. It challenges the technical, intellectual, and problem-solving skills of the anesthesiologist while building valuable bridges with our colleagues in other departments, such as radiology, gastroenterology, and interventional cardiology. By reading this text, you will familiarize yourself with many of the pitfalls and eccentricities of NORA, thereby smoothing your path as you gain experience in the field. Although the learning curve associated with NORA may appear great, so too are the rewards.

References

1. Adams K, Pennock N, Phelps B, Rose W, Peters M. Anesthesia services outside of the operating room. *Pediatr Nurs.* 2007;33(3): 232–237.
2. Bader AM, Pothier MM. Out-of-operating room procedures: preprocedure assessment. *Anesthesiol Clin.* 2009;27(1):121–126.
3. Cutter TW. Radiologists and anesthesiologists. *Anesthesiology Clin.* 2009;27(1):95–106.
4. Holzman RS, Cullen DJ, Eichorn JH, Phillip JH. Guidelines for sedation by nonanesthesiologists during diagnostic and therapeutic procedures. *J Clin Anesth.* 1994;6(4):265–276.
5. Pino RM. The nature of anesthesia and procedural sedation outside of the operating room. *Curr Opin Anaesthesiol.* 2007;20(4):347–351.
6. Lai YC, Manninen PH. Anesthesia for cerebral aneurysms: a comparison between interventional neuroradiology and surgery. *Can J Anaesth.* 2001;48(4). 397–395.
7. American Society of Anesthesiologists. Practice guidelines for sedation and analgesia by nonanesthesiologists: a report by the American Society of Anesthesiologists Task Force on sedation and analgesia by nonanesthesiologists. *Anesthesiology.* 2002;96(4):1004–1017.
8. Meyer S, Grundmann U, Gottschling S, Kleinschmidt S, Gortner L. Sedation and analgesia for brief diagnostic and therapeutic procedures in children. *Eur J Pediatr.* 2007;166(4):291–302.
9. Coté CJ, Notterman DA, Karl WH, Weinberg JA, McCloskey C. Adverse sedation events in pediatrics: a critical incident analysis of contributing factors. *Pediatrics.* 2000;105(4 Pt 1):805–814.
10. Joint Commission on Accreditation of Healthcare Organizations. *2006 Comprehensive accreditation manual for hospitals: the official handbook.* Oak Brook, Ill: Joint Commission Resources; 2005.
11. Schenker MP, Martin R, Shyn PB, Baum RA. Interventional radiology and anesthesia. *Anesthesiology Clin.* 2009;27(1):87–94.
12. Gozal D, Gozal Y. Pediatric sedation/anesthesia outside the operating room. *Curr Opin Anaesthesiol.* 2008;21(4):494–498.
13. Massanari M, Novitsky J, Reinstein LJ. Paradoxical reactions in children associated with midazolam use during endoscopy. *Clin Pediatr (Phila).* 1997;36(12):681–684.
14. Slatt KA. Crazy with chloral hydrate: a parent witnesses a paradoxical reaction. *Gastroenterol Nurs.* 2009;32(4):296–297.
15. Mancuso CE, Tanzi MG, Gabay M. Paradoxical reactions to benzodiazepines: literature review and treatment options. *Pharmacotherapy.* 2004;24(9):1177–1185.
16. McMorrow SP, Abramo TJ. Dexmedetomidine sedation: uses in pediatric procedural sedation outside the operating room. *Pediatr Emerg Care.* 2012;28(3):292–296.
17. Frankel A. Patient safety: anesthesia in remote locations. *Anesthesiol Clin.* 2009;27(1):127–139.
18. Feldman JM, Kalli I. Equipment and environmental issues for nonoperating room anesthesia. *Anesthesiol Clin.* 2006;19(4):450–452.
19. Melloni C. Anesthesia and sedation outside the operating room: how to prevent risk and maintain good quality. *Curr Opin Anaesthesiol.* 2007;20(6):513–519.
20. Wong AB, Moore MSR. Positioning of obese patients in out-of-operating room locations. *Anaesth Analg.* 2007;104(5):1306.
21. Caplan JP, Querques J, Epstein LA, Stern TA. Consultation, communication, and conflict management by out-of-operating room anesthesiologists: strangers in a strange land. *Anesthesiol Clin.* 2009;27(1):111–120.
22. Missant C, Van de Velde M. Morbidity and mortality related to anaesthesia outside the operating room. *Curr Opin Anaesthesiol.* 2004;17(4):323–327.
23. Eichorn V, Henzler D, Murphy MF. Standardizing care and monitoring for anesthesia or procedural sedation delivered outside the operating room. *Curr Opin Anaesthesiol.* 2010;23(4):494–499.

24. Van de Velde M, Roofthooft E, Kuypers M. Risk and safety of anaesthesia outside the operating room. *Curr Opin Anesthesiol.* 2008;21(4):486–487.
25. Girshin M, Shapiro V, Rhee A, Ginsberg S, Inchiosa Jr MA. Increased risk of general anesthesia for high-risk patients undergoing magnetic resonance imaging. *J Comput Assist Tomogr.* 2009;33(2):312–315.
26. Cheney FW. The American Society of Anesthesiologists Closed Claims Project: what have we learned, how has it affected practice, and how will it affect practice in the future? *Anesthesiology.* 1999;91(2):552–556.
27. Robbertze R, Posner KL, Domino KB. Closed claims review of anesthesia for procedures outside the operating room. *Curr Opin Anesthesiol.* 2006;19(4):436–442.
28. Metzner J, Posner KL, Domino KB. The risk and safety of anesthesia at remote locations: the US closed claims analysis. *Curr Opin Anesthesiol.* 2009;22(4):502–508.
29. Kannikeswaran N, Mahajan PV, Sethuraman U, Groebe A, Chen X. Sedation medication received and adverse events related to sedation for brain MRI in children with and without developmental disabilities. *Paediatr Anaesth.* 2009;19(3):250–256.
30. Deleted in page proofs.
31. American Society of Anesthesiologists Committee on Standards and Practice Parameters. Standards for basic anesthetic monitoring. Approved by the ASA House of Delegates on October 21, 1986, and last amended on October 20, 2010 with an effective date of July 1, 2011. http://www.asahq.org/For-Members/Standards-Guidelines-and-Statements.aspx.
32. Gan TJ. Pharmacokinetic and pharmacodynamic characteristics of medications used for moderate sedation. *Clin Pharmacokinet.* 2006;45(9):855–869.
33. Vargo JJ, Zuccaro GJR, Dumot JA, Conwell DL, Morrow JB, Shay SS. Automated graphic assessment of respiratory activity is superior to pulse oximetry and visual assessment for the detection of early respiratory depression during therapeutic upper endoscopy. *Gastrointest Endosc.* 2002;55(7):826–831.
34. Soto RG, Fu ES, Vila Jr H, Miguel RV. Capnography accurately detects apnea during monitored anesthesia care. *Anesth Analg.* 2004;99(2):379–382.
35. Qadeer MA, Vargo J, Dumot JA, et al. Capnographic monitoring of respiratory activity improves safety of sedation for endoscopic cholangiopancreatography and ultrasonography. *Gastroenterology.* 2009;136(5):1568–1576.
36. Galvango SM, Bhavani-Shankar K. Critical monitoring issues outside the operating room. *Anesthesiol Clin.* 2009;27(1):141–156.
37. Srinivasa V, Kodali BS. Capnometry in the spontaneously breathing patient. *Curr Opin Anesthesiol.* 2004;17(6):517–520.
38. Downs JB. Has oxygen administration delayed appropriate respiratory care? Fallacies regarding oxygen therapy. *Respir Care.* 2003;48(6):611–620.
39. Keidan I, Gravenstein D, Berkenstadt H, Ziv A, Shavit I, Sidi A. Supplemental oxygen compromises the use of pulse oximetry for detection of apnea and hypoventilation during sedation in simulated pediatric patients. *Pediatrics.* 2008;122(2):293–298.
40. Jense HG, Dubin SA, Silverstein PI, O'Leary-Escolas U. Effect of obesity on safe duration of apnea in anesthetized humans. *Anesth Analg.* 1991;72(1):89–93.
41. Külling D, Rothenbühler R, Inauen W. Safety of nonanesthetist sedation with propofol for outpatient colonoscopy and esophagogastroduodenoscopy. *Endoscopy.* 2003;35(8):679–682.
42. Leroy PL, Nieman FH, Blokland-Loggers HE, Schipper DM, Zimmermann LJ, Knape JT. Adherence to safety guidelines on paediatric procedural sedation: the results of a nationwide survey under general paediatricians in The Netherlands. *Arch Dis Child.* 2010;95(12):1027–1030.
43. Cravero JP, Beach ML, Blike GT, Gallagher SM, Hertzog JH. Pediatric Sedation Research Consortium. Incidence and nature of adverse events during pediatric sedation/anesthesia for procedures outside the operating room: report from the Pediatric Sedation Research Consortium. *Pediatrics.* 2006;118(3):1087–1096.
44. Cravero JP, Beach ML, Blike GT, Gallagher SM, Hertzog JH. Pediatric Sedation Research Consortium. The incidence and nature of adverse events during pediatric sedation/anesthesia with propofol for procedures outside the operating room: a report from the Pediatric Sedation Research Consortium. *Anesth Analg.* 2009;108(3):795–804.
45. Cravero JP. Risk and safety of pediatric sedation/anesthesia for procedures outside the operating room. *Curr Opin Anaesthesiol.* 2009;22(4):509–513.
46. Munro HM, Tirotta CF, Felix DE, et al. Initial experience with dexmedetomidine for diagnostic and interventional cardiac catheterization in children. *Paediatr Anaesth.* 2007;17(2):109–112.
47. Phan H, Nahata MC. Clinical uses of dexmedetomidine in pediatric patients. *Paediatr Drugs.* 2008;10(1):49–69.
48. Mason KP, Zurakowski D, Zgleszewski SE, et al. High dose dexmedetomidine as the sole sedative for pediatric MRI. *Paediatr Anaesth.* 2008;18(5):403–411.
49. Heard C, Burrows F, Johnson K, Joshi P, Houck J, Lerman J. A comparison of dexmedetomidine-midazolam with propofol for maintenance of anesthesia in children undergoing magnetic resonance imaging. *Anesth Analg.* 2008;107(6):1832–1839.
50. Mason KP, Zgleszewski S, Forman RE, Stark C, DiNardo JA. An exaggerated hypertensive response to glycopyrrolate therapy for bradycardia associated with high-dose dexmedetomidine. *Anesth Analg.* 2009;108(3):906–908.
51. Hammer GB, Drover DR, Cao H, et al. The effects of dexmedetomidine on cardiac electrophysiology in children. *Anesth Analg.* 2008;106(1):79–83.
52. Metzner J, Domino KB. Risks of anesthesia or sedation outside the operating room: the role of the anesthesia care provider. *Curr Opin Anaesthesiol.* 2010;23(4):523–531.
53. Patel KN, Simon HK, Stockwell CA, et al. Pediatric procedural sedation by a dedicated nonanesthesiology pediatric sedation service using propofol. *Pediatr Emerg Care.* 2009;25(3):133–138.
54. Schilling D, Rosenbaum A, Schweizer S, Richter H, Rumstadt B. Sedation with propofol for interventional endoscopy by trained nurses in high-risk octogenarians: a prospective, randomized, controlled study. *Endoscopy.* 2009;41(4):295–298.
55. Miner JR, Gray RO, Stephens D, Biros MH. Randomized clinical trial of propofol with and without alfentanil for deep procedural sedation in the emergency department. *Acad Emerg Med.* 2009;16(9):825–834.
56. Phillips WJ, Halpin J, Jones J, McKenzie K. Remifentanil for procedural sedation in the emergency department. *Ann Emerg Med.* 2009;53(1):163.
57. Department of Health and Human Services. Revised hospital anesthesia services interpretive guidelines. CMS Manual System, Department of Health and Human Services pub no. 100–07 State Operations Provider Certification, Centers for Medicare and Medicaid Services; 2011. http://www.asahq.org/for-members/advocacy/federal-legislative-and-regulatory-activities/interpretive-guidelines.aspx.
58. American Society of Anesthesiologists House of Delegates. Statement on granting privileges to nonanesthesiologist physicians for personally administering or supervising deep sedation. Approved on October 18, 2006, amended on October 17, 2012. http://www.asahq.org/For-Members/Standards-Guidelines-and-Statements.aspx.
59. Harris EA, Lubarsky DA, Candiotti KA. Monitored anesthesia care (MAC) sedation: clinical utility of fospropofol. *Ther Clin Risk Manag.* 2009;5:949–959.
60. Lubarsky DA, Candiotti K, Harris E. Understanding modes of moderate sedation during gastrointestinal procedures: a current review of the literature. *J Clin Anesth.* 2007;19(5):397–404.
61. Gibiansky E, Struys MM, Gibiansky L, et al. Retraction. AQUAVAN injection, a water-soluble prodrug of propofol, as a bolus injection: a phase I dose-escalation comparison with DIPRIVAN. Part 1. Pharmacokinetics. *Anesthesiology.* 2010;112(4):1058.
62. Struys MM, Vanluchene AL, Gibiansky E, et al. Retraction. AQUAVAN injection, a water-soluble prodrug of propofol, as a bolus injection: a phase I dose-escalation comparison with DIPRIVAN. Part 2. Pharmacodynamics and safety. *Anesthesiology.* 2010;112(4):1058.
63. Fechner J, Ihmsen H, Hatterscheid D, et al. Retraction. Pharmacokinetics and clinical pharmacodynamics of the new propofol prodrug GPI 15715 in volunteers. *Anesthesiology.* 2010;112(4):1058.
64. Fechner J, Ihmsen H, Hatterscheid D, et al. Retraction. Comparative pharmacokinetics and pharmacodynamics of the new propofol prodrug GPI 15715 and propofol emulsion. *Anesthesiology.* 2010;112(4):1058.
65. Külling D, Bauerfeind P, Fried M, Biro P. Patient-controlled analgesia and sedation in gastrointestinal endoscopy. *Gastrointest Endosc Clin N Am.* 2004;14(2):353–368.
66. Egan TD. Target-controlled drug delivery: progress toward an intravenous "vaporizer" and automated anesthetic administration. *Anesthesiology.* 2003;99(5):1214–1219.
67. Bader AM, Pothier MM. Out-of-operating room procedures: preprocedure assessment. *Anesthesiol Clin.* 2009;27(1):121–126.
68. Whittemore AD. Introduction: the challenge of anesthesia outside the operating room. *Anesthesiol Clin.* 2009;27(1):1.

9 Preoperative Evaluations

JENNIFER E. HOFER, MELISSA L. PANT and BOBBIEJEAN SWEITZER

The preoperative evaluation of the patient undergoing anesthesia is both a requirement of the Centers for Medicare and Medicaid Services and important in preparing an anesthetic plan. Certain parts of the anesthesia preoperative evaluation are standard, whereas other elements are individualized depending on the patient, timing of the evaluation, type of procedure, and location. Non–operating room procedures requiring anesthesia (NORA) present a unique set of challenges for the anesthesiologist. The anesthesiologist experiences pressure to evaluate the patient with limited information, start the procedure in a location where emergency equipment is not readily accessible, and provide an anesthetic that will allow for a short recovery period in a busy procedural suite. Although commonalities exist in the preoperative evaluation of patients regardless of their American Society of Anesthesiologists (ASA) classification (Table 9-1), many parts of the evaluation depend on a patient's comorbidities and symptoms and the location of the planned procedure.

When patients have routine medical care, their comorbidities are known and properly managed. Other patients, however, present on the day of the procedure without diagnoses or with symptoms that may be serious enough to require further evaluation.[1,2] The severity of the symptoms and the urgency of the procedure determine whether additional testing is required. It is the anesthesiologist's responsibility to obtain a patient medical history, perform a physical examination, and decide with the proceduralist and patient how to best proceed.

Procedures outside the operating room are challenging for the anesthesiologist because emergency equipment such as the airway cart, defibrillator, and transducer for an arterial line need to be planned for and obtained ahead of time. Nonanesthesia personnel in NORA locations may not be accustomed to the patient preparations needed by the anesthesiologist. Skilled anesthesia personnel may be far away from the procedure room. Recovery room personnel are often not familiar with caring for a patient recovering after a general anesthetic. The goals of the anesthesiologist, proceduralist, and staff are to provide the patient with the safest, highest quality care in a way that is compassionate and efficient. A thorough preoperative evaluation by the anesthesiologist helps caregivers prepare for potential complications such as a difficult airway or prolonged recovery. Contingency plans should be communicated among practitioners so that challenges can be anticipated rather than unexpected.

Preoperative Assessment

To begin, it is important to address the standard elements of the preoperative assessment—a discussion with the patient or guardian to review the medical, medication, and anesthesia history and a physical examination focused on the airway, heart, and lungs. Diagnostic studies, previous anesthetics, laboratory values, and consultation reports are routinely reviewed during this assessment. On the basis of this information an ASA physical status is assigned to the patient. After reviewing and obtaining all the information, the anesthesiologist creates the anesthetic plan and then discusses it with the proceduralist and patient.

It is useful to have a mechanism to obtain patient-specific information. This can be a standardized form that documents the patient's medical history online or on paper (Figure 9-1). The form can guide the anesthesiologist in completing the assessment and focuses on comorbidities, current medications, allergies, previous surgical and anesthetic history, and use of alcohol, tobacco, or other illicit substances. If the patient does not know the medications currently taken, a phone call to the patient's pharmacy can provide this information. With this medication list, other elements of the patient's medical history can be deciphered. A review of systems with questions pertinent to cardiovascular, pulmonary, or neurologic symptoms completes the necessary evaluation. A targeted interview can subsequently concentrate on elucidating comorbidities pertinent to anesthesia care, their severity, frequency of exacerbations, and previous and current management. The interviewer will determine the patient's functional capacity (Table 9-2) and assign the patient an ASA physical status classification that can stratify periprocedural risk.[3] A better cardiopulmonary reserve as evidenced by a metabolic equivalent (MET) greater than 4 or 5 predicts a lower risk for perioperative complications. Complications during previous anesthetics or any family complications with anesthesia are reviewed. Certain complications are more difficult to treat in NORA locations, where resources such as postoperative ventilator support are typically unavailable and the patient may need monitored transport to the nearest phase I postoperative anesthesia care unit.

Table 9-1 American Society of Anesthesiologists Physical Status Classification*

ASA 1	Normal healthy patient
ASA 2	Patient with mild systemic disease
ASA 3	Patient with severe systemic disease
ASA 4	Patient with severe systemic disease that is a constant threat to life
ASA 5	Moribund patient who is not expected to survive without the operation
ASA 6	Declared brain-dead patient whose organs are being removed for donor purposes

*An "E" classification added to the ASA status indicates emergency surgery.
From American Society of Anesthesiologists. http://www.asahq.org.

PHYSICAL EXAMINATION

During the physical examination, attention is given to the patient's venous vasculature to assess how quickly or easily access can be obtained. If an abnormality is found on routine auscultation of the heart and lungs, a consultation, call to the patient's cardiologist or pulmonologist, or further work may be necessary. Based on the information obtained in the interview, a more detailed examination may follow. For example, if a patient has had a stroke, a residual neurological deficit is documented. The airway examination is critical to the preoperative assessment. The Mallampati type found on the physical examination will help determine if an airway has the potential for a difficult intubation. If a

Patient's Name _____ Age ____ Sex _____ Date of Surgery _____
Proposed operation _____
Primary care physician name/phone # _____ Cardiologist/phone # _____

1. Please list all previous operations (and approximate dates).

a. _____   d. _____

b. _____   e. _____

c. _____   f. _____

2. Please list any Allergies to medications, latex, food or other (and your reactions to them).

a. _____   c. _____

b. _____   d. _____

3. Circle TESTS that you have already completed; list where and when you had them. Please bring all existing reports for your visit. We are NOT suggesting that you require (or need to have) these tests.

a. ECG   Date: d. BLOOD WORK   Date:
LOCATION: LOCATION:

b. STRESS TEST   Date: e. SLEEP STUDY   Date:
LOCATION: LOCATION:

c. ECHO/Ultrasound of heart   Date: f. Other   Date:
LOCATION: LOCATION:

4. Please list all Medications you have taken in the last month (include over-the-counter drugs, inhalers, herbals, dietary supplements, and aspirin).

Drug Name   Dose and how often (am or pm)   Drug Name   Dose and how often (am or pm)

a. _____   f. _____

b. _____   g. _____

c. _____   h. _____

d. _____   i. _____

e. _____   j. _____

(Please check YES or NO and circle specific problems)   YES NO
5. Have you taken steroids (prednisone or cortisone) in the last year? .... ☐   ☐
6. Have you ever smoked?   (Quantify in _____ packs/day for _____ years) .... ☐   ☐
   Do you still smoke?   (Quantify in _____ packs/day) .... ☐   ☐
   Do you drink alcohol? (If so, how much?)_____ .... ☐   ☐
   Do you use or have you ever used any illegal drugs? (we need to know for your safety) ☐   ☐
7. Can you walk up one flight of stairs without stopping? .... ☐   ☐
8. Have you had any problems with your heart? (circle all that apply) .... ☐   ☐
(Chest pain or pressure, heart attack, abnormal ECG, skipped beats, murmur, palpitations, heart failure)
9. Do you have high blood pressure? .... ☐   ☐

Figure 9-1 Patient medical history.

Continued

	YES	NO
(Please check YES or NO and circle specific problems)		
10. Do you have diabetes?	☐	☐
11. Have you had any problems with your lungs or your chest? (circle all that apply) .... (shortness of breath, emphysema, bronchitis, asthma, TB, abnormal chest x-ray)	☐	☐
12. Are you ill now or were you recently ill with a cold, fever, chills, flu or productive cough? Describe recent changes _____	☐	☐
13. Have you or anyone in your family had serious bleeding problems? (circle all that apply) .... (prolonged bleeding from nose, gums, tooth extractions, or surgery)	☐	☐
14. Have you had any problems with your blood? (circle all that apply) .... (anemia, leukemia, lymphoma, sickle cell disease, blood clots, transfusions)	☐	☐
15. Have you ever had problems with your: (circle all that apply)		
Liver (cirrhosis; hepatitis A, B, C; jaundice)?	☐	☐
Kidney (stones, failure, dialysis)?	☐	☐
Digestive system (frequent heartburn, hiatus hernia, stomach ulcer)?	☐	☐
Back, neck or jaws (TMJ, rheumatoid arthritis, herniation)?	☐	☐
Thyroid gland (underactive or overactive)?	☐	☐
16. Have you ever had: (circle all that apply)		
Seizures?	☐	☐
Stroke; facial, leg or arm weakness; difficulty speaking?	☐	☐
Cramping pain in your legs with walking?	☐	☐
Problems with hearing, vision or memory?	☐	☐
17. Have you ever been treated with chemotherapy or radiation therapy? (circle all that apply) List indication and dates of treatment: _____	☐	☐
18. Women: Could you be pregnant? Last menstrual period began: _____	☐	☐
19. Have you ever had problems with anesthesia or surgery? (circle all that apply) .... (severe nausea or vomiting, malignant hyperthermia [in blood relatives or self], breathing difficulties, or problems with placement of a breathing tube)	☐	☐
20. Do you have any chipped or loose teeth, dentures, caps, bridgework, braces, problems opening your mouth or swallowing, or choking while eating? (circle all that apply)	☐	☐
21. Do your physical abilities limit your daily activities?	☐	☐
22. Do you snore?	☐	☐
23. Do you have sleep apnea?	☐	☐
24. Please list any medical illnesses not noted above: _____ _____		
25. Additional comments or questions for the anesthesiologist? _____ _____		

Figure 9-1, cont'd

Table 9-2 Metabolic Equivalents of Functional Capacity Measured 1 Through 12

Eating, working at computer, getting dressed	1*
Walking down stairs at home, cooking	2
Walking 1-2 blocks	3
Gardening, raking leaves	4
Climbing one flight of stairs, cycling, dancing	5
Carrying clubs while playing golf	6
Playing singles tennis	7
Climbing stairs quickly, slow jogging	8
Moderate cycling, jumping rope slowly	9
Running, or swimming quickly	10
Cross-country skiing, playing basketball using a full court	11
Rapidly running for long distances	12

*One metabolic equivalent (MET) is equivalent to the consumption of 3.5 mL O_2/min/kg.
From Jette M, Blumchen G. Metabolic equivalents (METS) in exercise testing, exercise prescription, and evaluation of functional capacity. *Clin Cardiol.* 1990;13(8):555-565.

difficult airway is anticipated, preparations must be made in advance. Other pertinent elements of the airway examination appear in Box 9-1.

Although anesthesiologists often have to make treatment decisions with only partial information available, the preoperative assessment should not be abbreviated because the anesthetic is being delivered in a NORA location. The assessment still must be thorough, even for a minor procedure with monitored anesthesia care. Any procedure or anesthetic has the potential for complications and may require conversion to a general anesthetic. In NORA locations, the paucity of resources makes planning for contingencies for even a minor procedure important.

PREOPERATIVE EVALUATIONS

If a patient with a history of syncope previously not evaluated is to undergo a colonoscopy, should the procedure continue as planned? It depends on whether the case is

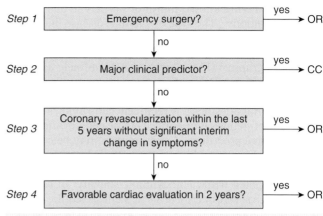

Figure 9-2 Cardiac evaluation algorithm.

elective or emergent, if there is a likely explanation for the syncope, or other factors. If the case is emergent or the syncope is not likely due to continued pathological issues, the anesthesiologist may choose to proceed and will take precautions for problems such as arrhythmias. If the case is elective, further evaluation of the syncope is warranted before proceeding, if there is any doubt to the precipitating cause.

Certain comorbidities require evaluation before an anesthetic is administered. Ischemic heart disease is common and associated with increased risk during anesthesia and certain procedures. Patients may have diagnosed and well-managed ischemic heart disease or symptoms suggestive of coronary artery disease (CAD) that have not been evaluated. Should the procedure proceed as planned? The American College of Cardiology Foundation and American Heart Association (ACC/AHA) have recommendations for testing and revascularization (Figure 9-2).[3] The anesthesiologist should stop at the first part of the algorithm that applies to the patient. For an emergency procedure such as thrombolytic therapy for an acute stroke, the focus is on risk reduction with beta-adrenergic blockers, statins, and perioperative surveillance with serial electrocardiograms (ECG), enzyme levels, and monitoring.[4] An emergent procedure should not be delayed for further testing. However, if the case is not emergent, a procedure should be postponed to have a patient's active cardiac condition stabilized or corrected. Active cardiac conditions include unstable angina, acute or recent myocardial infarction if other myocardium is at risk, decompensated heart failure, significant arrhythmias, or severe valvular disease. A patient without active cardiac symptoms who is undergoing a low-risk procedure proceeds without further testing. If the patient has a MET greater than 4 and is asymptomatic or stable, no additional testing is required, because the majority of NORA procedures would be considered low-risk procedures.

Coexisting Diseases

CORONARY ARTERY DISEASE

Patients with CAD are managed with medication regardless of whether they have had cardiac stenting or coronary artery bypass grafting. Evidence supports long-term benefits of statins and aspirin in all patients with vascular disease. Patients who have had a myocardial infarction benefit from beta-adrenergic blocking drugs unless contraindicated. These drugs typically need to be continued in the perioperative period, although acute initiation has been associated with increased risk. See the section on medications for a detailed discussion.

HEART FAILURE

Heart failure is associated with risk for perioperative complications.[5] Patients with heart failure may have fatigue, recent weight gain, dyspnea, orthopnea, or peripheral edema. Some patients may have new-onset heart failure, an exacerbation that needs additional evaluation, medication, or diet modification. For patients with decompensated heart failure, elective procedures are postponed until echocardiographic imaging is obtained and the patient's status has returned to baseline. Causes of heart failure are numerous, ranging from excessive circulating volume requiring diuretic therapy, to postchemotherapy cardiomyopathy, to worsening ischemic heart disease requiring evaluation. If the patient has symptoms compatible with undiagnosed, poorly managed, or decompensated heart failure, a cardiology evaluation is recommended for optimization of the patient's condition before the procedure. If a patient's symptoms are not significant and are stable, minor procedures may proceed as planned.

HEART MURMURS

Certain cardiac murmurs merit evaluation. Functional murmurs from turbulent flow across valves in high-output states such as pregnancy, hyperthyroidism, and anemia are not concerning.[6] Other murmurs may be pathological and need to be evaluated by echocardiography before an elective procedure. Valvular disease is suspected in patients with CAD, advanced age, a history of rheumatic fever, cardiomegaly, heart failure, or pulmonary disease. Some patients will report having known mitral or aortic valvular pathological conditions.[7] The type of valvular disease may affect the choice of anesthetic technique and may necessitate advanced monitoring via arterial line or transesophageal echocardiography (TEE), which are not routinely available in NORA locations. Delineation of conditions and communication are important. For example, if severe aortic stenosis is present, spinal anesthesia is relatively contraindicated and the degree of stenosis is quantified before general anesthesia for an elective procedure. Aortic stenosis may be confused for aortic sclerosis in older patients. Both have associated systolic murmurs, but aortic sclerosis is more prevalent and is not associated with hemodynamic stability. In contrast, patients with severe or critical aortic stenosis require a cardiology evaluation before elective procedures. These patients may be best managed by moving to an operating room setting where advanced support is available. If the case necessitates being done in NORA location, an anesthesiologist who can transport and use a TEE may be requested for the case.

ANTIBIOTIC PROPHYLAXIS

Guidelines by the American Heart Association that designate who requires antibiotic prophylaxis against infective endocarditis appear in Boxes 9-2 and 9-3.[8] Antibiotic recommendations depend on the patient's preexisting condition and the type of procedure. For patients with native valves, antibiotic prophylaxis is not routinely recommended even if an abnormality on the native valve is present. However, if a patient has a transplanted heart with valvular abnormalities, antibiotic prophylaxis is necessary for certain procedures. For a patient with a prosthetic cardiac valve, previous infective endocarditis, unrepaired congenital heart disease, or lifelong valvular defects after repair, antibiotic prophylaxis is also necessary after certain procedures, which are listed in Box 9-3. Antibiotic prophylaxis against infective endocarditis is no longer recommended for genitourinary and gastrointestinal procedures. For patients with abnormalities listed in Box 9-2 undergoing dental procedures that involve manipulation of gingival tissues or oral mucosa or for procedures on the respiratory tract or infected tissue, antibiotic prophylaxis is recommended.

STENTS AND ANTICOAGULATION THERAPY

Patients who have had percutaneous coronary intervention (PCI) should be identified before scheduling a procedure. The length of wait time before an elective noncardiac procedure after PCI is determined by the type of revascularization and the period of recommended dual antiplatelet therapy to prevent thrombosis.[9,10] For PCI without stenting, 2 weeks of dual antiplatelet therapy should be completed. If a drug-eluting stent is placed, 12 months of aspirin and thienopyridine therapy (clopidogrel or ticlopidine) is required. If a bare metal stent is placed, 1 month of dual antiplatelet therapy is indicated. The patient is considered high risk during the mandated period of dual antiplatelet therapy, and elective procedures requiring cessation of antiplatelets or with a risk for bleeding are delayed. However, if a procedure mandates the discontinuation of thienopyridine therapy during the high-risk period, aspirin is continued, with a plan to restart the thienopyridine postoperatively.[11] The preanesthetic visit

---

Box 9-2 Cardiac Conditions for Which Endocarditis Prophylaxis Is Indicated

Prosthetic cardiac valve or prosthetic material used for cardiac valve repair
Previous infective endocarditis
Congenital heart disease (CHD)
　Unrepaired cyanotic CHD (palliative shunts and conduits)
　Completely repaired congenital heart defect with prosthetic material or device, during the first 6 months after the procedure
　Repaired CHD with residual defects
Cardiac transplantation recipients who develop cardiac valvulopathy

From Wilson W, Taubert KA, Gewitz M, et al. Prevention of infective endocarditis: guidelines from the American Heart Association. Circulation. *2007;116(15):1736-1754.*

Box 9-3 Endocarditis Prophylaxis Indications

- Bacteremia resulting from daily activities is much more likely to cause infective endocarditis than bacteremia associated with a dental procedure.
- Only an extremely small number of cases of infective endocarditis might be prevented by antibiotic prophylaxis even if prophylaxis is 100% effective
- Limit recommendations for infective endocarditis prophylaxis to only those conditions listed in Box 9-2.
- Antibiotic prophylaxis is no longer recommended for any other form of congenital heart disease, except for the conditions listed in Box 9-2.
- Antibiotic prophylaxis is no longer recommended based solely on an increased lifetime risk for acquisition of infective endocarditis.
- Antibiotic prophylaxis is not recommended solely to prevent infective endocarditis for genitourinary or gastrointestinal tract procedures.

For patients with underlying cardiac conditions associated with the highest risk for adverse outcome from infective endocarditis (see Table 9-2), antibiotic prophylaxis is reasonable for the following:

- All dental procedures that involve manipulation of gingival tissues or periapical region of teeth or perforation of oral mucosa.
- Procedures on respiratory tract or infected skin, skin structures, or musculoskeletal tissue.

Although these guidelines recommend changes in indications for infective endocarditis prophylaxis with regard to selected dental procedures, the writing group reaffirms that those medical procedures listed as not requiring infective endocarditis prophylaxis in the 1997 statement remain unchanged and extends this view to vaginal delivery, hysterectomy, and tattooing. Additionally, the committee advises against body piercing for patients with conditions listed in Box 9-2 because of the possibility of bacteremia, while recognizing minimal published data exist regarding the risk for bacteremia or endocarditis associated with body piercing.

From Wilson W, Taubert KA, Gewitz M, et al. Prevention of infective endocarditis: guidelines from the American Heart Association. Circulation. *2007;116(15):1736-1754.*

offers the opportunity to identify the type of PCI and discuss the dual antiplatelet therapy with the patient's cardiologist. Premature discontinuation of antiplatelet therapy can have catastrophic consequences, such as stent thrombosis, myocardial infarction, or even death. The patient needs to be aware of the risks of discontinuation of these drugs (Box 9-4).

HYPERTENSION

Patients with hypertension who are to undergo NORA procedures may have elevated blood pressure on the day of a procedure as a result of chronically poor control, anxiety, or not taking morning medications.[12] Patients with severe hypertension commonly have comorbidities such as heart failure, renal insufficiency, ischemic heart disease, or history of stroke. The preoperative goal is to restore blood pressure to normal levels over a period of weeks before a procedure and to avoid intraoperative hypotension, which can result in an ischemic event.[13] Aggressive lowering of blood pressure on the day of a procedure is more dangerous than hypertension. Delaying procedures for patients with severe hypertension until a blood pressure of less than 180/110 mmHg is achieved is recommended.

CARDIOVASCULAR IMPLANTABLE ELECTRONIC DEVICES

Patients with pacemakers or implantable cardioverter-defibrillators (ICDs) have pathological arrhythmias, cardiomyopathies, or ischemic or valvular disease.[14] The patient's

wallet card will contain pertinent information regarding the device. Electrocautery can cause an ICD to discharge or inhibit pacemakers from pacing. A patient can be inappropriately defibrillated or not be paced adequately if he or she is pacemaker-dependent. All ICDs have backup pacing capabilities. Application of a magnet on an ICD inhibits antitachycardia therapies, but does not affect the pacing function. A magnet placed over a pacemaker converts the device to asynchronous pacing for the duration of magnet application. Suggestion has been made that if electrocautery is limited to below the umbilicus, it is highly unlikely to affect a pacemaker or ICD and use of a magnet or reprogramming the device is not necessary. If it is anticipated that electrocautery will be used above the umbilicus, it is prudent to contact someone who is familiar with such devices for recommendations on the use of a magnet or whether the device requires reprogramming. A defibrillator must be immediately available to deliver antitachycardia therapy or transcutaneous pacing whenever a patient with an ICD or a pacemaker who is pacemaker-dependent is having a procedure. Magnets may permanently disable antitachycardia therapies when applied to ICDs. If a magnet is used, the device was reprogrammed, or interference from electrocautery has occurred, these devices must be reinterrogated to establish previous settings before the patient leaves a monitored setting. A summary of the potential interactions between implanted cardiac devices and various procedures is provided in Box 9-5.

PULMONARY DISEASE

Postoperative pulmonary complications are more prevalent in patients with poor general health, older age, heart failure, a smoking history, obstructive sleep apnea (OSA), or poorly controlled pulmonary pathological conditions such as chronic obstructive pulmonary disease or asthma.[15]

Box 9-4 Summary of Recommendations from the 2007 Science Advisory and the 2007 American College of Cardiology and American Heart Association

- Premature discontinuation of dual antiplatelet therapy with new coronary stents increased risk for life-threatening stent thrombosis in the perioperative period.
- The time period for this risk is 4 to 6 weeks for bare metal stents and 12 months for drug-eluting stents.
- Timing of elective surgery with new coronary stents: Elective procedure should be deferred until patients complete an appropriate course of thienopyridine therapy.
- Elective noncardiac surgery is not recommended when thienopyridine therapy or thienopyridine and aspirin therapy needs to be continued during the perioperative period.
- The recommended period of thienopyridine therapy or thienopyridine and aspirin therapy is a minimum of 1 month or 4 to 6 weeks for bare metal stents and 12 months for drug-eluting stents.
- If surgery cannot be deferred and thienopyridine therapy must be interrupted in patients with new coronary stents, aspirin should be continued. The thienopyridine should be restarted as soon as possible after the surgical procedure.
- Dual antiplatelet therapy should be continued beyond the recommended time frame in any patient at high risk for stent thrombosis. Even after thienopyridine has been discontinued for a procedure, aspirin therapy should be continued perioperatively in any patient with a drug-eluting stent.

From American Society of Anesthesiologists Committee on Standards and Practice Parameters. Practice alert for the perioperative management of patients with coronary artery stents. Anesthesiology. 2009;110:22-23.

Box 9-5 Potential Problems with Cardiovascular Implantable Electronic Devices During Surgical Procedures

Bipolar electrocautery does not cause EMI unless applied directly to CIED; bipolar cautery should be used when possible.
EMI from monopolar electrocautery is common.
If monopolar cautery is used, bursts should be ≤5 seconds.
Pacemakers may oversense and be inhibited by EMI.
Device reset infrequently occurs with electrocautery.
Cardioversion can reset CIED.
Keeping the current path away from CIED decreases potential for CIED complications.
Gastrointestinal procedures using cautery can cause interference.
ECT causing tachycardia may prompt review of ICD tachycardia therapy zones.
TENS can cause EMI.

CIED, Cardiovascular implantable electronic device; ECT, electroconvulsive therapy; EMI, electromagnetic interference; ICD, implantable cardioverter-defibrillator; TENS, transcutaneous electrical nerve stimulation.
From Crossley GH, Poole JE, Rozner MA, et al. The Heart Rhythm Society (HRS)/American Society of Anesthesiologists (ASA) expert consensus statement on the perioperative management of patients with implantable defibrillators, pacemakers and arrhythmia monitors: facilities and patient management—executive summary. Heart Rhythm. 2011;8(7):e1-e18.

General anesthesia increases the risk of postoperative pulmonary complications. The bronchoscopy suite personnel are especially concerned about pulmonary complications. Preoperative administration of beta-adrenergic agonists and steroids can minimize bronchospasm with intubation for patients with obstructive or reactive airways disease. Methods to decrease postoperative pulmonary complications include treating pulmonary infections and heart failure, using pulmonary recruitment maneuvers such as incentive spirometry, using continuous positive airway pressure (CPAP), and avoiding general anesthesia when possible.

OBESITY

Obesity is a common disorder; 35% of adults in the United States are obese (body mass index [BMI] >30), 5% are severely obese (BMI >40), and 1% are superobese (BMI >50).[16] Obese patients have increased rates of chronic disease, including obstructive sleep apnea, CAD, pulmonary hypertension, diabetes, hypertension, and right and left heart failure. They also may be more difficult to ventilate by mask and intubate and desaturate more quickly after onset of apnea.[17] Special equipment is required to anesthetize extremely obese patients in a NORA location, including appropriate-sized operating or procedure room tables. Depending on the model, most interventional radiology fluoroscopic tables can support up to 350 to 400 lb (159-181 kg), and most standard gurneys can support 500 lb (227 kg). Computed tomography scanners have an internal diameter of 27.5 inches (70 cm) and circumference of 87 inches (221 cm) and can support up to 450 lb (204 kg). Magnetic resonance imaging (MRI) scanners have an internal diameter of 24 inches (60 cm) and circumference of 74 inches (188) and can support 350 to 400 lb (159-181 kg), again depending on model. Some obese patients will not fit into these devices, and measurement of their weight and abdominal girth should be performed before administering sedation or anesthesia.

DIABETES

Diabetes affects all major organ systems, especially the kidneys, heart, nervous system, and vasculature. Surgical and anesthetic risk both increase with poorly controlled diabetes, probably because of comorbid conditions such as cardiovascular disease, renal insufficiency, and increased susceptibility to infection. Patients with poorly controlled type 1 diabetes are at risk for ketoacidosis, even with glucose values less than 300 g/dL. Patients with poorly controlled type 2 diabetes are at risk for extreme hyperglycemia (>500 g/dL) and hyperosmolar hyperglycemic nonketotic syndrome. Despite this, no evidence supports cancellation of ambulatory surgery cases for hyperglycemia as long as no evidence of ketoacidosis, dehydration, or extreme hyperglycemia exists. Cases should be delayed for patients with severe hypoglycemia (glucose <50 g/dL). General preoperative goals for patients with diabetes are to avoid hypoglycemia by appropriately managing insulin during periods of fasting and prevent ketoacidosis and extreme hyperglycemia by ensuring proper glucose monitoring and medication management (Table 9-3). Perioperative glucose management has become a controversial topic, with literature supporting

Table 9-3   Preoperative Testing Guidelines for Procedures Performed Outside the Operating Room

Condition	Test
Potential for blood loss	Hemoglobin, hematocrit
Potential for transfusion	Hemoglobin, hematocrit
Administration of contrast media	Creatinine
Women of childbearing age	Offer human chorionic gonadotropin*
Diabetes	Glucose*
Cirrhosis	Prothrombin time, international normalized ratio, platelets
Active cardiac conditions†	Electrocardiogram

*Day of procedure.
†New onset or unstable angina, decompensated heart failure, new onset or significant arrhythmias, and severe valvular disease.

tight glycemic control in patients undergoing cardiac surgery but not in general and ambulatory patients.[18] The risk for hypoglycemia may outweigh any possible benefit of euglycemia, particularly in the NORA setting.

OBSTRUCTIVE SLEEP APNEA

OSA is a prevalent, often undiagnosed disorder characterized by intermittent apnea or hypopnea during sleep.[19] Patients with OSA have increased rates of chronic disease, including hypertension, arrhythmia, stroke, heart failure, pulmonary hypertension, and CAD.[20] Airway management, including mask ventilation and intubation, can be more challenging, and postoperative respiratory complications, including hypoxemia, atelectasis, pneumonia, and prolonged hospitalizations, occur more frequently in patients with moderate to severe OSA.[21] The ASA recommends screening for OSA as part of the preanesthetic assessment.[2] Many screening surveys exist; the STOP-BANG questionnaire is a previously validated eight-item survey (Figure 9-3).[22] Controversy exists over appropriate perioperative management of patients with OSA, in particular postoperative monitoring. The Society for Ambulatory Anesthesia consensus statement on OSA states that outpatient surgery is reasonable, providing the patient has otherwise good health or well-controlled comorbidities, will not receive opiates as the main source of pain control, and is willing to be compliant with CPAP therapy during any periods of rest for several days after surgery.[20] If a patient uses a CPAP or bilevel positive airway pressure (BiPAP) device, it should be brought to the procedure. In patients in whom moderate to severe OSA is suspected but not diagnosed, prolonged monitoring and empirical CPAP therapy may be indicated if obstruction occurs postoperatively. Patients with OSA may benefit from recovering in the main operating room postanesthesia care unit if possible.

RENAL DISEASE

Kidney disease is usually classified according to glomerular filtration rate (GFR), varying from stage 1 (kidney damage with normal GFR greater than 90 mL/min/1.73 m²) to stage 5 (kidney failure with GFR <15 mL/min/1.73 m²). Stage 3 and above chronic kidney disease is associated with cardiovascular disease and is one of the five major

---

STOP BANG Questionnaire

Age _____   Height _____ inches/cm   Weight _____ lb/kg   Male/Female

BMI _____   Neck circumference* _____ cm

1. Do you snore loudly (louder than talking or loud enough to be heard through closed doors)? Yes   No

2. Do you often feel tired, fatigued, or sleepy during daytime? Yes   No

3. Has anyone observed you stop breathing during your sleep? Yes   No

4. Do you have or are you being treated for high blood pressure? Yes   No

5. BMI more than 35 kg/m^2? Yes   No

6. Age over 50 yr old? Yes   No

7. Neck circumference greater than 40 cm? Yes   No

8. Gender male? Yes   No

* Neck circumference is measured by staff

High risk of OSA: answering yes to three or more items

Low risk of OSA: answering yes to less than three items

Figure 9-3 STOP BANG questionnaire.

---

clinical risk indicators identified in the ACC/AHA preoperative guidelines.[23,24] Kidney disease is also associated with disturbances in serum electrolytes, acid-base status, and intravascular volume, particularly in patients who require dialysis. Patients on chronic dialysis should be dialyzed the day before surgery to optimize volume status and electrolyte levels. Mild hyperkalemia (potassium 5.2-6.0) is common in patients on hemodialysis, and correction preoperatively is not usually necessary for procedures without expected long duration or need for transfusion, particularly if the potassium level is within the patient's baseline values. Patients with renal insufficiency are more susceptible to further renal injury with contrast media for interventional and imaging studies, and consideration is given to prehydration with normal saline or saline with sodium bicarbonate for those with creatinine greater than 2.0 or GFR less than 60 mL/min/1.73 m^2.[25] Nephrogenic systemic fibrosis can be caused by administration of gadolinium to patients with stage 4 or 5 chronic kidney disease. Most radiology and cardiology departments have specific protocols regarding administration of contrast to patients with renal insufficiency or failure.

ANEMIA

Anemia is often a marker of underlying disease. It is associated with increased perioperative mortality, possibly because anemic patients are more likely to receive blood products and incur the associated risks of transfusion.[26] In asymptomatic anemic patients without other major comorbidity undergoing outpatient procedures associated with minimal blood loss, preoperative transfusion is usually not indicated, but identification of the underlying source of their anemia may be beneficial. ASA practice guidelines state that patients should receive blood if their hemoglobin level is less than 6 g/dL.[27] Patients who are members of the Jehovah's Witness faith often refuse blood transfusion because of a religious belief that blood is sacred and should not leave the body or be stored outside of it. They may accept factor concentrates and are usually willing to accept cell-salvage blood as long as it remains in circuit. Clear delineation of their preferences is necessary before procedures associated with blood loss, and the assigned anesthesia team must be notified because some anesthesia providers will recuse themselves of caring for patients unwilling to accept transfusion. Iron can be prescribed preoperatively to increase hemoglobin, and some Jehovah's Witnesses will accept erythropoietin. Type and screen is not drawn on patients who will not accept blood products.

PREGNANCY

Pregnant patients should receive preoperative and postoperative fetal heart rate (FHR) assessment. Depending on the gestational age, procedure type, and anesthetic, continuous fetal monitoring may be indicated. The American College of Obstetrics and Gynecology recommends preprocedure and postprocedure FHR assessment by Doppler for previable fetuses with a gestational age of 24 weeks or under and electronic FHR and preprocedure and postprocedure contraction monitoring for viable fetuses.[28] They also support intraoperative fetal monitoring if it will guide intraoperative care, including oxygen delivery or blood pressure and positioning management, and if the patient will provide informed consent for cesarean delivery should sustained decompensation in FHR occur.[28] Coordination with obstetricians and obstetric nursing preoperatively is required to facilitate fetal monitoring. In particular, if continuous monitoring is planned, a member of the obstetric team will need to be present for the procedure. The second trimester of pregnancy is the safest time for patients to receive anesthesia because the risk for spontaneous abortion is lower than in the first trimester, and the risk for preterm labor is lower than in the third trimester.[28] After the first trimester, pregnant patients have decreased lower esophageal sphincter tone but gastric volumes and pH similar to those in nonpregnant individuals.[29] Therefore they may be at higher risk for aspiration, which should be considered during anesthetic planning, in particular with deep sedation. Pregnant patients with viable fetuses undergoing NORA procedures should be cared for in a center with an obstetric suite, neonatal services, and capability to perform emergency delivery.[28]

Prematurely born infants are at increased risk for postoperative apnea, and admission should be planned for observation for at least 12 hours if they are younger than 60 weeks' gestational age.[30] Gestational age is defined as the number of weeks the neonate is beyond the mother's last menstrual period or by considering the infant's due date as 40 weeks and adding or subtracting number of weeks from that date until the current day. Any neonate with a history of anemia or apnea or on home apnea monitoring is not an appropriate candidate for an outpatient procedure and may benefit from administration of caffeine to prevent apnea.[30,31] In healthy infants born at term, practice varies, but most centers discharge patients older than 44 weeks' gestational age, as long as no respiratory events are observed postoperatively. Young infants should be scheduled as the first case of the day, and appropriately sized monitors, supplies, a pediatric resuscitation cart, and a warming device should be present before anesthesia administration.

Preoperative Testing

Routine diagnostic testing not tailored to patients' specific comorbidities offers little value and has not been shown to affect outcome in patients undergoing low-risk ambulatory surgery.[32-34] In fact, pursuing abnormal results discovered on routine preoperative testing may lead to more harm than benefit, because further diagnostic tests may incur unwarranted risk to the patient.[1,32] However, patient-specific comorbidities may warrant further investigation or monitoring, such as assessing coagulation status in cirrhotic patients, because abnormal values may change both anesthetic and procedural plans. Type and screen should be ordered only for procedures in which blood loss is anticipated. Assessment of kidney function is recommended for patients receiving contrast media.

ELECTROCARDIOGRAMS

Routine requirement for preoperative resting 12-lead ECGs has not been shown to improve care in patients undergoing ambulatory surgery.[35,36] ECG abnormalities are very common, particularly in older patients, and are generally very poor predictors of postoperative cardiac events.[34] The ASA

Preoperative Evaluation Practice Advisory acknowledges that electrocardiography does not improve prediction of cardiac risk beyond risk factors identified by patient history.[2] The ACC/AHA guidelines state that "ECGs are not indicated in asymptomatic persons undergoing low-risk surgical procedures."[3] The vast majority of patients undergoing low-risk NORA procedures will not benefit from a preoperative resting ECG.

CHEST RADIOGRAPHS

Preoperative "routine" chest radiographs have not been shown to predict postoperative pulmonary complications and should not be ordered without indication.[15]

PREGNANCY TESTING

The effects of anesthesia on the developing fetus are unknown; therefore women of childbearing age should be offered pregnancy testing, particularly for elective procedures. Recommended preoperative testing guidelines are summarized in Table 9-3.

Perioperative Medications

Patients are often confused about which medications to continue or discontinue in the perioperative period, particularly on the day of surgery. Written instructions can help clarify which medications the patient should take. Medications need to be reconciled between the medical record and patient during the preoperative visit. Both comorbidities and the type of procedure should be considered when managing medications before NORA anesthesia.

CARDIOVASCULAR AND ANTIHYPERTENSIVE MEDICINES

Cardiovascular medications, including antihypertensive agents, are continued preoperatively. Cessation of beta blockade perioperatively is associated with adverse cardiovascular events and is not recommended.[37] Most patients undergoing ambulatory surgery do not need to be started on perioperative beta blockers because they are undergoing low-risk procedures. Specific abnormalities noted during the preoperative history and physical may warrant changes in preoperative medication instructions. Patients taking angiotensin-converting enzyme inhibitors or angiotensin-receptor blockers, especially in combination with diuretics, may have refractory hypotension during general anesthesia that is unresponsive to treatment with conventional vasopressors. The potential for hypotension should be balanced against the benefit of continuing these agents, especially for patients with heart failure. Patients with heart failure are continued on their diuretic dose unless hypovolemia is suspected.

ASPIRIN AND OTHER ANTIPLATELET DRUGS

Aspirin is commonly used to lower the risk for cardiac events in patients with cardiac disease, cerebrovascular disease, peripheral vascular disease, and diabetes. Although aspirin has traditionally been discontinued for the week before surgery, preoperative cessation of aspirin puts patients at increased risk for cardiovascular or cerebrovascular events preoperatively, possibly by creating a hypercoagulable state.[38,39] Aspirin should be continued in patients with atherosclerosis taking it for secondary prophylaxis against vascular events, except in procedures in which bleeding into closed spaces could cause severe injury, such as spinal surgery. Aspirin should usually be stopped in patients taking it for primary prophylaxis.[38] For secondary prophylaxis, 81-mg, or "baby," aspirin may be substituted for regular aspirin for the week before surgery. Aspirin can be continued at full dose for many superficial procedures not associated with blood loss, such as cataract extraction. Full-dose aspirin is also usually continued for patients with peripheral arterial disease undergoing revascularization surgery or arterial stenting. Neuraxial anesthesia is not contraindicated in patients taking aspirin.[40] The thienopyridines clopidogrel (Plavix) and ticlopidine (Ticlid) inhibit platelet function and should be discontinued before most procedures, with the exception of some vascular cases, including peripheral arterial stenting procedures. It is important to confirm with the proceduralists whether thienopyridines should be continued. Neuraxial anesthesia is contraindicated in patients taking thienopyridines; clopidogrel is discontinued for 7 days and ticlopidine 10 days before intrathecal or epidural anesthesia.[40,41]

ANTICOAGULANT THERAPY

Dabigatran (Pradaxa), a direct thrombin inhibitor used mainly for chronic anticoagulation in patients with atrial fibrillation, should be discontinued 1 to 5 days before procedures requiring normal coagulation, depending on creatinine clearance (CrCl) (1-2 days for those with CrCl >50 mL/min, 3-5 days for those with CrCl <50 mL/min). Of note, the anticoagulant activity of dabigatran cannot be assessed by prothrombin time and international normalized ratio (INR); activated partial thromboplastin time gives an estimate of effect, but thrombin time and ecarin clotting time give the most accurate assessment. Warfarin may increase bleeding except in very superficial procedures. If the INR is 2 to 3, warfarin should be held for 5 days before the procedure; if greater than 3, it should be held longer, with a goal INR of less than 1.5.[40] Neuraxial anesthesia is contraindicated with an INR greater than 1.3. Bridging of anticoagulation after warfarin discontinuation is necessary for some patients, in particular those with mechanical heart valves, history of atrial fibrillation–related embolic stroke or atrial thrombus, or recently diagnosed deep vein thrombosis. Therapeutic-dose low-molecular-weight heparin (LMWH) is commonly used for this purpose. Therapeutic LMWH is discontinued 24 hours before procedures or planned neuraxial anesthesia.[40] Subcutaneous unfractionated heparin 5000 units once or twice daily is not a contraindication to neuraxial anesthesia, although timing of a block 1 hour before next dose may be the safest.[40]

INSULIN AND ORAL DIABETES MEDICINES

Patients taking insulin usually have a basal insulin requirement that needs to be maintained, even during fasting. All patients taking long-acting glargine (Lantus) insulin should be continued on their usual dose perioperatively. Patients with insulin pumps should continue on their lowest basal rate. Patients with type 1 diabetes should take one third to half of their normal morning dose of intermediate-acting to long-acting insulin (Lente or neutral protamine Hagedorn [NPH]), and patients with type 2 diabetes can take up to half their dose of intermediate-acting to long-acting insulin or combination insulin on the date of their surgery. Taking half of the usual dose of intermediate, long-acting, or combination insulins on the day of surgery improves perioperative glycemic control in contrast to taking none on the day of surgery.[42] Short-acting insulins intended to provide coverage for meals are discontinued during fasting and on the day of surgery.

Sulfonylurea agents can cause hypoglycemia in fasting patients. Insulin sensitizers such as metformin and pioglitazone and agents that decrease intestinal carbohydrate absorption such as acarbose do not cause hypoglycemia during fasting. Metformin does not need to be discontinued before the date of surgery; the risk for lactic acidosis with metformin occurs only in patients with kidney and liver dysfunction. To avoid confusion, many centers hold all oral diabetic medications on the day of surgery.

STEROIDS

Steroids should be continued on the date of surgery. Patients taking chronic steroids may have suppression of their glucocorticoid production and are therefore unable to increase levels during physiological stress, causing acute adrenal insufficiency.[43,44] Patients who have taken more than 5 mg/day of prednisone or its equivalent for more than 3 to 4 weeks in the past year are at risk for adrenal suppression. Most NORA procedures are not physiologically stressful, and no increase in steroid dose is typically indicated if patients have taken their usual dosages on schedule. If a NORA procedure is anticipated to be stressful or acute adrenal insufficiency is suspected, a dose of 25 mg of intravenous hydrocortisone can be given to the patient.[45]

PSYCHIATRIC MEDICINES

Psychiatric drugs such as selective serotonin reuptake inhibitors, antipsychotics, and monoamine oxidase inhibitors (MAOIs) should be continued on the date of surgery because discontinuation puts patients at risk for relapse of their condition or suicide. MAOIs were previously discontinued before surgery for several weeks because of concern about serotonin syndrome or hypertensive crisis developing from their interaction with drugs commonly used during anesthesia. Provider awareness and avoidance of medications that perioperatively interact with MAOIs should negate the need for their discontinuation.

HERBAL SUPPLEMENTS

Herbals and supplements are discontinued at least 7 days before surgery. Garlic, ginseng, and gingko have mild anticoagulant activity.

CONTROLLED SUBSTANCES

Patients can continue opioid medications, benzodiazepines, and nicotine replacement therapy to avoid withdrawal symptoms and pain or anxiety.[46] Patients undergoing MRI scans need to remove transdermal patches before the study.

A summary of recommendations for perioperative medication management is listed in Box 9-6.

Box 9-6   Preoperative Medication Management

Continue Day of Surgery

Anxiolytics, psychiatric medications
Antihypertensives*
Aspirin for secondary prophylaxis
Asthma medications
Autoimmune medications
Cardiac medications
Clopidogrel (Plavix): Patients with drug-eluting stents <12 months or bare metal stents <1 month
Cyclooxygenase-2 inhibitors
Diuretics: Triamterene, hydrochlorothiazide
Eye drops
Estrogen compounds
Gastrointestinal reflux medications
Insulin
  Type 1 diabetes: Take less than one third to half of intermediate to long-acting (neutral protamine Hagedorn [NPH], Lente)
  Type 2 diabetes: Up to half of long-acting (NPH) or combination (70/30) *glargine (Lantus)*
  Insulin pump: Continue lowest basal rate
Opioids for pain or addiction
Oral contraceptives
Seizure medications
Statins
Steroids (oral or inhaled)
Thyroid medications

Discontinue

Aspirin for primary prophylaxis 5 to 7 days before surgery
Autoimmune
  Methotrexate (if risk of renal failure)
  Etanercept (Enbrel) 2 weeks before
  Infliximab (Remicade) 6 weeks before
  Adalimumab (Humira) 8 weeks before
Clopidogrel (Plavix): No recent stents, nonvascular surgery
Diuretics: Potent loop diuretics except for patients with heart failure
Estrogen compounds if not for cancer or contraception
Herbals and nonvitamin supplements: 7 to 14 days before surgery
Hypoglycemic agents, oral
Insulin: Short-acting insulin (except lowest basal rate for continuous pump therapy)
Nonsteroidal antiinflammatory drugs: 48 hours before day of surgery
Topical creams and ointments
Viagra or similar medications: 24 hours before surgery
Vitamins, minerals, iron
Warfarin: Discontinue 5 days before surgery (except for cataract surgery)

*Consider discontinuing angiotensin-converting enzyme inhibitors and angiotensin receptor blockers based on patient condition and procedure.

Fasting Guidelines

Current ASA guidelines for adult patients recommend fasting for 6 hours after a light meal or nonclear liquid and 8 hours after meals containing fatty foods or meat before procedures requiring anesthesia.[47] Most patients may continue clear liquids up to 2 hours before the procedure and take medications with water on the day of surgery. Patients with conditions that are associated with aspiration, such as hiatal hernia, long-standing diabetes mellitus, pregnancy, severe ascites, and bowel obstruction, should remain on nil per os (NPO) restriction for 8 hours, except for necessary medications with water. Pediatric patients follow the same instructions, except that infants may have breast milk up to 4 hours before the procedure or formula up to 6 hours before the procedure, and intake of clear liquids is encouraged up until 2 hours before the procedure to avoid dehydration.

Conclusion

Patients undergoing NORA require adequate preoperative evaluation and preparation, most importantly a comprehensive history and properly conducted physical examination and appropriate medication and fasting instructions. Most patients undergoing NORA will not require further cardiovascular testing unless an active cardiac condition is discovered during the preoperative assessment, and routine laboratory testing usually is not indicated. Ensuring access to appropriate anesthetic monitors, devices, and drugs, as well as adequate planning for patients with comorbidities, will lead to improved care and less frustration on the part of providers operating outside their usual environment.

References

1. Apfelbaum JL. Preoperative evaluation, laboratory screening, and selection of adult surgical outpatients in the 1990s. *Anesth Rev.* 1990;17(suppl 2):4–12.
2. Apfelbaum J, Connis RT, Nickinovich DG, et al. Committee on Standards and Practice Parameters. Practice advisory for preanesthesia evaluation: an updated report by the American Society of Anesthesiologists Task Force on Preanesthesia Evaluation. *Anesthesiology.* 2012;116(3):1–17.
3. Fleisher LA, Beckman JA, Brown KA, et al. ACC/AHA 2007 guidelines on perioperative cardiovascular evaluation and care for noncardiac surgery. *J Am Coll Cardiol.* 2007;50(17):1707–1732.
4. Grayburn PA, Hillis LD. Cardiac events in patients undergoing noncardiac surgery: shifting the paradigm from noninvasive risk stratification to therapy. *Ann Intern Med.* 2003;138(6):506–511.
5. Jessup M, Abraham WT, Casey DE, et al. 2009 Focused update: ACCF/AHA guidelines for the diagnosis and management of heart failure in adults. *J Am Coll Cardiol.* 2009;53(15):1343–1382.
6. Bonow RO, Carabello BA, Chatterjee K, et al. 2008 focused update incorporated into the 2006 ACC/AHA guidelines for the management of patients with valvular heart disease. *Circulation.* 2008;118(15):e523–e661.
7. Frogel J, Galusca D. Anesthetic considerations for patients with advanced valvular heart disease undergoing noncardiac surgery. *Anesthesiol Clin.* 2010;28(1):67–85.
8. Wilson W, Taubert KA, Gewitz M, et al. Prevention of infective endocarditis: guidelines from the American Heart Association. *Circulation.* 2007;116(15):1736–1754.
9. Newsome LT, Weller RS, Gerancher JC, et al. Coronary artery stents. II. Perioperative considerations and management. *Anesth Analg.* 2008;107(2):570–590.

10. Grines CI, Bonow RD, Casey Jr DE, et al. Prevention of premature discontinuation of dual antiplatelet therapy in patients with coronary artery stents: a science advisory from the American Heart Association/American College of Cardiology, Society for Cardiovascular Angiography and Interventions, American College of Surgeon, and American Dental Association with representation from the American College of Physicians. *J Am Coll Cardiol.* 2007;49:734–739.

11. Burger W, Chemnitius JM, Kneissl GD, et al. Low-dose aspirin for secondary cardiovascular prevention-cardiovascular risks after its perioperative withdrawal versus bleeding risks with its continuation: review and meta-analysis. *J Intern Med.* 2005;257(5):399–414.

12. Howell SJ, Sear JW, Foëx P. Hypertension, hypertensive heart disease and perioperative cardiac risk. *Br J Anaesth.* 2004;92(4):570–583.

13. Wax DB, Porter SB, Lin HM, et al. Association of preanesthesia hypertension with adverse outcomes. *J Cardiovasc Vasc Anesth.* 2012;24(6):927–930.

14. Crossley GH, Poole JE, Rozner MA, et al. The Heart Rhythm Society (HRS)/American Society of Anesthesiologists (ASA) expert consensus statement on the perioperative management of patients with implantable defibrillators, pacemakers and arrhythmia monitors: facilities and patient management—executive summary. *Heart Rhythm.* 2011;8(7):e1–e18.

15. Smetana GW, Lawrence VA, Cornell JE. American College of Physicians. Preoperative pulmonary risk stratification for noncardiothoracic surgery: systematic review for the American College of Physicians. *Ann Intern Med.* 2006;144(8):581–595.

16. Ogden CL, Carroll MD, Kit BK, Flegal KM. *Prevalence of obesity in the United States, 2009–2010. NCHS Data Brief No. 82.* Atlanta: National Center for Health Statistics; January 2012.

17. Gonzalez H, Minville V, Delanoue K, et al. The importance of increased neck circumference to intubation difficulties in obese patients. *Anesth Analg.* 2008;106(4):1132–1136.

18. Lipshutz AK, Gropper MA. Perioperative glycemic control. *Anesthesiology.* 2009;110(2):408–421.

19. Young T, Skatrud J, Peppard PE. Risk factors for obstructive sleep apnea in adults. *JAMA.* 2004;291(16):2013–2016.

20. Bradley TD, Floras JS. Sleep apnea and heart failure. I. Obstructive sleep apnea. *Circulation.* 2003;107(12):1671–1678.

21. Hwang D, Shakir N, Limann B, et al. Association of sleep-disordered breathing with postoperative complications. *Chest.* 2008;133(5):1128–1134.

22. Chung F, Yegneswaran B, Liao P, et al. STOP questionnaire: a tool to screen patients for obstructive sleep apnea. *Anesthesiology.* 2008;108(5):812–821.

23. Joshi GP, Ankichetty SP, Gan TJ, Chung F. Society for Ambulatory Anesthesia consensus statement on preoperative selection of adult patients with obstructive sleep apnea scheduled for ambulatory surgery. *Anesth Analg.* 2012;115(5):1060–1068.

24. Mathew A, Devereaux PJ, O'Hare A, et al. Chronic kidney disease and postoperative mortality: a systematic review and meta-analysis. *Kidney Int.* 2008;73(9):1069–1081.

25. Tepel M, Aspelin P, Lameire N. Contrast-induced nephropathy: a clinical and evidence-based approach. *Circulation.* 2006;113(14):1799–1806.

26. Beattie WS, Karkouti K, Wijeysundera DN, et al. Risk associated with preoperative anemia in noncardiac surgery. *Anesthesiology.* 2009;110(3):574–581.

27. American Society of Anesthesiologists Task Force on Perioperative Blood Transfusion and Adjuvant Therapies. Practice guidelines for perioperative blood transfusion and adjuvant therapies: an updated report. *Anesthesiology.* 2006;105(1):198–208.

28. American College of Obstetricians and Gynecologists. Nonobstetric surgery during pregnancy. Committee Opinion No. 474. *Obstet Gynecol.* 2011;117(2 Pt. 1):420–421.

29. Chesnut D, Polley L, Wong C, Tsen L. *Chestnut's obstetrics anesthesia principles and practice.* 4th ed. Philadelphia: Mosby; 2009.

30. Walther-Larsen S, Rasmussen LS. The former preterm infant and risk of post operative apnoea: recommendations for management. *Acta Anaesthesiol Scand.* 2006;50(7):888–893.

31. Coté CJ, Lerman J, Todres ID. *A practice of anesthesia for infants and children.* 4th ed. Philadelphia: Saunders; 2008.

32. Chung F, Yuan H, Yin L, et al. Elimination of preoperative testing in ambulatory surgery. *Anesth Analg.* 2009;108(2):467–475.

33. Narr BJ, Hansen TR, Warner MA. Preoperative laboratory screening in healthy Mayo patients: cost-effective elimination of tests and unchanged outcomes. *Mayo Clin Proc.* 1991;66(2):155–159.

34. Liu LL, Dzankic S, Leung JM. Preoperative electrocardiogram abnormalities do not predict postoperative cardiac complications in geriatric surgical patients. *J Am Geriatr Soc.* 2002;50(7):1186–1191.

35. Gold BS, Young ML, Kinman JL, et al. The utility of preoperative electrocardiograms in the ambulatory surgical patient. *Arch Intern Med.* 1992;152(2):301–305.

36. van Klei WA, Bryson GL, Yang H, et al. The value of routine preoperative electrocardiography in predicting myocardial infarction after noncardiac surgery. *Ann Surg.* 2007;246(2):165–170.

37. Fleischmann KE, Beckman JA, Buller CE, et al. 2009 ACCF/AHA focused update on perioperative beta blockade. *J Am Coll Cardiol.* 2009;54(22):2102–2128.

38. Chassot PG, Delabays A, Spahn DR. Perioperative antiplatelet therapy: the case for continuing therapy in patients at risk of myocardial infarction. *Br J Anaesth.* 2007;99(3):316–328.

39. Senior K. Aspirin withdrawal increases risk of heart problems. *Lancet.* 2003;362(9395):1558.

40. Horlocker TT, Wedel DJ, Rowlingson JC, et al. Regional anesthesia in the patient receiving antithrombotic or thrombolytic therapy: American Society of Regional Anesthesia and Pain Medicine evidence-based guidelines (3rd edition). *Reg Anesth Pain Med.* 2010;35(1):64–101.

41. Kearon C, Hirsh J. Management of anticoagulation before and after elective surgery. *N Engl J Med.* 1997;336(21):1506–1511.

42. Likavec A, Moitra V, Greenberg J, et al. Comparison of preoperative blood glucose levels in patients receiving different insulin regimens. *Anesthesiology.* 2006:A567.

43. Salem M, Tainsh RE, Bromberg J, et al. Perioperative glucocorticoid coverage: a reassessment 42 years after emergence of a problem. *Ann Surg.* 1994;219(4):416–425.

44. Udelsman R, Norton JA, Jelenich SE, et al. Responses of the hypothalamic-pituitary-adrenal and renin-angiotensin axes and the sympathetic system during controlled surgical and anesthetic stress. *J Clin Endocrinol Metab.* 1987;64(5):986–994.

45. Coursin DB, Wood KE. Corticosteroid supplementation for adrenal insufficiency. *JAMA.* 2002;287(2):236–240.

46. Spell III NO. Stopping and restarting medications in the perioperative period. *Med Clin North Am.* 2001;85(5):1117–1128.

47. American Society of Anesthesiologists Committee on Standards and Practice. Practice guidelines for preoperative fasting and the use of pharmacologic agents to reduce the risk of pulmonary aspiration: application to healthy patients undergoing elective procedures: an updated report. *Anesthesiology.* 2011;114(3):495–511.

10 Anesthesia in the Catheterization Laboratory: Valves and Devices

JACK S. SHANEWISE

The treatment of structural heart disease is undergoing a revolution reminiscent of the management of coronary artery disease 30 years ago—the development, evaluation, and application of catheter-based techniques of valve repair and replacement. Catheter deployed devices have also displaced surgical repair as the preferred treatment for several other cardiac conditions, such as patent ductus arteriosus, atrial septal defect, and patent foramen ovale. These procedures typically require radiological imaging and thus are usually performed in a catheterization laboratory rather than a conventional operating room. This chapter reviews the anesthetic considerations of adult patients undergoing these procedures in the interventional cardiology catheterization laboratory (ICCL) and examines in detail a new procedure, transcatheter aortic valve replacement (TAVR), which has been approved for use by the U.S. Food and Drug Administration (FDA) and will be performed at an increasing number of hospitals in the near future. No outcomes studies addressing these issues exist; therefore the information in this chapter is based on the author's experience and discussions with other practitioners.

Most patients having procedures in the ICCL do so without direct anesthesiologist involvement. Diagnostic catheterizations, percutaneous coronary interventions, and many other procedures, including balloon mitral valvuloplasty and closure of atrial septal defect and patent foramen ovale, are routinely managed with local anesthetic infiltration by the operator and conscious sedation with intravenous agents administered by specially trained registered nurses under the supervision of the operator, and only occasionally do patients who may be difficult to sedate or have a history of problems with sedation require anesthesia management. Guidelines are published regarding the use of moderate sedation by nonanesthesia personnel.[1] However, an increasing number of ICCL interventions call for general anesthesia because of the inherent nature of the procedure. Whether anesthesiologists are routinely involved with a particular procedure will vary from center to center, depending on how the procedure is performed, the comfort level of the operators with their ability to manage the sedation, and the hemodynamics while trying to perform the intervention. The most effective approach to these cases is probably for the interventional cardiologist and the anesthesiologist to discuss the needs of the procedure and the options for anesthetic management and come to a consensus of how best to manage them. The characteristics and needs of each individual patient must also be considered in making the final anesthesia plan.

Many ICCL procedures are performed using transesophageal echocardiography (TEE) to guide the operator and assess the results.[2] Although diagnostic TEEs are usually done with conscious sedation and topical anesthesia, many centers consider the need for TEE during an interventional procedure an indication for general anesthesia with endotracheal intubation to secure the airway because of the duration and intensity of the TEE manipulation and because the patient is supine. In some cases, the imaging needed for a procedure can be obtained with transthoracic or intracardiac echocardiography, eliminating the need for TEE and thus general anesthesia.

Hemodynamic Monitoring

By definition, ICCL procedures involve insertion and direct manipulation of catheters and devices within the heart, creating the continuous potential for arrhythmias, perforation, or rupture, causing sudden hemodynamic changes. Monitoring must be continuous and effective. Standard American Society of Anesthesiologists monitors are used for all cases requiring anesthesia, but additional hemodynamic monitors are needed as well. Because of the risk for arrhythmias, external defibrillator pads should be placed on the patient and connected to the defibrillator before starting.

Continuous invasive arterial pressure measurement is the most important hemodynamic parameter to monitor during ICCL procedures. The beat-to-beat blood pressure facilitates the immediate recognition of any significant perturbation, allowing an appropriate reaction to follow in a timely manner. If the patient has significant cardiovascular compromise and needs to be anesthetized, the arterial monitoring should be established before induction. Arterial cannulation for pressure monitoring may be accomplished by the anesthesiologist typically with radial artery cannulation or the cardiologist with a femoral artery sheath. The former allows induction of anesthesia to proceed without delay and has the advantage of being under the control of the anesthesiologist. A radial arterial cannula may be helpful after the procedure if continued monitoring is needed. Femoral artery cannulation may be necessary for access during the procedure and can provide essentially a central aortic pressure, but close communication with the cardiologist is needed to prevent the interruption of monitoring at a crucial time.

Central venous access during ICCL procedures is not as important for monitoring but is needed primarily for the rapid administration of vasoactive drugs to respond to hemodynamic aberrations. Again, this may be accomplished by the anesthesiologist, typically through internal jugular venous cannulation, or the cardiologist with a femoral venous sheath. Internal jugular access has the advantages of being under the control of the anesthesiologist and less dead space, both in the tubing and in the patient, but it may be considered unnecessary if reliable femoral venous access is available. Another important use of central venous access can be rapid administration of fluids in procedures where unexpected blood loss occurs.

If TEE is needed to guide the procedure, it can be used as a monitor as well. In patients for whom general anesthesia is planned, TEE may be used as a monitor even if it is not needed to guide the intervention. Placement of a pulmonary artery catheter may be considered helpful in some cases, such as patients with severe pulmonary hypertension or severe ventricular dysfunction, but these decisions will be influenced by local experience and practice.

When general anesthesia is anticipated for an ICCL procedure, the usual expectation is to emerge and extubate the patient at the end of the case, so the anesthetic plan is tailored to keep this option open whenever possible. On occasion, patients present for an interventional cardiology procedure in such severe respiratory or cardiovascular distress that it is decided to keep them intubated and sedated after the procedure. Patients may need to be kept intubated because of complications occurring during the procedure. Short-acting inhalation and intravenous anesthetics are available, and either technique may be used for ICCL cases, depending on the practitioner's experience and preference and the patient's needs.

Transcatheter Aortic Valve Replacement

Aortic valve replacement (AVR) for calcific aortic stenosis remains the most common valvular heart surgery, with 50,000 procedures performed annually in the United States.[3,4] Although percutaneous valvuloplasty provides temporary relief,[5] valvular stenosis and symptoms typically return within 6 months,[6] making valvular replacement the only definitive therapy.[7,8] Aortic stenosis prevalence and age-related comorbidities will only increase as the population ages.[9] Health care providers have been developing novel techniques for addressing symptomatic aortic stenosis, including transcatheter prosthetic valve implantation.[10]

Despite the clear benefits of AVR for patients with stenotic valves,[11] open AVR surgery in high-risk patients has an associated perioperative mortality of 4% to 18%, depending on patient comorbidities.[12,13] Consequently, despite the dismal prognosis of symptomatic aortic stenosis,[14] open-heart surgery is often withheld from high-risk patients. A less invasive management for valvular stenosis might benefit this patient population. Cribier and colleagues[15] first described transcatheter AVR (TAVR) after transcatheter valvuloplasty in 2002. He chose to approach the aortic valve by femoral venous cannulation, transatrial septal puncture, and antegrade

deployment through the left ventricular outflow tract by way of the mitral valve. Since then, prosthetic aortic valves have more commonly been deployed retrograde from the aorta by cannulation of the femoral artery and antegrade by puncture of the left ventricular apex by a small left thoracotomy.[16] The PARTNER (Placement of AoRTic TraNscathetER Valve) Trial is a multicenter, randomized study comparing TAVR to medical management (including balloon valvuloplasty) in patients not considered to be surgical candidates and to conventional AVR in high-risk surgical candidates. Published results showed improved survival with TAVR over medical management in patients not considered suitable candidates for conventional AVR[17] and equivalent midterm survival in contrast to AVR in high-risk surgical candidates.[18] Questions have been raised about the findings of these studies and the broad application of TAVR in place of conventional AVR.[19]

In 2011 the FDA approved TAVR in the United States with the Edwards SAPIEN valve for patients with severe aortic stenosis who are not surgical candidates. Ongoing trials are comparing TAVR to conventional AVR in high-risk patients with TAVR using two devices: the Edwards SAPIEN valve (Edwards Lifesciences, Irvine, Calif.) and the Medtronic Core-Valve (Medtronic, Minneapolis, Minn.). In 2007, both devices received the quality certificate needed for use in the European Union countries, and it is estimated that over 40,000 devices have been implanted in patients.[19] An expert consensus document addressing TAVR was recently published in a collaborative effort by the American Heart Association, American Society of Echocardiography, European Association for Cardio-Thoracic Surgery, Heart Failure Society of America, Mended Hearts, Society of Cardiovascular Anesthesiologists, Society of Cardiovascular Computed Tomography, and Society for Cardiovascular Magnetic Resonance.[20] It includes an extensive review of the development of TAVR and considerations in evaluating patients for the procedure and the team approach needed to have a successful TAVR program. TAVR is typically performed by a surgeon and an interventional cardiologist in a room that has imaging capabilities and where patients can be anesthetized and undergo surgery, so it is often referred to as a hybrid procedure. This may take place in the ICCL or an operating room, depending on the institution.

The decision to use the transfemoral, transapical, or transaortic approach is based on the size and disease state of the femoral and iliac vessels as assessed with preprocedure imaging. The transfemoral approach is preferred when possible, because it avoids the small thoracotomy needed for the transapical approach. In patients with vessels unsuitable for the transfemoral approach and pathological findings involving the left ventricular apex, such as previous thoracotomy or apical aneurysm, the TAVR may be accomplished through the mid–ascending aorta through a hemisternotomy, referred to as the transaortic approach.

TRANSFEMORAL APPROACH (Figure 10-1)

Percutaneous femoral venous access is obtained and a pacing catheter placed in the right ventricle. Small doses of heparin are used to prevent arterial thrombus formation on the arterial catheters. A femoral artery is percutaneously accessed, a 20- to 23-mm balloon-tipped catheter is placed retrograde across the stenotic aortic valve, and a balloon valvuloplasty is performed while rapid ventricular pacing

	Transfemoral approach	Transapical or Transaortic approach
Anesthetic technique	If no TEE, MAC with local/sedation. If TEE used, GA with intubation.	GA with intubation
		Consider local infiltration of bupiv or paravert block for post op analgesia.
	Blood pressure support typically needed with GA. Consider inotropic drug (e.g., epi or milr) if LV bad. Tailor GA to allow emergence and extubation if all goes well.	
Pacing wire	Femoral vein to RV	Femoral vein or epicardial
	Check threshold & rapid V pacing before proceeding.	
Monitoring	Pre-induction arterial pressure monitoring. Consider PAC if LV bad or pul htn. TEE (requires GA with intubation).	
Vascular access	Central venous access for vasoactive drugs (Int jug vein by anesthesia or femoral vein by cardiology)	
	Large bore IV with warmer for rapid volume infusion (crossmatched blood available)	
Defibrillator	External pads applied and connected before induction.	
Balloon aortic valvuloplasty	AV dilated with balloon-tipped catheter during brief burst of rapid V pacing. Restore stable hemodynamics before proceeding. Check for worse AR with TEE.	
Device positioning	AV annulus at midlevel of device checked with fluoro and/or TEE. Check position with rapid V pacing and ventilator off.	
Device deployment	If possible, restore stable hemodynamics before deployment. Deploy device with rapid V pacing and ventilator off. Be prepared to pace after deployment (e.g., heart block). Check for AR & myocardial ischemia after deployment. Be prepared to resuscitate after deployment.	
Postdeployment	Be prepared to treat hypertension after deployment (e.g., with nicardipine or NTG). Be prepared for vascular injury (i.e., bleeding). Check for hemopericardium with TEE if hypotensive. Check for hemiparesis after emergence.	

TAVR = transcatheter aortic valve replacement. TEE = transesophageal echocardiography. GA = general anesthesia. MAC = monitored anesthesia care. bupiv = bupivacaine. paravert = paravertebral. epi = epinephrine. milr = milrinone. LV = left ventricle. V pacing = ventricular pacing. PAC = pulmonary artery catheter. pul htn = pulmonary hypertension. Int jug = internal jugular. IV = intravenous. post op = post operative. RV = right ventricle. AV = aortic valve. AR = aortic regurgitation. fluoro = fluoroscopy. NTG = nitroglycerine.

Figure 10-4 Key anesthesia elements for transcatheter aortic valve replacement.

Despite all our efforts, there may be circulatory collapse during TAVR requiring cardiopulmonary resuscitation with chest compressions and large doses of resuscitation drugs. When possible, mechanical factors contributing to the circulatory collapse should be remedied. It may help to rapidly deploy the valve if the arrest occurs before that point. If the deployed valve is grossly incompetent, deploying another valve inside it may make the resuscitation successful. Hemopericardium should be identified and drained. If the resuscitation does not quickly restore stable and adequate hemodynamics, consideration should be given to starting mechanical support with cardiopulmonary bypass or extracorporeal membrane oxygenation. This possibility is best thought out before starting the procedure, so a clear course of action is agreed on among the caregivers and the patient should persistent hemodynamic collapse occur.

AORTIC REGURGITATION

Persistent moderate aortic regurgitation was associated with poor outcome in the 2-year follow-up in the

PARTNER trial.[25] Aortic regurgitation after deployment should be evaluated for severity and location. This evaluation is best done with TEE, but aortic root injection with contrast dye may be used to rule out significant aortic regurgitation. If aortic regurgitation is present, TEE can be used to determine whether it is transvalvular or paravalvular. Transvalvular aortic regurgitation is usually caused by overexpansion of the device as a result of improper sizing or malpositioning and may be remedied by deploying another valve within the first. Guidewires may contribute to transvalvular aortic regurgitation and should be pulled out of the valve before assessment. The prosthesis leaflets may (rarely) be damaged by crimping or not open properly after expansion, especially if the blood pressure is low and left ventricular function is poor. Paravalvular aortic regurgitation is common and may be treated with reexpansion of the balloon within the device if more than mild. Repeat expansions may increase the risk for annular rupture and systemic embolism, so judgment is needed to balance the risk with the potential benefit.

NEUROLOGICAL INJURY

TAVR has been associated with a higher incidence of neurological injury than conventional aortic valve replacement in the PARTNER trial.[26] Acute stroke resulting from systemic embolization during the procedure accounts for some of this, but the increase in risk may persist into the postoperative period. Patients should be checked for signs of stroke, such as hemiparesis, as soon as emerging from anesthesia, and, if present, immediate interventions considered such as imaging followed by thrombolysis or catheter retrieval of embolus material if indicated.

HEART BLOCK

TAVR has a higher incidence of heart block than conventional aortic valve replacement, especially with the self-expanding CoreValve device (Medtronic). This may occur immediately with valve deployment or hours, days, or weeks later. In the ICCL, it is treated with temporary pacing but, if persistent, may require permanent pacemaker implantation. The onset of a new first-degree heart block or bundle branch block after deployment of the valve may be a harbinger of more severe conduction problems to come and prompt consideration of leaving a temporary pacing wire in the patient after the procedure. Continuous monitoring of the electrocardiogram (ECG) after the procedure is essential.

PERIPHERAL VASCULAR INJURY

Peripheral vascular injury to the femoral and iliac arteries is the most common complication of transfemoral TAVR because of the size of the deployment sheath and the frequent presence of atherosclerosis in these vessels. This is often treated with endovascular stents but may require open exploration by a vascular surgeon.[27] Important consequences of these injuries may include hypovolemia from hemorrhage, both external and internal, and leg ischemia.

Type crossmatched blood should be available before starting the procedure.

CORONARY ARTERY OBSTRUCTION

Obstruction of the coronary artery ostium during TAVR is uncommon but has been reported. This obstruction may be somewhat predictable based on the distance measured from the aortic valve annulus to the right and left coronary ostia with TEE or computed tomography. The prosthesis consists of an open wire web that permits flow through the coronary arteries if it covers the ostium, but displacement of calcified native aortic valve leaflet with deployment may block the flow. Coronary artery obstruction is manifested by acute ECG ST-T changes and regional wall motion abnormalities on echocardiography, usually accompanied by hemodynamic compromise or collapse. Treatment includes support of the circulation as needed and attempts to restore flow with percutaneous coronary intervention techniques such as stents. In cases thought to be at high risk for coronary ostium obstruction, a guidewire may be passed into the coronary artery to facilitate access if problems develop with valve deployment.

HEMOPERICARDIUM

Perforation of the heart during TAVR may cause hemopericardium and hypotension as a result of acute cardiac tamponade. This perforation may be quickly diagnosed if TEE is in place; if not, sudden unexplained hypotension during TAVR should prompt a rapid echocardiographic examination. Initial management in the ICCL usually involves subxiphoid pericardiocentesis, aspiration of the pericardial blood, and insertion of a drainage catheter, which typically improves the hemodynamics. If the bleeding is venous (e.g., from the right ventricular pacing catheter), removal of the catheter, continued aspiration of the pericardial blood, and reversal of heparin may resolve the problem. If significant bleeding with hemodynamic compromise persists, more definitive surgical exploration of the pericardium and suturing of the perforation may be needed. Arterial pericardial bleeding after valve deployment may indicate aortic valve annular rupture, a rare but catastrophic complication that is difficult to overcome.

Transapical Closure of Mitral Prosthesis Paravalular Regurgitation

Cases of closing prosthetic paravalvular leaks using catheter-delivered closure devices have been reported in the literature.[28] The transapical approach as used with TAVR provides more direct access than the previously used transfemoral approach with transseptal puncture to access the left atrium (Figure 10-5) with invasive arterial pressure monitoring and central venous access.[29] TEE is critical to localize the paravalvular leak and assist with positioning and deploying the device and assessing the results. The potential advantages of this technique

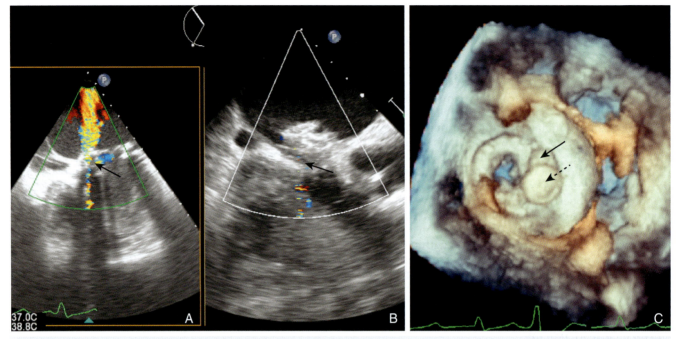

Figure 10-5 A, Transesophageal echocardiography (TEE) showing preoperative paravalvular leak (PVL). **B,** TEE showing postoperative PVL. **C,** Three-dimensional TEE showing postoperative double device closure *(solid and dashed arrows).* (From Thourani VH, Smith CM, Guyton RA, et al. Repair of prosthetic mitral valve paravalvular leak using an off-pump transapical approach. *Ann Thorac Surg.* 2012;94[1]:275-278.)

include a possibly higher success rate than the more indirect transfemoral approach and the avoidance of a repeat sternotomy and cardiopulmonary bypass with conventional surgery.

Left Atrial Appendage Closure Device

An investigational device is being percutaneously deployed in the ICCL to ligate the left atrial appendage (LAA) in patients with atrial fibrillation to prevent thromboembolic complications such as stroke (Figure 10-6).[30] General anesthesia with endotracheal intubation is required because TEE is used to guide the passage of a magnet-tipped endocardial guidewire into the LAA and because the epicardial suture ligation device is introduced through the pericardial space by a subxiphoid needle stick over another magnet-tipped guidewire. In one series of 89 patients, 2 developed hemopericardium during the procedure, which was successfully managed with pericardiocentesis and drainage. One was from inadvertent puncture of the right ventricle and the other from the transseptal puncture.[30]

Mitral Valve Edge-to-Edge Clip Repair

An investigational device has been used to percutaneously treat mitral regurgitation by clipping together portions of the anterior and posterior mitral valve leaflets similar to the edge-to-edge Alfieri surgical repair (Figure 10-7).[31] The technique is performed through femoral venous access

with the transseptal approach to the left atrium in the ICCL. Because TEE is critical in guiding the procedure and assessing the results, patients are anesthetized and intubated. Although results of this procedure have not been favorable in contrast to conventional surgical repair of the mitral valve, it is being evaluated in high-risk patients who are not considered candidates for surgery.[32] Many of these patients are extremely elderly, frail, and a challenge to manage. As with other procedures being performed in the ICCL, it is important to monitor the arterial blood pressure beat to beat and to have central venous access to give vasoactive drugs.

Conclusion

Development of new catheter-based techniques to treat valvular and structural heart disease has been rapid over the past 10 years. Many new devices are under investigation, and some will undoubtedly achieve widespread application. Many of these procedures call for the involvement of anesthesiologists during the procedure because of the need for TEE guidance or because access to the heart is obtained through a small apical or subxiphoid incision. Although these procedures are less invasive and stressful for the patient than conventional open-heart surgery with cardiopulmonary bypass, they nonetheless have the potential to cause acute, life-threatening hemodynamic disturbances and require the same concern, attention, and vigilance on the part of the anesthesiologist. One of the keys to success in the anesthetic management is close communication with the interventional cardiologist or surgeon performing the procedure before and during the procedure.

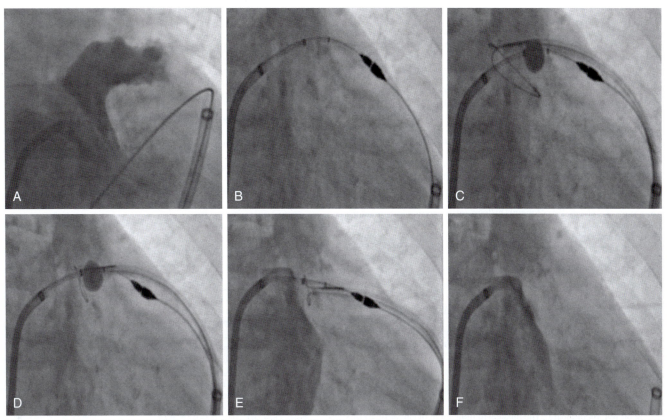

Figure 10-6 All images are in the right anterior oblique projection. Left atrial (LA) angiography identifies the ostium and body of the left atrial append-age (LAA) **(A)**. Attachment of the magnet-tipped endocardial and epicardial guidewires **(B)** allows for the LARIAT suture delivery device to be guided over the LAA by the magnet-tipped epicardial guidewire using an over-the-wire approach **(C)**. After verification of the correct position of the snare with the balloon catheter **(D)**, an LA angiogram is performed before release of the pre-tied suture to exclude the existence of a remnant trabeculated LAA lobe **(E)**. A final LA angiogram is performed to verify LAA exclusion **(F)**. (From Bartus K, Han FT, Bednarek J, et al. Percutaneous left atrial appendage suture ligation using the LARIAT device in patients with atrial fibrillation: initial clinical experience. *J Am Coll Cardiol.* 2013;62:108-118.)

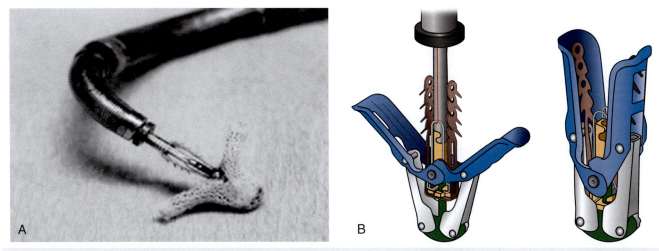

Figure 10-7 A, Photograph of the clip attached to the delivery system. The clip is covered with polyester fabric. The two arms are opened and closed by control mechanisms on the clip delivery system. The arms have an opened span of approximately 2 cm and a width of 4 mm. **B,** Schematic illustra-tion of the clip components. On the inner portion of the clip is a U-shaped gripper that matches each arm and helps stabilize the leaflets from the atrial aspect as they are captured during closure of the clip arms. Leaflet tissue is secured between the closed arms and each side of the gripper when the clip is closed and locked, to effect and maintain coaptation of the two leaflets. (From Silvestry FE, Rodriguez LL, Herrmann HC, et al. Echocardiographic guidance and assessment of percutaneous repair for mitral regurgitation with the Evalve MitraClip: lessons learned from EVEREST I. *J Am Soc Echocardiogr.* 2007;20[10]:1131-1140.)

References

1. Gross JB, Bailey PL, Connis RT, et al. Practice guidelines for sedation and analgesia by non-anesthesiologists: an updated report by the American Society of Anesthesiologists Task Force on Sedation and Analgesia by Non-anesthesiologists. *Anesthesiology.* 2002;96:1004–1017.

2. Zamorano JL, Badano LP, Bruce C, et al. EAE/ASE recommendations for the use of echocardiography in new transcatheter interventions for valvular heart disease. *J Am Soc Echocardiogr.* 2011;24:937–965.

3. Passik CS, Ackermann DM, Pluth JR, Edwards WD. Temporal changes in the causes of aortic stenosis: a surgical pathologic study of 646 cases. *Mayo Clinic Proc.* 1987;62(2):119–123.

4. Rosamond W, Flegal K, Friday G, et al. Heart disease and stroke statistics—2007 update: a report from the American Heart Association Statistics Committee and Stroke Statistics Subcommittee. *Circulation.* 2007;115:e69–e171.

5. Cribier A, Letac B. Percutaneous balloon aortic valvuloplasty in adults with calcific aortic stenosis. *Curr Opin Cardiol.* 1991;6:212–218.

6. Lieberman EB, Bashore TM, Hermiller JB, et al. Balloon aortic valvuloplasty in adults: failure of procedure to improve long-term survival. *J Am Coll Cardiol.* 1995;26(6):1522–1528.

7. Bonow RO, Carabello BA, Kanu C, et al. ACC/AHA 2006 guidelines for the management of patients with valvular heart disease: a report of the American College of Cardiology/American Heart Association Task Force on Practice Guidelines (writing committee to revise the 1998 Guidelines for the Management of Patients With Valvular Heart Disease), developed in collaboration with the Society of Cardiovascular Anesthesiologists, endorsed by the Society for Cardiovascular Angiography and Interventions and the Society of Thoracic Surgeons. *Circulation.* 2006;114:e84–e231.

8. Otto CM, Mickel MC, Kennedy JW, et al. Three-year outcome after balloon aortic valvuloplasty: insights into prognosis of valvular aortic stenosis. *Circulation.* 1994;89(2):642–650.

9. Boon NA, Bloomfield P. The medical management of valvar heart disease. *Heart.* 2002;87(4):395–400.

10. Leon MB, Kodali S, Williams M, et al. Transcatheter aortic valve replacement in patients with critical aortic stenosis: rationale, device descriptions, early clinical experiences, and perspectives. *Semin Thorac Cardiovasc Surg.* 2006;18:165–174.

11. Schwarz F, Baumann P, Manthey J, et al. The effect of aortic valve replacement on survival. *Circulation.* 1982;66:1105–1110.

12. Jamieson WR, Edwards FH, Schwartz M, et al. Risk stratification for cardiac valve replacement. National Cardiac Surgery Database. Database Committee of The Society of Thoracic Surgeons. *Ann Thorac Surg.* 1999;67:943–951.

13. Powell DE, Tunick PA, Rosenzweig BP, et al. Aortic valve replacement in patients with aortic stenosis and severe left ventricular dysfunction. *Arch Intern Med.* 2000;160:1337–1341.

14. Kennedy KD, Nishimura RA, Holmes DR Jr, Bailey KR. Natural history of moderate aortic stenosis. *J Am Coll Cardiol.* 1991;17:313–319.

15. Cribier A, Eltchaninoff H, Bash A, et al. Percutaneous transcatheter implantation of an aortic valve prosthesis for calcific aortic stenosis: first human case description. *Circulation.* 2002;106:3006–3008.

16. Ye J, Cheung A, Lichtenstein SV, et al. Transapical aortic valve implantation in humans. *J Thorac Cardiovasc Surg.* 2006;131:1194–1196.

17. Leon MB, Smith CR, Mack M, et al. PARTNER Trial Investigators. Transcatheter aortic-valve implantation for aortic stenosis in patients who cannot undergo surgery. *N Engl J Med.* 363(17):1597–1607.

18. Smith CR, Leon MB, Mack MJ, et al. PARTNER Trial Investigators. Transcatheter versus surgical aortic-valve replacement in high-risk patients. *N Engl J Med.* 2011;364(23):2187–2198.

19. Van Brabandt H, Neyt M, Hulstaert F. Transcatheter aortic valve implantation (TAVI): risky and costly. *BMJ.* 2012;345. e4710 doi: 10.1136/bmj.e4710.

20. Holmes Jr DR, Mack MJ, Kaul S, et al. 2012 ACCF/AATS/SCAI/STS expert consensus document on transcatheter aortic valve replacement. *J Am Coll Cardiol.* 2012;59(13):1200–1254.

21. Billings IV FT, Kodali SK, Shanewise JS. Transcatheter aortic valve implantation: anesthetic considerations. *Anesth Analg.* 2009;108(5):1453–1462.

22. Klein AA, Webb ST, Tsui S, et al. Transcatheter aortic valve insertion: anaesthetic implications of emerging new technology. *Br J Anaesth.* 2009;103(6). 792–729.

23. Guinot PG, Depoix JP, Etchegoyen L, et al. Anesthesia and perioperative management of patients undergoing transcatheter aortic valve implantation: analysis of 90 consecutive patients with focus on perioperative complications. *J Cardiothorac Vasc Anesth.* 2010;24(5):752–761.

24. Jayasuriya C, Moss RR, Munt B. Transcatheter aortic valve implantation in aortic stenosis: the role of echocardiography [Review]. *J Am Soc Echocardiogr.* 2011;24(1):15–27.

25. Kodali SK, Williams MR, Smith CR, et al. PARTNER Trial Investigators. Two-year outcomes after transcatheter or surgical aortic-valve replacement. *N Engl J Med.* 2012;366(18):1686–1695.

26. Miller DC, Blackstone EH, Mack MJ, et al. PARTNER Trial Investigators and Patients. PARTNER Stroke Substudy Writing Group and Executive Committee. Transcatheter (TAVR) versus surgical (AVR) aortic valve replacement: occurrence, hazard, risk factors, and consequences of neurologic events in the PARTNER trial. *J Thorac Cardiovasc Surg.* 2012;143(4):832–843.

27. Genereux P, Webb JG, Svensson LG, PARTNER Trial Investigators, et al. Vascular complications after transcatheter aortic valve replacement: insights from the PARTNER (Placement of AoRTic TraNscatheteER Valve) trial. *J Am Coll Cardiol.* 2012;60(12):1043–1052.

28. Latson LA. Transcatheter closure of paraprosthetic valve leaks after surgical mitral and aortic valve replacements. *Expert Rev Cardiovasc Ther.* 2009;7(5):507–514.

29. Thourani VH, Smith CM, Guyton RA, et al. Repair of prosthetic mitral valve paravalvular leak using an off-pump transapical approach. *Ann Thorac Surg.* 2012;94(1):275–278.

30. Bartus K, Han FT, Bednarek J, et al. Percutaneous left atrial appendage suture ligation using the LARIAT device in patients with atrial fibrillation: initial clinical experience. *J Am Coll Cardiol.* 2013;62:108–118.

31. Silvestry FE, Rodriguez LL, Herrmann HC, et al. Echocardiographic guidance and assessment of percutaneous repair for mitral regurgitation with the Evalve MitraClip: lessons learned from EVEREST I. *J Am Soc Echocardiogr.* 2007;20(10):1131–1140.

32. Whitlow PL, Feldman T, Pedersen WR, EVEREST II Investigators, et al. Acute and 12-month results with catheter-based mitral valve leaflet repair: the EVEREST II (Endovascular Valve Edge-to-Edge Repair) High Risk Study. *J Am Coll Cardiol.* 2012;59(2):130–139.

11 Anesthesia for Electrophysiology Procedures

JONATHAN W. TANNER, ROGER A. MOORE, and MARK S. WEISS

In the electrophysiology laboratory, procedures are performed to diagnose and treat abnormal cardiac rhythms. These procedures can be accomplished less invasively and more safely than major surgical procedures that were required in the past, especially with higher-risk, older, and sicker patients. Procedures commonly performed in electrophysiology laboratories to diagnose and treat abnormal cardiac rhythms include catheter-based ablations, device implants, lead extractions, noninvasive programmed stimulations (NIPS), and cardioversions (Table 11-1). A fuller understanding of these procedures and their potential complications will provide a better framework for planning a more rational and safer anesthetic approach. With the exception of cardioversion procedures, which are discussed in Chapter 12, the focus of this chapter will be the most common interventions, issues, and challenges for the anesthesiologist in the electrophysiology laboratory.

Before an anesthesia group considers extending anesthesia coverage to the electrophysiology laboratory, a review should be made of the availability of anesthesia personnel within the practice and the economics of providing the requested coverage. Procedures in the electrophysiology laboratory often involve anesthesia hands-on attendance for 12 hours or more. Because most of the anesthesia revenue will be derived from the relatively poor time unit accumulation, the cost of providing anesthesia coverage may be significantly more expensive than the final reimbursement that is realized. Because the electrophysiology laboratory is usually a positive revenue generator for the hospital and anesthesia is critical for sustaining this revenue source, a serious discussion needs to occur with the hospital administrators concerning the hospital's supplementing anesthesia services to cover any shortfall in revenue.

Role of the Anesthesiologist in the Electrophysiology Laboratory

In 2011 a statistical review of the incidence of cardiac arrhythmias in the United States revealed that over 14 million people suffered from some form of cardiac arrhythmia. Within this group of patients, more than 881,000 required hospitalization and 40,700 died as a result of the arrhythmia or associated comorbidities.[1] With this increase in the patient population diagnosed with arrhythmias, as well as the improvements that have occurred in the technological approaches for treating arrhythmias, the number of interventional procedures in electrophysiology laboratories has greatly increased over the past several years. Included in this increase is a trend toward greater use of anesthesiology services in the electrophysiology laboratory. A consensus document published in 1998[2] indicated that conscious sedation was standard for arrhythmia-specific procedures, particularly catheter ablations in adults. A survey of the task force members of a consensus statement group concerning catheter ablation of atrial fibrillation published in 2007[3] found that approximately two thirds of centers used conscious sedation for these procedures and reserved general anesthesia support for patients at higher risk. A more recent publication reported that approximately 50% of centers routinely employed general anesthesia for all their atrial fibrillation ablation procedures.[4]

Consistent with this trend, anesthesiology involvement in electrophysiology laboratories at the Hospital of the University of Pennsylvania increased significantly over the past several years (Figure 11-1). A decade ago, an anesthesiologist would occasionally be called to the electrophysiology laboratory for a cardioversion, often as part of a longer ablation procedure done mostly with sedation by cardiology nurses.

The role of anesthesiologists has rapidly changed in the last decade to one of active involvement in nearly every procedure except for straightforward venograms and tilt table testing. The primary reason mandating the presence of anesthesia personnel during nearly every electrophysiology procedure is that the use of anesthesiologists allows the electrophysiology procedures to be performed faster and more effectively.[5] The need for qualified anesthesia services is of particular benefit when dealing with an anxious patient who is difficult to sedate by ordinary means or a patient with airway concerns such as sleep apnea or a history of difficult intubation. In addition, it is the rare patient undergoing an electrophysiological procedure without other major comorbidities who would not benefit from the input and management of an anesthesiologist. An anesthesiologist brings other skill sets to the electrophysiology table in addition to airway and sedation management. The high-risk procedure of transvenous lead extraction can be more effectively and safely directed by an anesthesiologist using the findings from real-time transesophageal echocardiography (TEE). TEE allows early warning of events such as clot embolization, ischemic myocardial changes, and tamponade.[6]

Table 11-1   Common Electrophysiology Cases and Estimated Anesthesia Times

Category	Procedure	Usual Anesthetic Technique	Time
MAC in recovery unit	Cardioversion	A short period of deep sedation usually using a bolus dose of propofol (or etomidate if the ejection fraction is low)	15 min
—	TEE	Deeper sedation may be required for some patients undergoing TEE who are unable to tolerate the procedure with conscious sedation by the cardiology team	60 min
—	NIPS	Deep sedation may be required for cardioversion or defibrillation	30-45 min
MAC in electrophysiology laboratory	Pacemaker placement or battery change	Fentanyl/midazolam or infusions of propofol/remifentanil/midazolam	3-4 hr
—	ICD or biventricular ICD placements or battery changes	Fentanyl/midazolam or infusions of propofol/remifentanil/midazolam (defibrillator threshold testing will require a short period of deeper anesthesia similar to that in a cardioversion)	3-4 hr
—	Loop recorder placement in superficial anterior chest wall	Fentanyl/midazolam or infusions of propofol/remifentanil/midazolam	2-3 hr
—	Atrial flutter radiofrequency ablation*	Infusions of propofol/remifentanil/midazolam	6-10 hr
—	Ventricular tachycardia or ventricular fibrillation or premature ventricular contraction radiofrequency ablation*	Usually infusions of remifentanil only; discuss additional sedatives with cardiologist	6-10 hr
General anesthesia in electrophysiology laboratory	Atrial fibrillation radiofrequency ablation	General endotracheal anesthesia using jet ventilation and TIVA, which predominantly involves propofol and remifentanil infusions Radial arterial lines commonly placed	6-10 hr
—	Lead extraction (especially using laser)	General endotracheal anesthesia	3-4 hr
—	Ventricular tachycardia or ventricular fibrillation radiofrequency ablation using an epicardial approach	General endotracheal anesthesia	6-10 hr

*These cases may require conversion to general anesthesia on short notice.
ICD, Implantable cardioverter-defibrillator; *MAC,* monitored anesthesia care; *TEE,* transesophageal echocardiography; *TIVA,* total intravenous anesthesia.

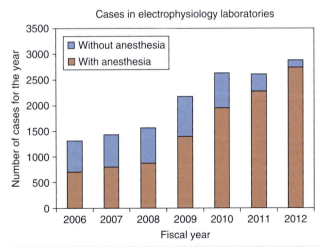

Figure 11-1 Growth of annual case load at the Hospital of the University of Pennsylvania electrophysiology laboratories over the past several years with particular emphasis on the caseload requiring anesthesia services.

Considerations in the Electrophysiology Laboratory

PREPROCEDURE TESTING

Before an electrophysiological procedure, an echocardiogram provides important information for the anesthesiologist concerning planned fluid management and left ventricular function, which is critical for determining the approach that will be used for induction and maintenance of anesthesia. In addition, the echocardiographic evaluation provides important information about the presence or absence of a thrombus. TEE is more sensitive than transthoracic echocardiography for determining the presence of thrombus. A thrombus can develop in the left atrial appendage in patients with atrial fibrillation and can lead to an embolic stroke on cardioversion. Therefore ruling out the presence of a left atrial thrombus before cardioversion is necessary. Echocardiography also can help define abnormal anatomy in patients with congenital heart disease who have right-to-left shunting of blood. These patients are at risk for systemic air embolization should air inadvertently be introduced into the venous circulation. Under these circumstances, extreme care must be given to ensure that all intravenous fluids provided are free of air (Box 11-1). The presence of specific congenital anatomical abnormalities also may be a root cause for long-term dysrhythmias in spite of surgical or electrophysiology intervention.

Blood laboratory testing is recommended before most electrophysiology procedures. Complications of invasive, as well as "just" percutaneous, procedures can include significant hemorrhage, so a baseline hemoglobin or hematocrit value and blood type and screen results should be obtained before all major procedures. In cases with a high risk for hemorrhage, such as lead extractions, ensuring that blood is crossmatched before

Box 11-1   Air Bubble Precautions With Right-to-Left Shunting of Blood

Intravenous

Ensure that all injection ports and tubing are free of air. If the intravenous is prepared and left in a cold environment for any time, recheck before use, because air bubbles can form in the tubing from dissolved air coming out of solution.

Syringe

Air bubbles adhere to the plunger and should be removed before giving a bolus of a drug. It is suggested that avoiding use of the last half a milliliter of drug in a syringe will prevent the injection of micro air bubbles that adhere to the plunger.

Syringe in Stopcock

When connecting a syringe to a stopcock to give a drug, make sure the air in the stopcock connector and air in the tip of the syringe have been flushed out before connecting the two for giving medication. Draw back half a milliliter of intravenous fluid into syringe to ensure no air is present before injecting.

Syringe in Injection Port

Recheck injection port to ensure it is free of air, and squirt some of the drug out of syringe needle to ensure no air in needle before putting the needle into the injection port. Draw back half a milliliter of intravenous fluid into syringe to ensure no air is present before injecting.

Central Venous Catheter

A central venous catheter is rarely placed by an anesthesiologist in the electrophysiology laboratory. If one is used during the placement procedure, extreme caution should be taken in the nonparalyzed patient to never let the catheter be open to room air, which would allow entrainment of air into the venous circuit should the patient develop a negative intrathoracic pressure with inspiration.

the start of the procedure and immediately available is recommended. Coagulation studies should be performed preoperatively, because many patients undergoing an electrophysiology procedure are medicated with anticoagulants in an attempt to reduce the risk for a thromboembolic event such as a stroke. Serum creatinine and blood urea nitrogen are good indirect methods for assessing renal function. The status of the kidneys becomes especially important in the electrophysiology laboratory for the longer ablation procedures because significant amounts of fluids are given by the electrophysiologist and intravenous contrast dye is often administered. Finally, serum electrolytes and thyroid function tests may help diagnose the underlying cause of some of the cardiac rhythm abnormalities.

A baseline electrocardiogram (ECG) should be obtained, with particular attention paid to the rhythm and any existing ischemic changes. During the ablation process, the coronary arteries and their branches, particularly on the right, can be harmed, and a baseline ECG for comparison is useful when trying to determine the cause for a sudden fall in blood pressure. Longer cardiac rhythm studies may have been performed on many of the patients undergoing electrophysiology procedures with such modalities as 24-hour

Holter monitoring. A chest radiograph may be helpful in demonstrating cardiomegaly, heart failure, implanted devices, and preexisting pulmonary conditions.

ANESTHETIC MANAGEMENT

Procedures in electrophysiology laboratories are performed with either monitored anesthesia care (MAC) or general anesthesia. Some procedures, such as atrial flutter radiofrequency ablation, may start out as a MAC case and then convert to a general anesthetic (see Table 11-1). One commonly accepted approach to general anesthesia is the use of continuous infusions of propofol and remifentanil. The combination of propofol 50 to 100 mcg/kg/min and remifentanil 0.08 to 0.14 mcg/kg/min usually causes a fall in blood pressure, so once the infusions of anesthetics begin, an infusion of phenylephrine at a baseline rate of 25 to 75 mcg/min is also added. The infusion of phenylephrine is adjusted based on the patient's individual response to the anesthetics, but it is rare that phenylephrine is not needed at all. In patients with poor left ventricular function, 1 to 2 mcg/min of epinephrine may be a better approach than phenylephrine. Succinylcholine is used by some anesthesiologists to facilitate endotracheal intubation, but other paralytics are not often used. The reason for avoiding long-acting muscle relaxation is to allow the electrophysiologist to determine the path of the phrenic nerve during the mapping procedure on the posterior endocardial wall and thereby avoid harming it during the ablation process. The reason for avoiding an inhalational agent is outlined in the section concerning the effect of anesthetics on electrophysiological function.

The anesthesia plan in electrophysiology will depend on the nature of the procedure and patient-specific considerations. Most procedures performed in electrophysiology laboratories are not as painful as invasive surgical procedures. However, some parts of the procedures are associated with pain, particularly if tunneling is necessary, if the patient experiences the burning sensation associated with ablation, or if cardioversion or defibrillation is necessary. Potential hemodynamic instability or the length of a procedure may be indications for general anesthesia with a secured airway. Although the procedures themselves may not be especially painful, patients with preexisting skeletal or joint injuries, especially spine issues, may have significant postprocedure pain as a result of remaining in one position for an extended period.

AIRWAY MANAGEMENT

Airway management in the electrophysiology laboratory may be extremely difficult because of the large, bulky equipment in the room. During intubation, it is not uncommon for the anesthesiologist to contort his or her body, straddle one arm of an x-ray machine, and duck under another arm in an effort to gain a reasonable position from which to intubate (Figures 11-2 and 11-3).

For intubation, a video laryngoscope may be less traumatic than conventional laryngoscopy and reduces the number of repeat laryngoscopies.[7] Many patients undergoing electrophysiology procedures have received anticoagulation, so minor trauma during airway management can result in a major hematoma.[8] Likewise, placement of a soft bite block between the teeth is recommended to decrease

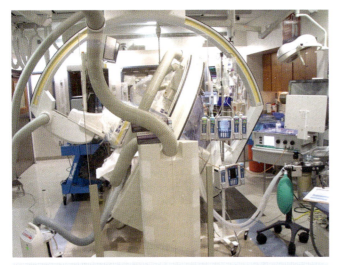

Figure 11-2 An illustration of the cramped space at the head of the table in the typical electrophysiology laboratory. The equipment required for the procedure envelops the patient, often leaving the anesthesia provider limited access during intubation. Note the distance of the anesthesia machine from the patient's head. In addition, the anesthesia provider must be prepared to move the infusion pumps out of the way as the cardiology x-ray equipment moves.

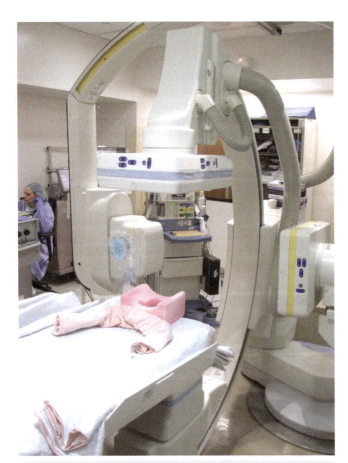

Figure 11-3 Another view of the space allowed the anesthesia provider. Note that it will be necessary to straddle the lower arm of the x-ray equipment while ducking under the upper arm during intubation. Once again, the distance of the anesthesia machine from the patient's head can be appreciated.

the chance of the patient biting the tongue or cheek during cardioversion and defibrillation.[8]

POSITIONING AND PADDING

Procedures in electrophysiology laboratories are generally performed with the patient in the supine position with arms tucked and padded. This position grants the interventionist better access to the patient and facilitates biplane fluoroscopy, but having the arms tucked makes detecting intravenous and arterial catheter problems (e.g., infiltration or disconnection) more difficult. Proper positioning and padding are important to avoid patient injury, particularly during longer procedures. Procedures in the electrophysiology laboratories may last 8 hours or longer. Maintaining a well-padded patient who is comfortable throughout the procedure is the key to a pain-free postprocedure recovery (Figure 11-4). After padding is complete, the arms of the patient must be restrained to prevent movement and injury during cardioversion and defibrillation. Because patients are not usually paralyzed after induction of anesthesia, cardioversion during the procedure may produce injury from flail movement of the limbs. Restraining the arms is important for patients receiving MAC and general anesthesia. If an arterial catheter is placed for the procedure, the arm to be used may be left unrestrained until the catheter is placed, usually after intubation and securing of the airway.

MONITORING

American Society of Anesthesiologists (ASA) standard monitoring[9] should be used for patients anesthetized in

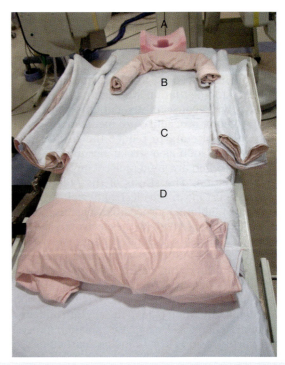

Figure 11-4 An illustration of the typical techniques used for padding the patient. These measures include a headrest **(A)**, a horseshoe-shaped roll placed under the shoulders and then covered by soft padding **(B)**, arm padding **(C)**, and a large roll or pillow **(D)** placed under the knees to help alleviate pressure on the spine.

electrophysiology laboratories. For electrophysiology procedures in which rapid changes in blood pressure might occur as a result of changes in cardiac rhythm or bleeding complications, blood pressure should be monitored by either a radial artery catheter or a femoral artery catheter. In most patients, these catheters may be placed after induction of anesthesia. An arterial cannula is useful for sampling blood for arterial blood gas, glucose, and electrolyte levels; titration of anticoagulation therapy; and helping with the differential diagnosis of a hypotensive episode. A urinary bladder catheter should be placed for longer procedures to monitor urine output, to guide fluid management, and to keep the bladder from becoming distended while the patient must remain motionless in the supine position for an extended period.

FLUID MANAGEMENT

Intravenous fluids must be actively managed by the anesthesiologist for all patients undergoing electrophysiology procedures. These patients often have a delicate cardiac status, and judicious management of fluids is mandatory. Liters of fluid may often be infused by the electrophysiologist during the ablation process. It is not unusual that by the end of the procedure the patient may have a positive fluid balance of over 3 L. Many patients undergoing electrophysiology procedures have cardiomyopathies and are prone to congestive heart failure; thus the anesthesiologist's attention must be directed at both limiting the amount of fluids provided during the anesthesia and performing a continuous careful evaluation for signs of volume overload. This ongoing evaluation of fluids translates into not only monitoring the patient's fluid intake and output but also periodically communicating the fluid status to the interventionist. Diuretics are often used when a large positive fluid balance exists, especially if signs of congestive failure appear.

TEMPERATURE CONTROL

Electrophysiology laboratories are often cold, and patients are within this cold environment for hours under anesthesia. To prevent hypothermia, active warming devices should be used. However, based on the type of procedure, limitations exist concerning modalities such as full-body forced air heaters. Often, partial body warmers and fluid warmers are the extent to which the anesthesiologist can prevent hypothermia. In addition, core temperature measurements using an esophageal probe serve the dual purpose of providing guidance in regard to effectiveness of warming devices and providing warning when the ablating is being performed near the esophagus.

ENVIRONMENTAL FACTORS

Most procedures in electrophysiology laboratories involve fluoroscopy, so it is necessary for staff to take protective precautions, such as working behind lead shielding and wearing lead aprons and protective glasses. Placement and orientation of x-ray machines may present a challenge in airway management because they can limit access to the patient, as discussed earlier. Some electrophysiology laboratories also use a magnetic system for positioning ablation catheters. In such laboratories, it is important to keep ferromagnetic objects away from the magnetic system to prevent common metallic objects from turning into projectiles that may harm the patient, staff, or equipment. In addition, special magnet-compatible monitoring equipment and anesthesia machines may be needed.

COMMUNICATION AND TEAMWORK

Communication between the electrophysiology and anesthesiology teams is critical, regardless of whether the case proceeds uneventfully or during a time of complicated crisis. Both groups perform actions that affect the patient's heart rate and blood pressure. For example, the electrophysiologist should be made aware if the anesthesiologist needs to administer additional inotropic medications or vasopressors, because this may be an early indicator of a cardiac chamber perforation. The anesthesiologist needs to be informed when drug challenges or rapid pacing is being initiated by the electrophysiologist, because these will produce significant hemodynamic responses. The electrophysiologist also should be informed of any changes in the patient's mental status when conscious sedation is being used. If the patient is not following verbal commands, all of the parties involved in the patient's care must know if this change is related to the patient's anesthetic medications or if it is a change in the patient's condition that would indicate a neurological insult. The anesthesiologist should communicate with the electrophysiologist when the phrenic nerve is tested for diaphragm contraction, which is the key reason neuromuscular blockade is avoided. Acid-base and fluid status should be periodically reviewed to ensure adequate ventilation and the prevention of volume overload. Clear communication is most important during times of crisis, such as ventricular perforation or cardiac arrest. Every member of the care team needs to work together and communicate clearly to improve patient safety and outcome.

Because of the extensive amount of equipment present in the typical electrophysiology laboratory (Figure 11-5), one method for rapid and clear communication is the use of headphones, which allow all parties to hear and understand each other. In this manner, errors based on inaccurate or missed information can be kept to a minimum.

PHARMACOPEIA

The drugs most commonly used for an electrophysiology procedure fall into three main categories: anesthetic agents, cardiovascular drugs, and medications aimed at improved postoperative comfort. Table 11-2 provides a listing of the drugs commonly used and the manner in which they are provided.

BASIC DRUG EFFECTS

Understanding the concept of electrophysiological actions of drugs and how they might affect an electrophysiological procedure requires a consideration of the cardiac conduction system action potential. Anesthetic drugs may act directly on the action potential, indirectly by changing sympathetic and parasympathetic tone, or by modulating humoral or environmental effects.

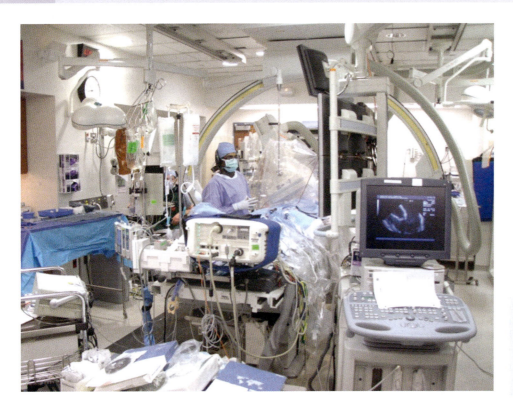

Figure 11-5 An illustration of the physical barriers that can obstruct oral and visual communication in the electrophysiology laboratory. Headphones are worn by the electrophysiologist, anesthesiologist, and nursing staff to facilitate communication.

Table 11-2 Drugs Commonly Used in Electrophysiology Procedures

Category	Concentrations
ANESTHETIC AGENTS	
Muscle Relaxants	
Succinylcholine	Bolus: 100 mg
Opioids	
Remifentanil	Infusion: 0.01-0.2 mcg/kg/min
Fentanyl	Bolus: 50-100 mcg
Induction Agents	
Propofol	Bolus: 2 mg/kg
	Infusion: 5-150 mcg/kg/min
Etomidate	Bolus: 0.1-0.3 mg/kg
Benzodiazepines	
Midazolam	Bolus: 1-2 mg
Alpha-2 (α_2) Adrenergic Receptor Agonists	
Dexmedetomidine	Loading dose: 1 mcg/kg over approximately 10 min
	Infusion: 0.2-1 mcg/kg/hr
CARDIOVASCULAR AGENTS	
Phenylephrine	Bolus: 100 mcg
	Infusion: 10 to 500 mcg/min
Epinephrine	Bolus: 8 mcg
	Infusion: 1 to 8 mcg/min
Atropine	Bolus: 0.5 to 1 mg
Isoproterenol	Infusion: 3 to 40 mcg/min
COMFORT AGENTS	
Dexamethasone	Bolus: 4 to 10 mg
Ondansetron	Bolus: 4 to 8 mg
Acetaminophen	Bolus: 1 g if normal liver function
Ketorolac	Bolus: 15-30 mg if normal renal function

THE ACTION POTENTIAL

Although the shape of the action potential changes depending where it is measured in the cardiac conduction system, the basic features remain the same. However, striking differences exist in the action potentials between those that serve as pacemakers and those that serve simply as conductors of the impulse. Figure 11-6 illustrates the differences between an action potential taken from the pacing cells of the sinoatrial node and those taken from an impulse-conducting cell in the distal Purkinje fibers. These action potentials are also shown in relationship to the timing of a surface electrocardiogram.

The primary characteristics of all action potentials are as follows:

■ *Phase 0—depolarization phase:* In the sinoatrial node, the upstroke is less steep than in the general cardiac conduction system represented by the Purkinje fiber action potential in Figure 11-6. The primary reason for this difference is that the upstroke in the sinoatrial node is due to a slow inward leak of ionized calcium, whereas the upstroke or development of a positive intracellular ionic state is due to the more rapid influx of ionized sodium throughout the rest of the cardiac conduction system. In the general cardiac conduction system without pacer activity, the slow upstroke caused by calcium leak is missing and only the steep upward depolarization from rapid sodium influx is observed.

■ *Phase 1—early repolarization phase:* The slight drop in the action potential in the Purkinje fiber represents initial repolarization mediated by an outward flow of potassium ions. This is not seen in cells that serve as pacemakers.

■ *Phase 2—plateau phase:* This phase of the action potential occurring in nonpacemaker cardiac conduction cells represents a combination of slow but significant exchanges in ions across the cell membrane. The move-

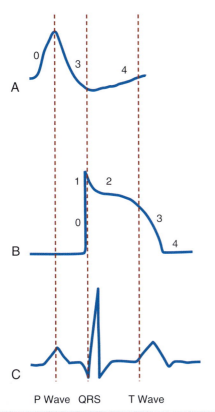

Figure 11-6 The action potential taken from a cell in the sinoatrial node **(A)** and from a Purkinje fiber **(B)** in relationship to the surface electrocardiogram **(C)**. Note that the temporal components of the electrocardiogram differ for the action potentials depending on where the action potential originates.

ment of calcium ions into the cell and potassium ions out of the cell and a decrease in sodium ion influx leads to a relative steady state. This phase is absent in the action potentials of pacemaker cells.

■ *Phase 3—repolarization phase:* The drop in the slope of the action potential of impulse conducting cells is due primarily to an outward flow of potassium ions. The same is occurring in pacemaker cells but at a slower rate than in the conducting cells.

■ *Phase 4—resting phase:* Ionic equilibrium has been achieved in impulse-conducting cells. However, no period of quiescence occurs in the pacemaker cells; rather, a slow flow of calcium ions into the pacer cells will again begin the cycle that will trigger depolarization, or phase 0.

ACTION POTENTIAL MODULATION

Any variety of factors can affect the action potential, and it is not surprising that these factors play a significant role in either suppressing or inducing cardiac arrhythmias.

SYMPATHETIC AND PARASYMPATHETIC NERVOUS SYSTEMS

The heart has significant innervation by both sympathetic and parasympathetic nerves. The parasympathetic system's effects on the heart are mediated primarily by the vagus nerve, with acetylcholine acting as the

neurotransmitter at muscarinic receptors. Stimulation of the vagus nerve slows depolarization of the pacing cells within the sinoatrial node, thereby decreasing chronotropy. Similarly, as a result of vagal nerve connections to the atrial myocardium and the atrioventricular node, negative dromotropic and inotropic effects occur. These effects are opposite to those observed with sympathetic nerve stimulation. Sympathetic innervation occurs throughout the heart, with norepinephrine serving as the neurotransmitter. Beta-1 (β_1) receptors mediate the sympathetic nervous system effects. Sympathetic nerve stimulation leads to an increase of chronotropy, dromotropy, and inotropy. As might be expected, drugs used for noncardiac reasons, such as anesthetics, which change the tone of either the sympathetic or parasympathetic nervous systems, can have significant secondary effects on impulse conduction in the heart. Studies into whether a specific anesthetic drug has a direct effect on inducing or suppressing an arrhythmia are confounded by this secondary action, whereby the sedation from the drug may be altering the arrhythmia by reducing sympathetic tone or stimulating parasympathetic activity.

HUMORAL AND ENVIRONMENTAL EFFECTS ON CARDIAC CONDUCTION

In addition to direct innervation of the cardiac conduction system and secondary effects from the sympathetic and parasympathetic nervous systems, a drug's observed action may also be based on humoral influences. The sympathetic nervous system's transmission is mediated by norepinephrine, and thus a release of humoral norepinephrine or epinephrine by the adrenal glands can clearly increase sympathetic tone. The myriad factors that cause the adrenals to secrete norepinephrine and epinephrine also might influence cardiac conduction, with the possibility of either suppressing or stimulating the induction of an arrhythmogenic state. Because the adrenal glands react to stress, pain, hypercarbia, hypoxia, hypovolemia, and many other stimuli within the electrophysiology laboratory, it is difficult to control all factors that might avoid interference with the planned procedure. Although direct effects of anesthetic agents are often blamed for the inability to induce premature ventricular contractions, ventricular tachycardia, or atrial arrhythmias, there is no question that other neuronal, humoral, and environmental conditions serve as compounding factors.

EFFECTS OF ANESTHETIC DRUGS

Much of the clinical research performed to evaluate the cardiac effects of anesthetic drugs is confounded by the many secondary influences that may exist with a specific drug. For instance, patients receiving propofol for sedation may have decreased arrhythmogenesis, but separating the direct effect of propofol from its secondary indirect effects to produce this result is difficult. In the electrophysiology laboratory, many different types of anesthetic drugs and techniques have been used to allow the electrophysiologist to successfully perform procedures. Because of the sensitivity of the heart to both the direct and indirect effects of a drug, the search for the ideal drug for the electrophysiology laboratory continues. If one could design the perfect anesthetic for use in these procedures, it would have no effect on the action potential originating from either the intrinsic pacemaker or any of the arrhythmogenic foci within the heart. The ideal drug also should not change the overall autonomic tone or refractoriness of the heart.[10] Although an ideal drug should not prevent an impulse change, it should also not prevent the reoccurrence or triggering of reentrant arrhythmias, which is required for targeting the active arrhythmogenic site during the ablative procedure. At the same time, the ideal agents should be both rapidly reversible and have minimal residual effects.

Some of the anesthetic agents presently used in the electrophysiology laboratory will be discussed, with emphasis on the rarely used inhalational agents, as well as the more commonly used propofol, opioids, benzodiazepines, and muscle relaxants.

INHALATIONAL AGENTS

Various mechanisms exist by which inhalational agents might alter impulse conduction through the heart. Halothane, enflurane, and isoflurane all have been found to stimulate activation of wandering atrial pacemakers, as well as to allow the induction of ectopic atrial rhythm disorders, which are mediated through the enhancement of automaticity in secondary atrial pacemakers.[11,12] All inhalational agents have varying effects on the atrioventricular node and the His-Purkinje system. In general, the volatile agents cause both a dose-dependent reduction in myocardial contractility and a prolongation of the Q-T interval.[13,14]

Halothane, although essentially unavailable in present practice, is noted for its significant depressive effect on impulse formation within the sinoatrial node. This depression can result in the development of a junctional or a wandering atrial pacemaker.[14] Secondarily, halothane has a profound central effect in suppressing the release of catecholamines from the adrenal glands. This suppression of humoral activity leads to the parasympathetic predominance, which in turn can result in the occurrence of sinus bradycardia and junctional rhythms.[15-17] Further effects of halothane are mediated by a reduction of automaticity (phase 4 depolarization [see Figure 11-6]) in the atrioventricular node and His-Purkinje system.[15-17] Finally, while decreasing the release of humoral catecholamines, halothane also sensitizes the heart to catecholamines. This increased sensitivity, combined with the observed decrease of automaticity, may facilitate atrioventricular nodal reentry arrhythmias. In fact, the potentiation of atrioventricular nodal reentry may be the primary mechanism by which halothane produces tachydysrhythmias.[18-20]

Isoflurane has been observed to differ from halothane by not inducing bradycardia. In contrast to the intravenous anesthetic agent propofol, isoflurane causes faster atrioventricular nodal conduction while also producing a slower repolarization, at least in one group of pediatric patients undergoing electrophysiological procedures.[21] The conclusion was that both propofol and isoflurane could be used without suppression of supraventricular tachycardia (SVT). The ability of isoflurane to maintain a relatively steady heart rate is due primarily to its lack of impulse conduction suppression through the atrioventricular node.[22-24]

Others have substantiated the lack of significant clinical difference between propofol and isoflurane on sinoatrial or atrioventricular node function, although the findings are not conclusive, because an anesthetic base of alfentanil and midazolam had been provided before the evaluations.[25] However, others have found isoflurane or other inhalational anesthetic agents to suppress the occurrence of supraventricular reentrant tachycardia, so they argue against their use in situations in which induction of atrial or supraventricular reentry is needed to identify a focus for ablation.[22]

Sevoflurane has been found in some studies to be suitable for use in electrophysiology studies because of minimal observed effects on sinoatrial node, atrioventricular node, or accessory pathways conduction. In spite of the lack of direct effects on impulse generation or conduction, sevoflurane has secondary effects, as do all inhalational agents, through suppression of the autonomic nervous system.[26,27] In addition, sevoflurane has been observed to increase the corrected QT interval in the normal pediatric population.[28]

Nitrous oxide causes mild sympathetic activation, which in turn can sensitize a myocardium at risk for catecholamine stimulation to the development of a dysrhythmia. In spite of the potential for inducing a dysrhythmia with nitrous oxide, clinical studies indicate that this is rarely a problem.[29-31]

In regard to atrioventricular node refractoriness within accessory pathways, it has been demonstrated that enflurane, followed by isoflurane and then halothane, has the greatest effect. Therefore if these agents are used for electrophysiology ablation studies, the evaluation of the trigger sites of reentry needed to direct the ablation procedure may be problematic. The one exception may be sevoflurane, but further evaluation needs to be directed at the electrophysiological effects of this agent before recommendations for routine use can be made. In addition, one study has found that both sevoflurane and desflurane have a suppressive effect on postinfarction arrhythmias; this could interfere with locating the ablation targets during ventricular tachyarrhythmia ablation procedures.[32] In patients with preexcitation syndrome requiring a general anesthetic, all volatile agents, because of their effect on refractoriness, should be avoided.[33]

PROPOFOL

Propofol is widely used in many electrophysiology laboratories because of the reduced effect it has on impulse conduction. Another advantage of propofol is that patients rapidly recover from its effects; this makes it ideal for both short procedures, such as cardioversion, and lengthy interventions, such as atrial ablations. In the electrophysiology laboratory it is mainly used as one component of a total intravenous anesthetic (TIVA). Propofol is associated with inducing both bradycardia and tachycardia.[34-39] Some have found no effect from propofol on cardiac conduction, whereas others have observed it to produce slowing in a dose-dependent manner as a result of conduction delays or depression of sinoatrial nodal, atrioventricular nodal, and His-Purkinje system functions.[40-42] Propofol has been noted to enhance epinephrine-induced arrhythmias in a dose-dependent manner in dogs.[43] The hypotension associated with propofol use is thought to be a result of impaired regulation of the baroreflex—part of its overall inhibition of the sympathetic nervous system.[44]

Of significance for the electrophysiology laboratory, propofol infusions seem to have little or no direct effect on accessory pathway conduction, nor on normal atrioventricular nodal or accessory pathway conduction in patients with Wolff-Parkinson-White (WPW) syndrome.[27] Propofol does not appear to trigger SVT or ventricular tachyarrhythmias in the electrophysiology laboratory. At least in children undergoing radiofrequency ablations for SVTs, propofol does not appear to alter sinoatrial or atrioventricular node function.[25] However, significant concerns do exist for using propofol in the presence of the long QT syndrome, because it can result in cardiac standstill.[45]

OPIOIDS

Opioids generally produce bradycardia, especially if given in large doses.[46-49] The observed bradycardia is a result of a central vagotonic effect. These drugs prolong the action potential by affecting both the potassium and calcium ion channels in the heart. The prolonged action potential is similar to the action of class 3 antiarrhythmic agents.[50-52] Opioids prolong the Q-T interval, but whether this is due to a direct effect on the myocardial membrane or to actions from myocardial opioid receptors in the heart has not been demonstrated.[10]

Remifentanil has properties that allow a rapid change in the depth of anesthesia, thus making it well suited for cases in the electrophysiology suite. This drug has a rapid time to peak effect of approximately 90 seconds and a half-life of 3 to 4 minutes, regardless of how long it has been administered.[53] Remifentanil, like the other mu-opioid (μ-opioid) agonists, acts synergistically with other sedatives to potentiate anesthetic effects. This synergy allows lower doses of midazolam or propofol to be used, with the key advantage being a more rapid return to consciousness once the drugs are discontinued.[54] For cardioversion, remifentanil has allowed the use of a lower dose of hypnotic drugs such as propofol and midazolam.

However, like other opioids, remifentanil can produce bradycardia, although it has relatively little effect on arrhythmogenesis.[55] Remifentanil has been demonstrated to prolong the impulse conduction from the atrium to the His bundle and increase both the QRS duration and the sinoatrial node recovery time.[56,57] Significant bradycardia is often seen with remifentanil use for this reason.[58] One very positive aspect of remifentanil in the electrophysiology laboratory is that it does not appear to alter the ability to induce ventricular tachycardia that results from structural heart disease. For instance, in one study in dogs, the dose of epinephrine required to induce ventricular dysrhythmias was not affected by remifentanil.[58,59] In children, remifentanil appears to slow both sinoatrial and atrioventricular nodal function in patients undergoing ablation of SVT. Therefore it may not be the best drug of choice in pediatric patients undergoing electrophysiology procedures in which atrioventricular nodal function must be preserved.[60] Bolus doses of remifentanil have been associated with attenuation of a corrected QT interval prolongation under sevoflurane anesthesia, although the clinical significance of this observation is yet to be defined.[61] One fascinating area of current research is directed at evaluating variations in individual patient electrophysiological responses to anesthetic agents based on genetic variations. For instance, remifentanil will provide a positive synergistic anesthetic effect when used with propofol for patients with one genetic variation but will have minimal synergistic effects for patients without this genetic variation.[62] As future studies better define the genetic factors influencing the anesthetic and electrophysiological effects of each drug used in the electrophysiology laboratory, the decisions made in regard to the best drug selections for any particular patient undergoing a specific procedure will be more rational but decidedly more complex.

Hypotension associated with remifentanil use is most likely due primarily to noncardiac factors.[55] Remifentanil was found to directly vasodilate arterial beds in the forearm; this resulted in increased regional blood flow.[63] Thus hypotension associated with remifentanil is due to a combination of bradycardia and vasodilation, conditions easily remedied in the electrophysiology suite. Because of its unique profile, remifentanil is a reasonable anesthetic choice for use in adults.

BENZODIAZEPINES

All benzodiazepines reduce blood pressure by decreasing both cardiac contractility and peripheral vascular resistance. As a result of the decreased contractility and vasodilation, a reflex tachycardia may result. These effects are dose-dependent but similar in overall effect for all benzodiazepines, varying only in the speed of onset and the duration of action. Other than the hemodynamic responses, this class of drugs has no known specific direct effects on cardiac conduction, including the QT interval.[64]

As a result of the slower onset of action and the higher doses needed to provide sedation, benzodiazepines in the electrophysiology laboratory may not be the best choice. In a retrospective review of patients undergoing electrophysiology procedures, 40% of the patients receiving a benzodiazepine for sedation required advanced airway support.[65] For most ventricular arrhythmia interventions, ventricular tachycardias or ventricular fibrillation may be induced, and sedation for the cardioversion or defibrillation must be provided on very short notice. Drugs used for sedation must have a rapid onset but at the same time be rapidly metabolized to allow assessment of the patient's neurological function. Benzodiazepines are not suitable for this situation. In addition, during ventricular tachyarrhythmia ablation procedures when ventricular tachycardia is being initiated as part of the procedure, suppression of the autonomic nervous system by the benzodiazepines can interfere with the induction of the ventricular arrhythmias. A retrospective study of midazolam and diazepam use for elective cardioversion during atrial ablation procedures showed that the time needed to provide adequate sedation for the electric shock averaged 5 minutes.[66] In addition, hypotension occurred in 20% of these patients. The dose to achieve adequate sedation averaged 12.5 mg of midazolam, a dosage that would negate rapid recovery. In the electrophysiology laboratory, even without the hypotensive instability, a 5-minute delay for performing cardioversion in a patient with an atrial arrhythmia is impractical and is more so for the patient with a ventricular tachyarrhythmia.

ETOMIDATE

Etomidate has a rapid onset and a rapid recovery; these are both highly desirable features for the provision of sedation in the electrophysiology laboratory. Its ability to maintain the blood pressure also makes it desirable for patients in a compromised cardiac state or with low left ventricular ejection fraction. In fact, etomidate serves as an excellent substitute for propofol as an anesthesia induction agent in the presence of cardiovascular instability. Nearly 40% of patients may experience myoclonic jerking after administration, and concern has been expressed that this could interfere with interpretation of the ECG during elective cardioversion,[67] but in practice this is rarely a problem. Although relatively free of adverse hemodynamic effects, etomidate has been used to suppress electrical storm in a patient; however, separating out the contribution of any direct electrophysiological effects from secondary autonomic nervous system effects was not determined.[68]

DEXMEDETOMIDINE

Dexmedetomidine has been considered a possible anesthetic agent for adults and children undergoing electrophysiology procedures. The drug has attractive properties in that it is short-acting and preserves respiratory function. However, bradycardia associated with the use of dexmedetomidine has been reported. The incidence of bradycardia is unknown when dexmedetomidine is used in infants and children. However, Hammer et al[69] reported that dexmedetomidine significantly decreased sinus and atrioventricular nodal function in pediatric patients and resulted in the unusual combination of bradycardia and increased arterial blood pressure. Because of this result, it was suggested that the use of dexmedetomidine may not be desirable for electrophysiology studies in pediatric patients. In studies that focused on adults, bradycardia has been cited to occur in 9% to 40% of the population.[70-73] Although Peden et al[74] reported sinus arrest after a patient received an initial dose of dexmedetomidine over 15 minutes, the bradycardia noted in the majority of adults was rarely hemodynamically significant and usually well-tolerated.

NEUROMUSCULAR BLOCKERS

Neuromuscular blockers can affect cardiac impulse conduction through several mechanisms. As with sedative and hypnotic anesthetic agents, muscle relaxants can have indirect effects on the sympathetic and parasympathetic nervous systems, and, depending on the agent, this effect may be stimulatory or depressive to impulse conduction. The muscle relaxants may act directly at sympathetic nerve terminals and as a result increase heart rate. In addition, an increased heart rate might be an indirect effect caused by vasodilation from histamine, which results in reflex tachycardia.[75] Succinylcholine has acetylcholine-like activity on receptors mediated by cholinergic neurotransmission, as found in the parasympathetic nervous system. The value of succinylcholine in the

electrophysiology laboratory primarily rests with its short duration of action. Because phrenic nerve assessment during the ablation procedure requires a nonparalyzed patient, the advantage of using succinylcholine for anesthesia induction and intubation is obvious. Pancuronium increases the heart rate both by its vagolytic properties and by releasing norepinephrine at cardiac sympathetic nerve terminals. Vecuronium and atracurium may produce bradycardias, especially when other vagotonic drugs such as propofol and opioids have been given.[76-78] Mivacurium and rocuronium have been found to be essentially free of cardiac conduction effects.[10]

The Physiology of Cardiac Arrhythmias

Cardiac rhythm disturbances are typically described in terms of the speed of cardiac impulse generation and conduction. By definition, any cardiac rhythm slower than 60 beats per minute is a bradyarrhythmia. Similarly, any rhythm over 100 beats per minute is a tachyarrhythmia. Although hemodynamic instability can be observed with both bradyarrhythmias and tachyarrhythmias, similar instability can be observed even in sinus rhythms when the heart rate is not stable (see Box 11-2[79] for a listing of common bradyarrhythmias and tachyarrhythmias).

Many types of arrhythmias are seen and treated in the electrophysiology laboratory. A bradyarrhythmia is seen either when the sinoatrial node is malfunctioning with an impulse being generated less than 60 times/min or from a defect in the conduction of a properly generated impulse leading to less than 60 beats/min. The most common type of bradyarrhythmia seen by electrophysiologists is a sinus bradyarrhythmia, which is due to disease of the sinus node. Many sinus bradyarrhythmias are asymptomatic and require no treatment, but some may progress to a point at which cardiac function and hemodynamic stability are

---

Box 11-2 Common Bradyarrhythmias and Tachyarrhythmias

Bradyarrhythmias

1. Abnormal sinoatrial impulse formation: Sick sinus syndrome
2. Abnormal impulse conduction: Atrioventricular block

Tachyarrhythmias

1. Normal complex QRS
   a. Sinus tachycardia
   b. Atrial flutter
   c. Atrioventricular nodal reentry tachycardia
2. Narrow complex QRS
   a. Atrial fibrillation
   b. Multifocal atrial tachycardia
3. Wide complex QRS
   a. Monomorphic ventricular tachycardia
   b. Polymorphic ventricular tachycardia
   c. Supraventricular tachycardia with bundle branch block

From Chua J, Patel K, Neelankavil J, Mahajan A. Anesthetic management of electrophysiology procedures. Curr Opin Anaesthesiol. *2012;25(4): 470-481.*

Protocol for Anesthesia for Ablation of Atrial Fibrillation—cont'd

3. Confirm Yankauer suction, airway supplies, medications (listed earlier)
4. Connect intravenous line to multiport manifold (for infusion of propofol, remifentanil, phenylephrine, epinephrine)
5. Pad and secure patient's arms, with attention to pressure points
6. Denitrogenate the patient with 100% oxygen by mask
7. Induction typically with intravenous lidocaine (1 to 2 mg/kg), propofol (~2 mg/kg) or etomidate (0.2 to 0.3 mg/kg), fentanyl (1 to 2 mcg/kg), and succinylcholine (1 mg/kg)
8. Intubate patient (video laryngoscope may be used if patient has received anticoagulation therapy or in anticipated difficult laryngoscopy); cardiologist can check endotracheal tube position fluoroscopically
9. Esophageal temperature probe; cardiologist can check position fluoroscopically
10. Bite block
11. Forced-air warming blanket
12. Foley catheter placed typically by cardiology nurse
13. Place arterial catheter

E. Maintenance
  1. Typical drug infusions
    a. Propofol (50 to 75 mcg/kg/min)
    b. Remifentanil (~0.12 mcg/kg/min)
    c. Phenylephrine (20 to 100 mcg/min) to maintain blood pressure
  2. Jet ventilation (coordinate with the cardiologist). If initiated, an arterial blood gas (ABG) sample should be sent to the laboratory approximately 30 minutes later. The jet ventilator settings should be adjusted on the basis of the laboratory results to achieve a normal Pa_{CO_2}; ABGs should be checked 30 minutes after each adjustment or at least every 2 hours if no adjustment is made.
  3. Once atrial fibrillation ablation has occurred, the cardiologist may wish to test ablation with an infusion of isoproterenol. Phenylephrine infusion should be immediately available to treat isoproterenol-induced hypotension.

F. After the procedure
  1. Consider antiemetic prophylaxis
  2. Consider analgesic longer-acting than remifentanil (e.g., fentanyl, hydromorphone, ketorolac, or meperidine)
  3. Extubation may proceed when criteria have been met. Infusion of vasopressor(s) may be discontinued based on the hemodynamic status of the patient.
  4. Patient should be transported to cardiology recovery unit with appropriate monitors and oxygen.
  5. Appropriate report (including medications given, fluid balance, etc.) must be made to the recovery nurse.

HYBRID ABLATION PROCEDURE

A hybrid "convergent" procedure for ablation of atrial fibrillation has recently been developed, in which a surgeon does epicardial ablation using an endoscopic, closed-chest, subthoracic approach (Figures 11-10 and 11-11) to the beating heart and the electrophysiologist ablates endocardially similar to standard electrophysiology procedures.[86] The combined effort can greatly reduce the overall length of the procedure, but if the surgeon works in the operating room and the cardiologist in the electrophysiology laboratory, transporting an anesthetized, intubated patient from one location to the

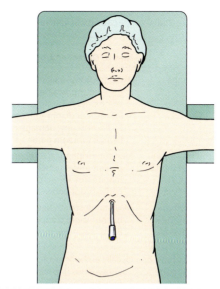

Figure 11-10 Placement of an endoscope for epicardial catheter ablation technique using a closed subthoracic approach.

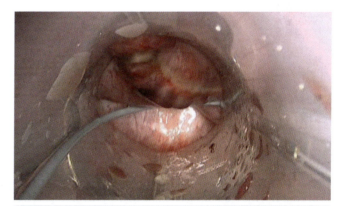

Figure 11-11 Epicardial lesions seen endoscopically between the pericardium and the atrium during a subthoracic epicardial catheter ablation. (Courtesy of nContact, Morrisville, NC, with permission.)

other is required. Furthermore, more analgesic medication may be needed than for a strictly endovascular procedure.

COMPLICATIONS OF ATRIAL FIBRILLATION ABLATION FROM DAMAGE TO ADJACENT STRUCTURES

Potential complications of atrial fibrillation ablation procedures are listed in Table 11-3. Some relate to injury from structures adjacent to the heart, such as the phrenic nerve and esophagus.

The phrenic nerve may sustain damage during an ablation procedure because of its close proximity to the area being ablated on the posterior surface of the atrium. The risk for damage to the nerve increases as the distance to the ablated area decreases. To identify the phrenic nerve for decreasing the risk for damage, the electrophysiologist will often stimulate the posterior surface of the right atrium and check for diaphragm motion on fluoroscopy. Neuromuscular blockade is undesirable at this point in the

Table 11-3 Potential Complications of Catheter Ablation of Atrial Fibrillation

Complication	How to Detect and/or Avoid
Phrenic nerve damage	Avoid neuromuscular blockade so that the electrophysiologist can identify the nerve by stimulating it and looking for diaphragm contraction by fluoroscopy; damage could cause hemidiaphragm paralysis.
Esophageal thermal injury (ulceration, atrioesophageal fistula)	Monitor esophageal temperature in patient under general anesthesia; monitor for severe chest pain in patients not under general anesthesia.
Complications of femoral access (retroperitoneal bleeding, arteriovenous fistula, pseudoaneurysm)	May manifest with back pain, anemia, hypotension; computed tomography helps diagnose; may need surgery.
Transient ischemic attack or cerebrovascular accident	Usually embolic; avoid air bubbles in intravenous line with transseptal puncture; neurological deficit will probably not be apparent until emergence from general anesthesia.
Myocardial infarction	Monitor for electrocardiogram changes, most commonly in right coronary distribution.
Pulmonary vein stenosis	Typically presents months after the procedure; may be diagnosed with computed tomography, treated with balloons and/or stents.
Anaphylaxis	Hypotension, wheezing; not unique to electrophysiology
Tamponade from cardiac or aorta perforation	Hypotension; pericardial effusion can be seen on echocardiogram; effusion can be tapped, anticoagulation reversed; sometimes requires surgery.

procedure. This can be accomplished by avoiding long-acting muscle relaxants to facilitate tracheal intubation and instead using succinylcholine or an intubating dose of a short-acting muscle relaxant. Communication should be initiated with the electrophysiologist before induction of anesthesia concerning the use of any muscle relaxant that might have residual effects during the evaluation of phrenic nerve function.

The cardiologist will also ablate near the esophagus. Thermal injury to the esophagus resulting in ulceration or atrioesophageal fistula is another potential complication. Monitoring esophageal temperature may help avoid this complication in the patient under general anesthesia. A rapid increase recorded by the esophageal temperature probe should be communicated to the cardiologist.

Another major complication in the electrophysiology laboratory is the uncommon but not rare perforation of the atrium or ventricle that can lead to a cardiac tamponade. Once the diagnosis is established, usually by echocardiography, the patient may be stabilized by increasing preload and use of vasoconstrictors. Inotropic support may be necessary to maintain adequate blood pressure. If the patient becomes unstable and the blood pressure cannot be maintained, subxyphoid drainage of the tamponade may be needed. If that fails, emergency surgical intervention is required.

OTHER COMPLICATIONS OF ATRIAL FIBRILLATION ABLATION

Major complications of ablation can arise from attempting to gain femoral access, such as retroperitoneal bleeding, arteriovenous fistulas, and pseudoaneurysms. Transient ischemic attacks or cerebrovascular accidents can occur, because the procedure involves a transseptal puncture through the fossa ovalis membrane to cross into the left atrium. It is imperative during these transseptal procedures to avoid air bubbles in the intravenous lines because of potential air embolism (see Box 11-1). Embolism of particulate matter formed by heat coagulation is even more common. Other major complications include myocardial infarction (most commonly along the right coronary artery distribution), pulmonary vein stenosis, and anaphylaxis.

The risk for major complications of ablation, as listed in Table 11-3, is approximately 2%. Treatment of these complications varies according to each case. Treatment can range from supportive to pharmacologic, all the way up to major surgical intervention. It is important to plan for emergencies. The ability to call for and obtain help is essential. A well-stocked code cart should be nearby, as well as a rapid infuser. Resuscitation scenarios need to be in place. Surgical backup must be available. The method of transportation, monitoring, and transfer of care of the patient from the electrophysiology laboratory to the operating room should be in place before the start of any procedure.

When deciding the value of performing an atrial ablation, the risks for potential complications must be balanced against the risks to the patient of continued atrial fibrillation. Complications of atrial fibrillation include heart failure, decreased quality of life, increased risk for stroke, and death. The first line of treatment of atrial fibrillation is the use of a variety of medications, but they often fail over time. This failure has led to the rise in ablation procedures.

ABLATION OF OTHER DYSRHYTHMIAS

Catheter ablation of dysrhythmias other than atrial fibrillation is usually performed with sedation, rather than general anesthesia. It is important to consider the impact of certain drugs for patients presenting for an electrophysiology study to diagnose dysrhythmias, such as supraventricular or ventricular tachycardia and premature ventricular contractions. For example, drugs affecting the autonomic nervous system should be avoided, because they may affect the ability of the cardiologist to reproduce the offending arrhythmia. Some sedatives may also suppress arrhythmias (see the earlier discussion on the effects of anesthetic drugs).

Patients who present for ablation of ventricular tachycardia in the setting of structural heart disease can be severely compromised, with poor cardiac output resulting in multiorgan failure. Inotropic or mechanical support such as extracorporeal membrane oxygenation, intraaortic balloon pump, or an Impella device (AbioMed, Danvers, Massachusetts) may be necessary for the patient to tolerate the procedure. Cardioversion may be necessary if organ perfusion is compromised by ventricular arrhythmia. The hemodynamic effects of ventricular dysrhythmias are easily evaluated with arterial catheter monitoring. The anesthesia provider typically works near the patient's head, so is often the person best able to assess the patient's mental status as an indicator of cerebral perfusion. Cerebral oximetry also can be used as a surrogate measurement of cerebral perfusion, particularly in patients whose mental status is already compromised by sedative or anesthetic medications. It can be challenging to avoid oversedation with a resultant suppression of arrhythmias but at the same time provide adequate sedation so that the patient can tolerate the procedure.

The cardiologist's approach for ventricular tachycardia can be endocardial, as described earlier, or epicardial, in which catheters are inserted through the chest wall. The latter can be particularly painful. Temporary suspension of respiration is sometimes desirable during this procedure, so general anesthesia with an endotracheal tube may be the preferred anesthesia plan for epicardial ablations. However, at least one case of successful use of remifentanil and midazolam for sedation for this procedure in a young patient has been reported.[55]

Device Implantation

Electrophysiologists will place pacemakers and defibrillators in patients when indicated. Anesthesia is not necessarily needed for pacemaker implants, so the present discussion will focus only on ICD implantation. Patients presenting for ICD placement often have cardiomyopathy with a low left ventricular ejection fraction (typically ≤35%), with published guidelines[87] recommending ICD therapy for such patients. Studies have shown that long-term mortality is reduced when ICDs are implanted in these patients with either ischemic[88] or nonischemic[89] cardiomyopathies. Prophylactic ICD placement is warranted in these patients, as a primary preventive measure, even if no previous ventricular tachyarrhythmia has been identified. Although some of these patients may have nonischemic cardiomyopathy, many of them will have coronary disease, so it is important to consider the risk for myocardial ischemia and its sequelae as part of the anesthesia plan. Many patients are having an ICD placed for secondary prevention; in other words, they have already had a ventricular tachycardia or ventricular fibrillation arrest. These patients have multiple comorbidities and will usually have physical status of ASA 3 or greater.

The device implant can usually be performed with local anesthesia and mild to moderate sedation.[90-93] Rarely is general anesthesia required.[94] One suggested anesthetic approach is the use of a thoracic epidural, but experience with this technique is limited.[95] The cardiologist typically tests the ICD near the end of the procedure, and testing may require deeper sedation or brief general anesthesia.[96] For testing, the ICD is programmed to deliver a shock on a T-wave, to induce ventricular fibrillation. If the new device works properly, it will discharge and defibrillate; if not, external pads are used for defibrillation. The shock is painful. Cardiologists usually wait 5 minutes after a test before performing a second test, although in patients with sicker hearts they may test only once or not at all. Personnel should be clear of any contact with the patient before electrical discharge to avoid getting shocked.

Protocol for Anesthesia for Defibrillator Implantation

A. Preprocedural assessment of the patient
1. Verify patient identity and procedure consent.
2. Assess airway, verify NPO status
3. Cardiac status
   a. Arrhythmias
   b. Left ventricular function
   c. Pacing, previous defibrillator
   d. Ischemic heart disease
   e. Congenital heart disease
4. Chest radiograph
5. Allergies and medication regimen
6. Laboratory results
7. Obtain consent for anesthesia
B. Airway checklist
1. Anesthesia machine checked out
2. Oxygen sources (wall/tank) verified
3. Suction available with Yankauer catheter
4. Mapleson circuit
5. Masks, soft bite blocks
6. Working end-tidal carbon dioxide monitor with gas sampling tubing
7. Emergency supplies
   a. Laryngoscopes
   b. Endotracheal tubes
   c. Stylets
   d. Laryngeal, oral, and nasal airways
C. Medication checklist
1. Etomidate or propofol
2. Succinylcholine
3. Midazolam
4. Fentanyl or remifentanil
5. Phenylephrine
6. Atropine
7. Ephedrine
8. Antibiotic (typically cefazolin, if the patient is not allergic)
D. Induction
1. Standard monitors (electrocardiograph, blood pressure cuff, pulse oximeter)
2. Confirm freely flowing intravenous line (preferably at least 18 gauge)
3. Confirm Yankauer suction, airway supplies, medications (listed earlier)
4. Pad and secure patient's arms, with attention to pressure points
5. "Cage" is helpful to protect patient's face, though may impede airway access
6. Supplemental oxygen to patient (mask or cannula), end-tidal carbon dioxide monitoring
7. Consider risk for fire from high oxygen concentration, electrocautery, and alcohol-based skin preparation
8. Give antibiotic
9. Usually mild-to-moderate intravenous sedation (midazolam, fentanyl, and/or low-dose propofol and/or remifentanil infusions) for device placement, to supplement local anesthetic infiltrated by cardiologist
E. If device is to be tested
1. Place soft bite block before device testing
2. Titrate intravenous agent to loss of consciousness (eyelash reflex) before testing
3. Notify cardiologist to proceed when titration is complete
4. Avoid contact with patient when shocks are delivered
5. Check pulse oximeter or carotid pulse after sinus rhythm is restored
6. Often testing will be repeated after 5 minutes

Protocol for Anesthesia for Defibrillator Implantation—cont'd

F. After the procedure
   1. Patient should be transported to cardiology recovery unit with appropriate monitors and oxygen.
   2. Appropriate report (including medications, fluid balance, etc.) must be made to the recovery nurse.

Potential complications of ICD placement include pneumothorax; tamponade, which can result from coronary sinus or cardiac perforation; and embolic events, such as a transient ischemic attack or stroke. These patients tend to have low ejection fractions, and putting them in and out of ventricular fibrillation can further compromise cardiac output. After the test, promptly check for a pulse to make sure that the patient has not suffered an episode of pulseless electrical activity.

Lead Extractions

Pacemaker or defibrillator leads may need to be removed because of infection, breakage, or other problems. Lead extraction carries a risk because of the potential for perforation of the heart or major blood vessel when the lead is removed. The difficulty in removing the lead often depends on the amount of scarring that holds the lead to the patient's tissue. The degree of scarring in turn depends on multiple factors, including how long the wire has been in place and the age of the patient. Younger patients scar faster and more thoroughly. The ease of extraction can range from simply pulling out a loose wire to the use of a laser to remove a wire surrounded by heavy scar tissue. The use of a laser indicates a higher risk for complications for a lead removal, and the electrophysiologist may prudently request that general anesthesia be given with an endotracheal tube. The electrophysiologist will typically place a femoral arterial line for continuous blood pressure measurement and a femoral venous line for access in case blood and vasopressors are required. Crossmatched blood and a rapid infuser, as well as surgical instruments and an echocardiographic machine, should be readily available.

Because of the potential for hemorrhage as a result of rupture of a blood vessel, this procedure is done in a cardiac or hybrid operating room at many institutions, although some institutions continue to perform lead extractions in the catheterization or electrophysiology laboratory. Regardless, a cardiothoracic surgical team should be on call for backup. Constant attention must be paid to the patient's arterial blood pressure during the lead extraction. A rapid fall in blood pressure may indicate a complication. Echocardiography is useful for determining the cause of hypotension, such as hypovolemia resulting from bleeding from a major vessel or tamponade from cardiac perforation. In case of a major bleed, the patient should go to the operating room immediately.

Protocol for Anesthesia for Lead Extraction

A. Preprocedural assessment of the patient
   1. Verify patient identity and procedure consent.
   2. Assess airway, verify NPO status
   3. Patient status
      a. Is the patient septic because of infected lead? If so, hemodynamic support?
      b. Left ventricular function
      c. Is the patient pacemaker-dependent?
      d. Ischemic heart disease
      e. Congenital heart disease
   4. Chest radiograph
   5. Allergies and medication regimen
   6. Laboratory results (starting hemoglobin and hematocrit, coagulation studies)
   7. Obtain consent for anesthesia
B. Airway checklist
   1. Anesthesia machine checked out
   2. Oxygen sources (wall/tank) verified
   3. Suction available with Yankauer catheter
   4. Mapleson circuit
   5. Working end-tidal carbon dioxide monitor with gas sampling tubing
   6. Appropriate-size endotracheal tube and mask
   7. Appropriate-size oral and nasal airways
   8. Stylet
   9. Laryngoscopes
   10. Laryngeal mask airways
   11. Temperature probe
C. Medication checklist
   1. Lidocaine
   2. Propofol or etomidate
   3. Neuromuscular blocker to facilitate intubation
   4. Anesthesia maintenance agent (e.g., inhaled)
   5. Phenylephrine
   6. Epinephrine
   7. Dopamine, dobutamine, and/or norepinephrine, depending on patient's condition
   8. Ephedrine
   9. Atropine
D. Induction
   1. Standard monitors (electrocardiograph, blood pressure cuff, pulse oximeter)
   2. Confirm freely flowing intravenous line (preferably at least 18 gauge)
   3. Confirm Yankauer suction, airway supplies, medications (listed above)
   4. Pad and secure patient's arms, with attention to pressure points
   5. Discuss anticipated ease of procedure with cardiologist; if the lead has been in a long time and the patient is young, extraction may be more difficult because of scarring, and general anesthesia with an endotracheal tube may be appropriate so that the airway is secured in case of hemodynamic collapse.
   6. In case of general anesthesia
      a. Standard induction is appropriate, subject to the patient's condition
      b. Intubate patient's trachea; cardiologist can check tube position fluoroscopically
      c. Insert temperature probe
E. Prepare for possible perforation of heart or major vessel
   1. Arterial and central venous lines
   2. Crossmatched blood and a rapid infuser
   3. Surgical backup, instruments
   4. Echocardiography machine

Continued

Protocol for Anesthesia for Lead Extraction—cont'd

F. Maintenance
1. Standard maintenance is appropriate
2. Monitor blood pressure closely; communicate with cardiologist immediately in case of decline
G. After extraction
1. Extubation may proceed when criteria have been met.
2. Patient should be transported to cardiology recovery unit with appropriate monitors and oxygen.
3. Appropriate report (including medications given, fluid balance, etc.) must be made to the recovery nurse.

The risk for major complications, such as myocardial avulsion, vascular tear, pneumothorax, hemothorax, pulmonary embolism, cardiac tamponade, arteriovenous fistula, and death, is approximately 1.9%. Other complications, including pericardial effusion, hematoma, venous thrombosis, and arrhythmia also may occur.

Noninvasive Programmed Stimulation

In the NIPS procedure, the cardiologists program the ICD to stimulate the patient's heart to see if ventricular tachycardia can be elicited and then determine whether the ICD fires appropriately. Anesthetic considerations are similar to those for cardioversion, although the patients usually have a more severe cardiomyopathy, and these procedures can be longer than simple cardioversion. In cardioversion, typically a single shock lasting a fraction of a second is all that is required, whereas a NIPS procedure can last for 20 minutes or more, while the electrophysiologist tries a variety of different patterns of electrical stimulation. Oxygen by face mask and short-acting intravenous agents are usually appropriate. Etomidate may be a better choice than propofol in patients with poor left ventricular function. Many electrophysiologists prefer to avoid use of intravenous lidocaine given before propofol or etomidate to reduce the burning sensation during injection, because lidocaine may affect the ventricular arrhythmia threshold.

Protocol for Anesthesia for Noninvasive Programmed Stimulations

A. Preprocedural assessment of the patient
1. Verify patient identity and procedure consent
2. Assess airway, verify NPO status
3. Cardiac evaluation
   a. Device
   b. Arrhythmia and ablation history
   c. Left ventricular function
   d. Ischemic heart disease
   e. Congenital heart disease
4. Allergies and medication (particularly antiarrhythmic) regimen
5. Laboratory and chest radiograph results
6. Obtain consent for anesthesia

Protocol for Anesthesia for Noninvasive Programmed Stimulations—cont'd

B. Airway checklist
1. Oxygen sources (wall/tank) verified
2. Suction available with Yankauer catheter
3. Mapleson circuit
4. Masks, soft bite blocks
5. Working end-tidal carbon dioxide monitor with gas sampling tubing
6. Emergency supplies
   a. Laryngoscopes, endotracheal tubes, stylets
   b. Laryngeal, oral, and nasal airways
C. Medication checklist
1. Etomidate or propofol
2. Emergency medications: succinylcholine, lidocaine, phenylephrine, epinephrine, atropine, ephedrine
D. Induction and maintenance
1. Standard monitors (electrocardiograph, blood pressure cuff, pulse oximeter)
2. Confirm freely flowing intravenous line (preferably at least 18 gauge)
3. Confirm Yankauer suction, airway supplies, medications (listed above)
4. Supplemental oxygen to patient (mask or cannula), end-tidal carbon dioxide monitoring
5. Place soft bite block
6. Titrate intravenous agent to loss of consciousness (eyelash reflex)
7. Notify cardiologist to proceed when titration is complete
8. Avoid contact with patient when shocks are delivered
9. Check pulse oximeter or carotid pulse after defibrillation if it occurs
10. Titrate additional intravenous anesthetic agent as needed until the procedure is completed
E. After the procedure, appropriate report (including medications given, fluid balance, etc.) must be made to the recovery nurse.

Postoperative Care and Pain Management

Anesthesia personnel should remain with the patient until the patient's care is transferred to the recovery nursing staff. Patients who use a continuous positive airway pressure machine for sleep apnea at home may benefit from using it in the recovery unit. Most patients having undergone femoral arterial cannulation will need to have supine bed rest for several hours. Considering that they have been in that position for some 6 to 12 hours, significant discomfort may result.

Many of the patients are in the electrophysiology laboratory for many hours, so those with preexisting back, shoulder, or joint ailments will often awaken in significant pain. In addition, the groin catheters removed after the patient emerges from anesthesia are another source for significant postprocedure pain. Therefore planning for postprocedure pain should begin before the patient enters the electrophysiology laboratory. Adequate padding of the neck, arms, back, knees, and heels will help reduce the pain from prolonged skeletal inactivity (see Figure 11-4). In addition, sensitivity to the level of postprocedure pain that many of these patients experience should direct the anesthetic management near the end of the procedure. Ketorolac 15 to 30 mg should be given routinely, if no renal or other contraindication exists. Intravenous acetaminophen 1 g should be considered for patients with normal liver function. In addition, because remifentanil is very short acting, consideration should be given to incorporating a longer-acting opioid, such as hydromorphone or morphine, as part of the emergence sequence. Finally, frequent postextubation assessments of the patient's pain level should be performed as the anesthetic agents continue to wear off.

Conclusion

The number of patients treated in the electrophysiology laboratory continues to grow nationwide. Improvements in noninvasive medical technology allow sick patients, who just a few years ago would have been excluded from care, to be treated effectively with decreased risk in the electrophysiology laboratory. Opinions[65,97-99] and practices[100] differ as to the extent to which anesthesiologists should be involved in cases in electrophysiology laboratories and whether those anesthesiologists should be cardiac anesthesiologists,[101] but as the procedures in that venue become more complex for patients who are sicker, the trend of increasing anesthesiology involvement will undoubtedly continue.

Acknowledgments

The authors thank Drs. David Callans, Lee Fleisher, and Sean Kennedy for their comments on a draft of this chapter.

References

1. Roger VL, Go AS, Lloyd-Jones DM, et al. Heart disease and stroke statistics 2011 update: a report from the American Heart Association. *Circulation*. 2011;123:e18–e209.
2. Bubien RS, Fisher GD, Gentzel JA, et al. NASPE expert consensus document: use of IV (conscious) sedation/analgesia by nonanesthesia personnel in patients undergoing arrhythmia specific diagnostic, therapeutic, and surgical procedures. *PACE*. 1998;21:375–385.
3. Calkins H, Brugada J, Packer DL, et al. HRS/EHRA/ECAS expert consensus statement on catheter and surgical ablation of atrial fibrillation: recommendations for personnel, policy, procedures and follow-up. *Heart Rhythm*. 2007;4:816–861.
4. Calkins H, Kuck KH, Cappato R, et al. 2012 HRS/EHRA/ECAS expert consensus statement on catheter and surgical ablation of atrial fibrillation: recommendations for patient selection, procedural techniques, patient management and follow-up, definitions, endpoints, and research trial design. *Heart Rhythm*. 2012;9:632–696.
5. DiBiase L, Conti S, Mohanty P, et al. General anesthesia reduces the prevalence of pulmonary vein reconnection during repeat ablation when compared with conscious sedation: results from a randomized study. *Heart Rhythm*. 2011;8:368–372.
6. Shillcutt SK, Schulte TE. Transesophageal echocardiography findings associated with transvenous lead extraction. *Anesth Analg*. 2012;115(6):1282–1285.
7. Kory P, Guevarra K, Mathew JP, et al. The impact of video laryngoscopy use during urgent endotracheal intubation in the critically ill. *Anesth Analg*. 2013;117(1):144–149.
8. Yan Z, Tanner JW, Lin D, et al. Airway trauma in a high patient volume academic cardiac electrophysiology laboratory center. *Anesth Analg*. 2013;116(1):112–117.
9. American Society of Anesthesiologists. Standards for basic anesthetic monitoring. Available at: http://www.asahq.org/For-Members/~/media/For%20Members/documents/Standards%20 Guidelines%20Stmts/Basic%20Anesthetic%20Monitoring%20 2011.ashx.
10. Renwick J, Kerr C, McTaggart R, Yeung J. Cardiac electrophysiology and conduction pathway ablation. *Can J Anaesth*. 1993;40(11):1053–1064.
11. Bosnjak ZJ, Kampine JP. Effects of halothane, enflurane, and isoflurane on the SA node. *Anesthesiology*. 1983;58(4):314–321.
12. Marshall BE, Longnecker DE. General anesthetics. In: Gilman AG, Rail TW, Nies AS, Taylor R, eds. *The pharmacological basis of therapeutics*. 8th ed. New York, NY: Permagon; 1990:285–310.
13. Riley DC, Schmeling WT, Al-Wathiqui MH, Kampine JP, Warltier DC. Prolongation of the QT interval by volatile anesthetics in chronically instrumented dog. *Anesth Analg*. 1988;67(8):741–749.
14. Atlee III JL, Alexander SC. Halothane effects on conductivity of the AV node and His-Purkinje system in the dog. *Anesth Analg*. 1977;56(3):378–386.
15. Eger II EI, Smith NT, Stoelting RK, et al. Cardiovascular effects of halothane in man. *Anesthesiology*. 1970;2(3):396–409.
16. Lynch III C, Vogel S, Sperelakis N. Halothane depression of myocardial slow action potentials. *Anesthesiology*. 1981;55(4):360–368.
17. Polic S, Atlee III JL, Laslo A, Kampine JP, Bosnjak ZJ. Anesthetics and automaticity in latent pacemaker fibers. II. Effects of halothane and epinephrine or norepinephrine on automaticity of dominant and subsidiary atrial pacemakers in the canine heart. *Anesthesiology*. 1991;75(2):298–304.
18. Reynolds AK. On the mechanism of myocardial sensitization to catecholamines by hydrocarbon anesthetics. *Can J Physiol Pharmacol*. 1984;62(2):183–198.
19. Maze M, Smith CM. Identification of receptor mechanism mediating epinephrine-induced arrhythmias during halothane anesthesia in the dog. *Anesthesiology*. 1983;59(4):322–326.
20. Gallagher JD, McClernan CA. The effects of halothane on ventricular tachycardia in intact dogs. *Anesthesiology*. 1991;75(5):866–875.
21. Erb TO, Kanter RJ, Hall JM, et al. Comparison of electrophysiologic effects of propofol and isoflurane-based anesthetics in children undergoing radiofrequency catheter ablation for supraventricular tachycardia. *Anesthesiology*. 2002;96(6):1386–1394.
22. Atlee 3rd JL, Yeager TS. Electrophysiologic assessment of the effects of enflurane, halothane, and isoflurane on properties affecting supraventricular re-entry in chronically instrumented dogs. *Anesthesiology*. 1989;71(6):941–952.
23. Blitt CD, Raessler KL, Wightman MA, et al. Atrioventricular conduction in dogs during anesthesia with isoflurane. *Anesthesiology*. 1979;50(3):210–212.
24. Skovsted P, Sapthavichaikul S. The effects of isoflurane on arterial pressure, pulse rate, autonomic nervous activity, and barostatic reflexes. *Can Anaesth Soc J*. 1977;24(3):304–314.
25. Lavoie J, Walsh EP, Burrows FA, et al. Effects of propofol or isoflurane anesthesia on cardiac conduction in children undergoing radiofrequency catheter ablation for tachydysrhythmias. *Anesthesiology*. 1995;82(4):884–887.
26. Pérez ER, Bartolomé FB, Carretero PS, et al. Electrophysiological effects of sevoflurane in comparison with propofol in children with Wolff-Parkinson-White syndrome. *Rev Esp Anestesiol Reanim*. 2008;55(1):26–31.
27. Sharpe MD, Cuillerier DJ, Lee JK, et al. Sevoflurane has no effect on sinoatrial node function or on normal atrioventricular and accessory pathway conduction in Wolff-Parkinson-White syndrome during alfentanil/midazolam anesthesia. *Anesthesiology*. 1999;90(1):60–65.
28. Whyte SD, Booker PD, Buckley DG. The effects of propofol and sevoflurane on the QT interval and transmural dispersion of repolarization in children. *Anesth Analg*. 2005;100(1):71–77.
29. Eisele JH, Smith NT. Cardiovascular effects of 40 percent nitrous oxide in man. *Anesth Analg*. 1972;51(6):956–963.
30. Smith NT, Eger 2nd EI, Stoelting RK, et al. The cardiovascular and sympathomimetic responses to the addition of nitrous oxide to halothane in man. *Anesthesiology*. 1970;32(5):410–421.
31. Lampe GH, Donegan JH, Rupp SM, et al. Nitrous oxide and epinephrine-induced arrhythmias. *Anesth Analg*. 1990;71(6):602–605.
32. Novalija E, Hogan QH, Kulier AH, et al. Effects of desflurane, sevoflurane and halothane on postinfarction spontaneous dysrhythmias in dogs. *Acta Anaesthesiol Scand*. 1998;42(3):353–357.
33. Sharpe MD, Dobkowski WB, Murkin JM, et al. The electrophysiologic effects of volatile anesthetics and sufentanil on the normal atrioventricular conduction system and accessory pathways in Wolff-Parkinson-White syndrome. *Anesthesiology*. 1994;80:63–70.

34. Thomson SJ, Yate PM. Bradycardia after propofol infusion. *Anaesthesia*. 1987;42(4):430.

35. Colson P, Barlet H, Roquefeuill B, Eledjam JJ. Mechanism of propofol bradycardia. *Anesth Analg*. 1988;67(9):906–907.

36. Guise PA. Asystole following propofol and fentanyl in an anxious patient. *Anaesth Intensive Care*. 1991;19(1):116–118.

37. Dorrington KL. Asystole with convulsion following a subanesthetic dose of propofol plus fentanyl. *Anaesthesia*. 1989;44(8):658–659.

38. Ebert TJ, Muzi M, Berens R, Goff D, Kampine JP. Sympathetic responses to induction of anesthesia in humans with propofol or etomidate. *Anesthesiology*. 1992;76:725–733.

39. Muñoz R, Goldberg ME, Cantillo J, Subramoni J, Nemiroff MS. Perioperative arrhythmias with a propofol-based anesthetic. *J Clin Anesth*. 1991;3(2):149–152.

40. Ikeno S, Akazawa S, Shimizu R, et al. Propofol does not affect the canine cardiac conduction system under autonomic blockade. *Can J Anaesth*. 1999;46(2):148–153.

41. Liu Q, Chen R, Quin C, et al. Propofol and arrhythmias: two sides of the coin. *Acta Pharmacol Sin*. 2011;32(6):817–823.

42. Pires LA, Haung SK, Wagshal AB, Kulkami RS. Electrophysiological effects of propofol on the normal cardiac conduction system. *Cardiology*. 1996;87(4):319–324.

43. Kamibayashi T, Hayashi Y, Sumikawa K, et al. Enhancement by propofol of epinephrine-induced arrhythmias in dogs. *Anesthesiology*. 1991;75(6):1035–1040.

44. Cullen PM, Turtle M, Prys-Roberts C, Way WL, Dye J. Effect of propofol anesthesia on baroreflex activity in humans. *Anesth Analg*. 1987;66(11):1115–1120.

45. Nathan AT, Antzelevitch C, Montenegro LM, Vetter VL. Case scenario: anesthesia-related cardiac arrest in a child with Timothy syndrome. *Anesthesiology*. 2012;117(5):1117–1126.

46. Gautret B, Schmitt H. Cardiac slowing induced by peripheral kappa-opiate receptor stimulation in rats. *Eur J Pharmacol*. 1984;102(1):159–163.

47. Maryniak JK, Bishop VA. Sinus arrest after alfentanil. *Br J Anaesth*. 1987;59(3):390–391.

48. Sebel PS, Bovill JG, van der Haven A. Cardiovascular effects of alfentanil anaesthesia. *Br J Anaesth*. 1982;54(11):1185–1190.

49. Schmeling WT, Bernstein JS, Vucins EJ, Cody R. Persistent bradycardia with episodic sinus arrest after sufentanil and vecuronium administration: successful treatment with isoproterenol. *J Cardiothorac Anesth*. 1990;4(1):89–94.

50. Pruett JK, Blair JR, Adams RJ. Cellular and subcellular actions of opioids in the heart. In: Estafanous FG, ed. *Opioids in anesthesia*. Boston: Butterworth-Heinemann; 1991.

51. Blair JR, Pruett JK, Introna RP, Adams RJ, Balser JS. Cardiac electrophysiologic effects of fentanyl and sufentanil in canine cardiac Purkinje fibers. *Anesthesiology*. 1989;71(4):565–570.

52. Dashwood MR, Spyer KM. Autoradiographic localization of alpha-adrenoceptors, muscarinic acetylcholine receptors and opiate receptors in the heart. *Eur J Pharmacol*. 1986;127(3):279–282.

53. Glass PS, Gan TJ, Howell S. A review of the pharmacokinetics and pharmacodynamics of remifentanil. *Anesth Analg*. 1999;89(4 suppl):S7–S14.

54. Yildirim V, Doganci S, Bolcal C, et al. Combination sedoanalgesia with remifentanil and propofol versus remifentanil and midazolam for elective cardioversion after coronary artery bypass grafting. *Adv Ther*. 2007;24(3):662–670.

55. Mandel JE, Hutchinson MD, Marchlinski FE. Remifentanil-midazolam sedation provides hemodynamic stability and comfort during epicardial ablation of ventricular tachycardia. *J Cardiovasc Electrophysiol*. 2010;22:464–466.

56. Leite SS, Firme EBP, Bevilaqua MS, Pereira LS, Atié J. Prospective study on the repercussions of low doses of remifentanil on sinoatrial function and in cardiac conduction and refractory period. *Rev Bras Anestesiol*. 2007;57(5):465–475.

57. Fujii K, Iranami H, Nakamura Y, Hatano Y. High dose remifentanil suppresses sinoatrial node conduction and sinus node automaticity in pediatric patients under propofol-based anesthesia. *Anesth Analg*. 2011;112(5):1169–1173.

58. Zaballos M, Jimeno C, Almendral J, et al. Cardiac electrophysiological effects of remifentanil: study in a closed-chest porcine model. *Br J Anaesth*. 2009;103(2):191–198.

59. Garofalo NA, Teixeira-Neto FJ, Schwartz DS, Vailati Mdo C, Steagall PV. Effects of the opioid remifentanil on the arrhythmogenicity of epinephrine in halothane-anesthetized dogs. *Can J Vet Res*. 2008;72(4):362–366.

60. Niksch A, Liberman L, Clapcich A, et al. Effects of remifentanil anesthesia on cardiac electrophysiologic properties in children undergoing catheter ablation of supraventricular tachycardia. *Pediatr Cardiol*. 2010;31(7):1079–1082.

61. Kim ES, Chang HW. The effects of a single bolus of remifentanil on corrected QT interval changes during sevoflurane induction. *Yonsei Med J*. 2011;52(2):333–338.

62. Borrat X, Troconiz IF, Valencia JF, et al. Modeling the influence of the A118G polymorphism in the *OPRM!* gene and the noxious stimulation on the synergistic relation between propofol and remifentanil. *Anesthesiology*. 2013;118(6):1395–1407.

63. Noseir RK, Ficke DJ, Kundu A, Arain SR, Ebert TJ. Sympathetic and vascular consequences from remifentanil in humans. *Anesth Analg*. 2003;96(6):1645–1650.

64. Michaloudis DG, Kanakoudis FS, Petrou AM, et al. The effects of midazolam or propofol followed by suxamethonium on the QT interval in humans. *Eur J Anaesthesiol*. 1996;13(4):364–368.

65. Trentman TL, Fassett SL, Mueller JT, Altemose GT. Airway interventions in the cardiac electrophysiology laboratory: a retrospective review. *J Cardiothorac Vasc Anesth*. 2009;23(6):841–845.

66. Mitchell AR, Chalil S, Boodhoo L, et al. Diazepam or midazolam for external DC cardioversion (the DORM Study). *Europace*. 2003;5(4):391–395.

67. Schulman MS, Edelmann R. Use of etomidate for elective cardioversion. *Anesthesiology*. 1988;68:656.

68. King S, Banker D. Etomidate as an antiarrhythmic. *Br J Anesth*. 2005;95(3):425.

69. Hammer GB, Drover DR, Cao H, et al. The effects of dexmedetomidine on cardiac electrophysiology in children. *Anesth Analg*. 2008;106(1):79–83.

70. Bhana N, Goa KL, McClellan KJ. Dexmedetomidine. *Drugs*. 2000;59(2):263–268.

71. Aho M, Erkola O, Kallio A, Scheinin H, Korttila K. Dexmedetomidine infusion for maintenance of anesthesia in patients undergoing abdominal hysterectomy. *Anesth Analg*. 1992;75:940–946.

72. Scheinin H, Jaakola ML, Sjövall S, et al. Intramuscular dexmedetomidine as premedication for general anesthesia: a comparative multicenter study. *Anesthesiology*. 1993;78(6):1065–1075.

73. Taittonen MT, Kirvelä OA, Aantaa R, Kanto JH. Effect of clonidine and dexmedetomidine premedication on perioperative oxygen consumption and haemodynamic state. *Br J Anaesth*. 1997;78(4):400–406.

74. Peden CJ, Cloote AH, Stratford N, Prys-Roberts C. The effect of intravenous dexmedetomidine premedication on the dose requirement of propofol to induce loss of consciousness in patients receiving alfentanil. *Anaesthesia*. 2001;56(5):408–413.

75. Harrah MD, Way WL, Katzung BG. The interaction of d-tubocurarine with antiarrhythmic drugs. *Anesthesiology*. 1970;33(4):406–410.

76. Saarnivaqara L, Klemola UM, Lindgren L. QT interval of the ECG, heart rate and arterial pressure using five non-depolarizing muscle relaxants for intubation. *Acta Anaesthesiol Scand*. 1988;32(8):623–628.

77. Hardy PA. Atracurium and bradycardia. *Anaesthesia*. 1985;40(5):504–405.

78. Cozanitis DA, Lindgren L, Rosenberg PH. Bradycardia in patients receiving atracurium or vecuronium in conditions of low vagal stimulation. *Anaesthesia*. 1989;44(4):303–305.

79. Chua J, Patel K, Neelankavil J, Mahajan A. Anesthetic management of electrophysiology procedures. *Curr Opin Anaesthesiol*. 2012;25(4):470–481.

80. Neumar RW, Otto CW, Link MS, et al. 2010 American Heart Association guidelines for cardiopulmonary resuscitation and emergency cardiovascular care science. VIII. Adult advanced cardiovascular life support. *Circulation*. 2010;122:S729–S767.

81. Faillace RT, Kaddaha R, Bikkina M, et al. The role of the out-of-operating room anesthesiologist in the care of the cardiac patient. *Anesthesiol Clin*. 2009;27(1):29–46.

82. Needleman M, Calkins H. The role of obesity and sleep apnea in atrial fibrillation. *Curr Opin Cardiol*. 2011;26(1):40–45.

83. Severgnini P, Selmo G, Lanza C, et al. Protective mechanical ventilation during general anesthesia for open abdominal surgery improves postoperative pulmonary function. *Anesthesiology*. 2013;118:1307–1321.

84. Goode JS, Taylor RL, Buffington CW, Klain M, Schwartzman D. High-frequency jet ventilation: utility in posterior left atrial catheter ablation. *Heart Rhythm*. 2006;3(1):13–19.

85. Hutchinson MD, Garcia FC, Mandel JE, et al. Efforts to enhance catheter stability improve atrial fibrillation ablation outcome. *Heart Rhythm*. 2013;10(3):347–353.

86. Gersak B, Pernat A, Robic B, Sinkovec M. Low rate of atrial fibrillation recurrence verified by implantable loop recorder monitoring following a convergent epicardial and endocardial ablation of atrial fibrillation. *J Cardiovasc Electrophysiol.* 2012;23:1059–1066.

87. Epstein AE, DiMarco JP, Ellenbogen KA, et al. ACA/AHA/HRS 2008 guidelines for device-based therapy of cardiac rhythm abnormalities: executive summary. *Circulation.* 2008;117:2820–2840.

88. Moss AJ, Zareba W, Hall WJ, et al. Prophylactic implantation of a defibrillator in patients with myocardial infarction and reduced ejection fraction. *N Engl J Med.* 2002;346(12):877–883.

89. Desai AS, Fang JC, Maisel WH, Baughman KL. Implantable defibrillators for the prevention of mortality in patients with nonischemic cardiomyopathy: a meta-analysis of randomized controlled trials. *J Am Med Assoc.* 2004;292(23):2874–2879.

90. Tung RT, Bajaj AK. Safety of implantation of a cardioverter-defibrillator without general anesthesia in an electrophysiology laboratory. *Am J Cardiol.* 1995;75(14):908–912.

91. Pacifico A, Cedillo-Salazar FR, Nasir Jr N, Doyle TK, Henry PD. Conscious sedation with combined hypnotic agents for implantation of implantable cardioverter-defibrillators. *J Am Coll Cardiol.* 1997;30(3):769–773.

92. Bollmann A, Kanuru NK, DeLurgio D, et al. Comparison of three different automatic defibrillator implantation approaches: pectoral implantation using conscious sedation reduces procedure times and cost. *J Intervent Card Electrophysiol.* 1997;1:221–225.

93. Manolis AS, Maounis T, Vassilikos V, Chiladakis J, Cokkinos DV. Electrophysiologist-implanted transvenous cardioverter defibrillators using local versus general anesthesia. *PACE.* 2000;23:96–105.

94. Conlay LA. Special concerns in the cardiac catheterization lab. *Int Anesthesiol Clin.* 2003;41:63–67.

95. Gilbert TB, Kent JL, Foster AH, Gold MR. Implantable cardioverter/defibrillator placement in a patient with amiodarone pulmonary toxicity under thoracic epidural anesthesia. *Anesthesiology.* 1993;79:608–611.

96. Shook DC, Savage RM. Anesthesia in the cardiac catheterization laboratory and electrophysiology laboratory. *Anesthesiol Clin.* 2009;27(1):47–56.

97. Geiger MJ, Wase A, Kearney MM, Brandon MJ, Kent V, et al. Evaluation of the safety and efficacy of deep sedation for electrophysiology procedures administered in the absence of an anesthetist. *PACE.* 1997;20(7):1808–1814.

98. Kezerashvili A, Fisher JD, DeLaney J, et al. Intravenous sedation for cardiac procedures can be administered safely and cost-effectively by non-anesthesia personnel. *J Interv Card Electrophysiol.* 2008;21(1):43–51.

99. Goldner BG, Baker J, Accordino A, et al. Electrical cardioversion of atrial fibrillation or flutter with conscious sedation in the age of cost containment. *Am Heart J.* 1998;136(6):961–964.

100. Gaitan BD, Trentman TL, Fassett SL, Mueller JT, Altemose GT. Sedation and analgesia in the cardiac electrophysiology laboratory: a national survey of electrophysiologists investigating the who, how, and why? *J Cardiothorac Vasc Anesth.* 2011;25:647–659.

101. Elkassabany NM, Mandel JE. Con: a general anesthesiologist with a certain skill set is qualified to provide services in the interventional cardiology and electrophysiology laboratory. *J Cardiothorac Vasc Anesth.* 2011;25:557–558.

12 Anesthesia for Cardioversion

MAX KANEVSKY

Direct-current cardioversion is a common cardiological procedure, consisting of delivering an electric shock to the patient's heart with the goal of restoring normal sinus rhythm. The common indication for the procedure is atrial fibrillation or flutter and less commonly other supraventricular arrhythmias or ventricular tachycardia. The shock is usually delivered by a pair of conductive pads applied to the patient's skin on the anterior and posterior chest or, if the patient already has an implanted cardioverter-defibrillator (ICD), by discharge from the internal device. In either case, the electric shock is painful and provokes anxiety in conscious patients. An anesthetic is usually administered in conjunction with the cardioversion. The main challenge to the anesthesiologist involved with a cardioversion is that although the procedure is simple and short, the patient often has comorbid cardiac and pulmonary conditions that require careful titration of anesthetic depth and duration against circulatory and respiratory embarrassment. Transesophageal echocardiogram (TEE) is often obtained just before direct-current cardioversion to discern the presence of a left atrial (LA) thrombus, which may be dislodged by the shock or subsequent resumption of synchronized atrial contractions. Both procedures are performed under the same anesthetic at many institutions, significantly extending its length and the likelihood of hypotension, hypoventilation, or oxygen desaturation episodes.

Cardioversion became a method of restoring normal sinus rhythm in the early 1960s after Lown and colleagues[1] published a report of successful treatment of patients with atrial fibrillation with a synchronized direct-current shock by a device they termed a cardioverter. Their innovation featured the synchronization of the discharge to the R-wave of the electrocardiogram (ECG) to avoid inducing ventricular fibrillation during the vulnerable portion of the cardiac cycle.[2] In the years since, electric cardioversion has been accepted for use as a treatment of all cardiac arrhythmias except ventricular fibrillation, which requires asynchronous defibrillation. More recently, devices using biphasic current waveform have supplanted the older monophasic cardioverters, allowing greater success rates at lower energies.[3] TEE has an excellent ability to visualize the left atrium and atrial appendage in detail to exclude the presence of atrial thrombus. Such information is valuable in patients with symptomatic arrhythmia or hemodynamic compromise but uncertain duration of atrial fibrillation and inadequate state of anticoagulation. For this reason, TEE extended the therapeutic reach of cardioversion to patients who would otherwise face a delay in treatment of several weeks to establish proper anticoagulation.[4] The proportion of TEE-guided cardioversions is growing and now exceeds 30% in some large centers.[5]

Over the last half century, the majority of intravenous sedative-hypnotic drugs, alone and in combination, have been used for procedural sedation and anesthesia in conjunction with direct-current cardioversion with or without TEE. Overall, anesthetic goals have remained the same—elimination of pain from the shock and blunting of recall of this unpleasant event. Early observations[6,7] led to speculation whether electric shock might be tolerated by patients without anesthesia, but subsequent experience convinced physicians this was not the case. Considering the need in many patients for repeat cardioversions over their lifetime, the anxiety engendered by recalling a prior painful shock likely would act as a deterrent to obtaining the necessary treatment. Many patients with atrial dysrhythmias currently receive cardioversion on an outpatient basis, on a prearranged date after a 3- to 4-week period of anticoagulant therapy, and with emphasis on the briefest duration of preprocedure stay and prompt discharge thereafter. In this setting, sedative premedication is usually impractical, the use of all but the shortest-acting opiates is inadvisable, and neuromuscular blockade is contraindicated. Therefore the intravenous anesthetics suitable for the procedure are the short-acting barbiturate methohexital, etomidate, and, most commonly today, propofol. However, prospective studies supporting a decisive advantage for any of these agents during cardioversion are lacking.[8]

Preoperative Assessment

In addition to the usual preanesthetic history, full review of systems, and a physical examination, several issues typically need to be addressed. First, the anesthesiologist should inquire about prior cardioversion attempts and the patient's satisfaction with the associated anesthetic. Old anesthetic records are a good guide to selecting anesthetic medications and dosages and can help anticipate postprocedure cardiorespiratory problems. Physicians' stated concern for suppressing recall is reassuring to most patients, but a possibility of recall should be frankly discussed with patients with complex cardiac or pulmonary problems.

Second, patients should be questioned about their compliance with an anticoagulation regimen, if any. For patients on warfarin, the absence of weekly International Normalized Ratio (INR) measurements in the therapeutic range (usually 2-3 or over >2.5 in the presence of mechanical heart valves[9]) over 3 to 4 weeks is an indication for pre-cardioversion TEE to exclude LA thrombus or sludge. Many patients on newer anticoagulants will not have a record of INR measurements and do not need TEE if they are compliant. These medications include the oral direct thrombin inhibitor dabigatran (Pradaxa)[10] and direct factor Xa inhibitors rivaroxaban (Xarelto)[11] and apixaban.[12]

Third, a careful review of medications may point to potential issues arising during the procedure. Many patients will be on antiarrhythmic and heart rate control medications. Among them, those taking calcium-channel and beta-adrenergic blockers will exhibit an early tendency toward hypotension and bradycardia with the restoration of sinus rhythm. Patients in atrial fibrillation on the newer antiarrhythmic drug dronedarone (Multaq) also may become bradycardic after cardioversion. Additionally, concern exists over QT prolongation if these patients are given some of the common antiemetic drugs, such as ondansetron (Zofran).

Fourth, a history of cardiomyopathy, congestive heart failure, ischemic heart disease, or dyspnea with mild exertion should alert the anesthesiologist to the need for a cautious induction of anesthesia with ample time for circulating the drug between incremental bolus doses. Patient history of obstructive sleep apnea correlates with the need to provide positive-pressure mask ventilation during the anesthesia. Head and neck and airway examinations will predict the difficulty of mask ventilation and prepare the physician for a potentially challenging intubation.

Necessary laboratory data include a recent potassium level; significant hypokalemia will need correction before cardioversion. If the patient is on warfarin, the INR over the preceding 3 to 4 weeks should be reviewed. In patients on digoxin (now uncommon), its levels must not exceed therapeutic range because of concern for cardioversion triggering ventricular tachyarrhythmias. The patient's electrocardiographic activity on the monitor should be reviewed just before starting the anesthetic. Not infrequently, patients can undergo spontaneous reversion to sinus rhythm during preparations for cardioversion.

Intraoperative Management

Cardioversions take place in established outpatient procedure areas, emergency wards, and at the bedside of hospitalized patients. Anesthesia machines typically are not available in these locations, and the anesthesiologist is usually expected to bring in the supplies and medications—both those likely to be used during the procedure and those reserved for emergency treatment. Regardless of location, the patient should be monitored according to the American Society of Anesthesiologists guidelines. Cuff blood pressure measurements must be reliably obtained. Insertion of an arterial line is rarely necessary. Audible variable-tone pulse oximetry is most helpful, because a monitor may not be directly facing the anesthesiologist. A primary and a backup supply of oxygen and a working suction line must be present. A single reliable intravenous catheter is sufficient for the procedure. If multiple clinical services are involved—for example, one for TEE and another performing the cardioversion—all practitioners must be on hand before induction of anesthesia to minimize the duration of anesthetic.

Echocardiographers skilled in TEE often have a routine for topical administration of local anesthetics in the oropharynx and conscious sedation before insertion of the TEE probe. For TEE expected to be followed immediately by a cardioversion, the anesthesiologist has two alternatives. The first is the topical and conscious sedation routine of the echocardiographer during the TEE portion, followed by the induction of a brief general anesthetic for the cardioversion portion. The advantages of this approach are potentially avoiding general anesthesia altogether, if TEE finding of a thrombus precludes immediate cardioversion, and minimizing the duration and depth of general anesthesia in high-risk patients. Patients with significantly compromised myocardial function, pulmonary diseases, morbid obesity, a history of obstructive sleep apnea, and especially the combination of several of these conditions, will benefit from the first approach. The second approach is the induction of a general anesthetic of somewhat longer duration and sufficient depth to cover both portions of the combined procedure. Patients with intact cardiac and pulmonary reserve and reassuring airway features are best served by receiving general anesthesia from the beginning, because this option is more comfortable to the patient, it does not impair protective airway reflexes during recovery secondary to topical anesthesia of the tongue and hypopharynx, and the procedure is briefer and less labor-intensive.

For direct-current cardioversion, as for all surgical procedures, a time-out protocol is a useful tool for avoiding preventable errors in treatment. At time-out, the patient and procedure are identified, all staff make their introductions, and the presence of adequate rescue supplies is confirmed. For both external and internal (by ICD) cardioversion, positioning is the same: conductive pads are placed anteriorly and posteriorly (or laterally) on the patient's chest, such that the vector of the current passes maximally through the atria (for atrial fibrillation or flutter); the patient is positioned supine, with all pressure points padded; and the arms are lightly tucked next to the body to avoid being thrown in the air by the energy of the shock.

General anesthesia is induced, after several minutes of thorough preoxygenation by tight-fitting mask at fraction of inspired oxygen (FiO_2) 1.0, by gradual titration of an intravenous hypnotic agent, typically propofol (initial bolus dose 1 mg/kg). Further 10- to 20-mg boluses of propofol may be given until the eyelash reflex is abolished. These are timed at longer intervals for patients with impaired myocardial performance. Patient readiness for the shock (or TEE probe introduction, if done under the same general anesthetic) can be ascertained by an absence of response to a firm mandibular thrust. If precardioversion TEE is performed under general anesthesia, the examination is typically brief and focused on excluding LA thrombus. The midesophageal two-chamber view (near 90 degrees) usually affords the best visualization of the left atrial appendage, but additional views should be sought by changing the probe angle from 0 to 120 degrees and by withdrawing and advancing the probe to scan the full height of the left atrium. The finding of spontaneous echo contrast ("smoke") in the left atrium and measuring pulsed-wave Doppler velocities less than 40 cm/second in the LA appendage further increase the suspicion for thrombus or sludge.

Once the patient is sufficiently deeply anesthetized and the decision is made to proceed with the cardioversion, the device's capacitor is charged and everyone at the bedside is reminded to stay clear and not touch the patient. The only exception is the person who will (optionally) apply firm pressure to the anterior chest pad through a dry towel, which serves to decrease the chest wall impedance and enable higher energy delivery to the myocardium for a given cardioverter setting. If the anesthesiologist is providing positive-pressure ventilation to the patient, the device discharge should take place after allowing a full exhalation to minimize impedance due to pulmonary air. The presence of a groan or a grimace in the patient receiving a shock, while often disconcerting to the physicians and nurses present at cardioversion, does not correlate with the recall of the event.[13] After the direct-current shock, the patient's ECG is closely monitored for the return of sinus rhythm. Failure to convert may necessitate another attempt at a higher energy setting or with a different pad position. In this case, care must be taken to provide adequate respiratory support between the shocks, assess hemodynamic stability, and reconfirm the depth of anesthesia before proceeding.

If cardioversion is successful, the uncomfortable step of removing the conductive pads is best performed while the patient is still under general anesthesia. Whereas some patients will maintain a patent airway and spontaneous respirations under adequate general anesthesia, a large proportion will need maneuvers to open the airway and require intermittent positive-pressure ventilation. This is quite problematic during the TEE portion of the procedure, when bag-mask ventilation of the patient is not an option. The three-pronged approach to this problem is to (1) thoroughly preoxygenate the patient; (2) communicate to the echocardiographer the need for a speedy, highly focused examination; and (3) use an oral airway device compatible with TEE. Especially promising are the multifunctional devices now becoming available that combine the features of a bite block, an oral airway, and a conduit for oxygen insufflation. The use of a nasopharyngeal airway is relatively contraindicated because of the possibility of epistaxis resulting from the anticoagulated state in most patients.

Postoperative Course

The cardioversion is, by itself, very brief, and therefore the induction medications, with minimal repeated boluses, will provide for the maintenance of anesthesia and have a strong bearing on the postoperative course. The most common challenge to the anesthesiologist is to manage cardiac depression in the wake of general anesthesia, exacerbated by temporary myocardial stunning as a result of the direct-current shock. The foundation for a stable postoperative course and timely discharge is laid by the judicious administration of a short-acting hypnotic drug, taking into account the patient's cardiopulmonary reserve. Immediately after cardioversion, the first step is to ascertain an appropriate rhythm and rate on the monitor. New-onset ventricular tachyarrhythmias must be treated according to the Advanced Cardiac Life Support protocols. Sinus bradycardia may initially emerge after cardioversion. Typically, an improved heart rate response occurs spontaneously; if delayed, it can be obtained with a dose of the vagolytic drug glycopyrrolate of 0.2 to 0.4 mg intravenously. Patients with pacemakers, particularly ICDs, should have their device interrogated after cardioversion for possible malfunction.[14] If the patient's heart rhythm and rate are reassuring, hypotension often will resolve in response to an administration of an intravenous fluid bolus of normal saline 250 mL, because many patients are hypovolemic from fasting. A steep head-up position should be avoided because it impedes venous return and exacerbates hypovolemia. Until fully awake, in many patients the vasomotor tone may be low, worsening hypotension. Treat cautiously with a vasopressor (e.g., phenylephrine 50 to 100 mcg). Note that with phenylephrine, sinus bradycardia may worsen unless already treated with a vagolytic. Infrequently, high-energy shocks produce significant myocardial stunning and globally depressed contractility. This may be assessed rapidly in unstable patients with transthoracic echo (TTE) if the machine is still at the bedside. A single dose of the indirect-acting inotrope ephedrine 5 to 10 mg intravenously will support cardiac output and blood pressure during myocardial recovery from stunning. Support the patient's airway and breathing until full wakeup to ensure optimal myocardial oxygen delivery.

Emergence from general anesthesia is usually rapid in neurologically intact patients given only a short-acting hypnotic without premedication. The areas of concern for the anesthesiologist are to ensure a stable cardiac rhythm and hemodynamics, which are a precondition for a speedy wakeup. In patients who are unexpectedly very slow to wake or emerge with new abnormal neurological findings, the physician must suspect a neurological event resulting from cerebral embolization of an intracardiac thrombus. Stroke specialists must be contacted immediately and stroke workup initiated. Most patients will experience only mild, if any, myalgia from the cardioversion, making opioid administration unnecessary and counterproductive to the goal of rapid emergence.

Conclusion

Most anesthesiologists will be called on to care for a patient who is to have a cardioversion. Careful preparation, including thoughtful preoperative examination, adequate monitoring, and judicious selection of drugs, help ensure successful treatment of the patient.

References

1. Lown B, Perlroth MG, Kaidbey S, Abe T, Harken DE. "Cardioversion" of atrial fibrillation: a report on the treatment of 65 episodes in 50 patients. *N Engl J Med.* 1963;269:325–331.
2. Lown B, Amarasingham R, Neuman J. New method for terminating cardiac arrhythmias: use of synchronized capacitor discharge. *JAMA.* 1962;182:548–555.
3. Mittal S, Ayati S, Stein KM, et al. Transthoracic cardioversion of atrial fibrillation: comparison of rectilinear biphasic versus damped sine wave monophasic shocks. *Circulation.* 2000;101(11):1282–1287.
4. Grewal GK, Klosterman TB, Shrestha K, et al. Indications for TEE before cardioversion for atrial fibrillation: implications for appropriateness criteria. *JACC Cardiovasc Imaging.* 2012;5(6):641–648.
5. Yarmohammadi H, Klosterman T, Grewal G, et al. Transesophageal echocardiography and cardioversion trends in patients with atrial fibrillation: a 10-year survey. *J Am Soc Echocardiogr.* 2012;25(9):962–968.
6. Lown B, Bey SK, Perlroth MG, Abe T. cardioversion of ectopic tachycardias. *Am J Med Sci.* 1963;246:257–264.
7. Usubiaga JE, Sardinas AA. Cardioversion and the anesthesiologist: anesthesia and analgesia. 1970;49(5):818–826.
8. Wood J, Ferguson C. Best evidence topic report: procedural sedation for cardioversion. *Emerg Med J.* 2006;23(12):932–934.
9. Fuster V, Ryden LE, Cannom DS, et al. 2011 ACCF/AHA/HRS focused updates incorporated into the ACC/AHA/ESC 2006 guidelines for the management of patients with atrial fibrillation: a report of the American College of Cardiology Foundation/American Heart Association Task Force on practice guidelines. *Circulation.* 2011;123(10):e269–e367.

10. Connolly SJ, Ezekowitz MD, Yusuf S, et al. Dabigatran versus warfarin in patients with atrial fibrillation. *N Engl J Med*. 2009;361(12):1139–1151.

11. Patel MR, Mahaffey KW, Garg J, et al. Rivaroxaban versus warfarin in nonvalvular atrial fibrillation. *New Engl J Med*. 2011;365(10):883–891.

12. Granger CB, Alexander JH, McMurray JJ, et al. Apixaban versus warfarin in patients with atrial fibrillation. *New Engl J Med*. 2011;365(11):981–992.

13. Swann A, Williams J, Fatovich DM. Recall after procedural sedation in the emergency department. *Emerg Med J*. 2007;24(5):322–324.

14. Crossley GH, Poole JE, Rozner MA, et al. The Heart Rhythm Society (HRS)/American Society of Anesthesiologists (ASA) expert consensus statement on the perioperative management of patients with implantable defibrillators, pacemakers and arrhythmia monitors: facilities and patient management. Document was developed as a joint project with the American Society of Anesthesiologists (ASA), and in collaboration with the American Heart Association (AHA), and the Society of Thoracic Surgeons (STS). *Heart Rhythm*. 2011;8(7):1114–1154.

13 High-Frequency Ventilation for Respiratory Immobilization

JEFF E. MANDEL

As imaging technology improves, it is increasingly possible to perform procedures with noninvasive or minimally invasive techniques that would have once required an operating room. Specialized suites such as cardiac electrophysiology, interventional radiology, and radiation oncology have arisen to support these new approaches. A common feature of these techniques is the desire for a motionless field that allows the proceduralist to perform his or her tasks. As anesthesiologists, we are called on to assist in providing immobility. Although lack of voluntary movement is easily produced with general anesthesia, safely eliminating respiratory movement for extended periods requires high-frequency ventilation (HFV).

This chapter will review the physics and physiology of HFV, with emphasis on the most commonly employed modality—high-frequency jet ventilation (HFJV). It will discuss the practical aspects of anesthetic management and examine some of the previous uses of HFV in non–operating room anesthesia (NORA). Finally, it will consider some of the emerging areas of use of the technique.

Uses of High-Frequency Ventilation for Respiratory Immobilization

Respiration imparts motion to numerous structures that proceduralists wish to maintain in their crosshairs. One of the earliest examples is extracorporeal shockwave lithotripsy. The initial reports were presented as American Society of Anesthesiologists abstracts,[1,2] but subsequent reports provided greater detail and demonstrated significantly lower stone movement and shock requirements in contrast to conventional mechanical ventilation[3] and spontaneous ventilation.[4] Canty and Dhara[5] described successful use of HFJV by a laryngeal mask airway (LMA).[5] The applicability of HFJV with narrow blast path lithotripters was described by our group.[6] Although it is clear from multiple reports that stone movement is markedly reduced and permits stone fragmentation with fewer shocks, the full implications of this have not been studied. It is known that renal oxidative stress is correlated with shock wave number,[7] but no studies have addressed whether HFJV results in less renal injury.

Another important application of respiratory immobilization is in pulmonary vein isolation for atrial fibrillation. The technique was first described by Goode et al.[8]

We adopted the technique at the University of Pennsylvania in 2007 and have expanded our practice to over 500 cases annually. In an analysis of the impact of measures to improve catheter stability,[9] 100 consecutive patients were identified in three groups—our baseline practice, the addition of steerable sheaths and electroanatomical mapping, and the addition of HFJV. The addition of all three measures improved freedom from atrial fibrillation at 1 year from 52% to 74%, as depicted in Figure 13-1. This improvement was seen despite significant increases in body mass index, atrial dimension, the proportion of persistent versus paroxysmal atrial fibrillation, all of which are independent predictors of failure of atrial fibrillation ablation.

HFJV was also associated with a significant decrease in fluoroscopy time. HFJV has been embraced by the electrophysiology community. More than half of the Monsoon ventilators sold in the United States since 2010 have been placed in electrophysiology laboratories (Travis Schaztberger, Susquehana Micro, personal communication, 2011), suggesting that the technique is becoming more prevalent.

Imaging of the coronary arteries and pulmonary circulation can be affected by respiratory motion. We reported a case in which HFJV was used to eliminate respiratory motion in a patient whose respiration was too chaotic to permit imaging of the coronary arteries.[10] This technique may hold promise for computed tomography (CT) and magnetic resonance angiography; although not approved for use in the United States, the Hayek MRI-RTX system (United Hayek Medical Industries) is available in Europe.

Respiratory motion may affect the cerebral circulation as well. Chen et al[11] described a case in which respiratory motion made coiling of a cerebral aneurysm problematic and suggested that HFJV may have been beneficial.

Liver movement also can be problematic during ablative procedures. Yin et al[12] demonstrated a 75% reduction in movement of implanted clips in the livers of dogs with HFJV in contrast to conventional ventilation. Fritz et al[13] implanted gold markers in proximity to liver tumors in 10 patients and demonstrated that motion was restricted to 3 mm during HFJV. Biro et al[14] reported use of HFJV to minimize tumor movement during CT-guided radiofrequency ablation of hepatic metastases and also found a 75% reduction in movement from 1.2 cm to 3 mm, in contrast to positive-pressure ventilation. This group also reported a significant reduction in fluoroscopic exposure during radiofrequency ablation of hepatic and renal masses using HFJV rather than conventional ventilation.[15] HFJV is not as commonly employed during ablation of liver masses, although it is clearly an area poised for growth.

Finally, the lung is the organ most affected by respiratory motion. Lara-Guerra et al,[16] in an ex vivo porcine lung model, demonstrated equivalent detection of artificial lesions averaging 6 mm with HFJV in contrast to inflation to 20 cm H_2O or total deflation. Fritz et al[17] found a 25% reduction in planned treatment volume for stereotactic irradiation of small lung lesions with HFJV in contrast to spontaneous ventilation. With advances in technologies such as stereotactic body radiation therapy and proton beam therapy, reduction of respiratory motion in radiation oncology is another promising area.

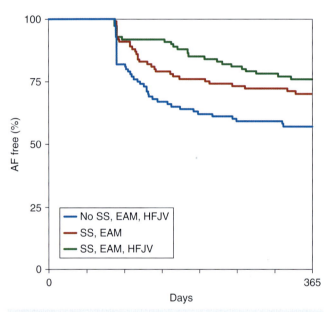

Figure 13-1 Kaplan-Meir survival plot for freedom from atrial fibrillation. *Blue* depicts baseline practice (conscious sedation without steerable sheaths or electroanatomical mapping), *red* indicates the addition of steerable sheaths and electroanatomical mapping, and *green* shows the addition of high-frequency jet ventilation.

Types of Ventilators

Respiratory rates above 60 breaths per minute are considered to constitute HFV.[18] Although conventional anesthesia ventilators can deliver rates of 30 breaths per minute, corrugated anesthesia circuits are not capable of transmitting higher rates, because most of the tidal volume simply expands the circuit rather than being delivered to the patient. Small variations in airway resistance and lung compliance will alter the fraction of delivered gas that reaches the patient, making consistent ventilation at high respiratory rates with conventional systems problematic. The following types of HFV were developed to address this issue:

1. *High-frequency jet ventilators.* These ventilators use a high-pressure source, typically the oxygen supply line, to generate a brief pulse of high-velocity gas during inspiration with expiration typically being passive. The Acutronic Monsoon Universal Ventilator (Susquehanna Micro, Windsor, Pa.) (Figure 13-2) is an example of this class of ventilator.
2. *Dual-frequency jet ventilators.* This HFJV and low-frequency jet[19] modality provides more efficient carbon dioxide elimination but causes larger fluctuations in lung volume. The Carl Reiner TwinStream ventilator (Wien, Austria) (Figure 13-3) is an example of this class of ventilator. It has never been marketed in the United States.
3. *High-frequency oscillators.* Oscillators use a piston or loudspeaker to create a bidirectional flow in the airway. The Sensormedics 3100B (CareFusion, San Diego, Calif.) (Figure 13-4) is an example of this class of ventilator. Although this ventilator has been employed in NORA settings, the higher cost of consumables may be a barrier to wide acceptance.
4. *High-frequency percussive ventilators.* The Percussionaire line of ventilators (Sandpoint Idaho) (Figure 13-5) uses a valve termed the Phasitron to create high-frequency oscillations that are superimposed on conventional volume control, principally for lung recruitment.[20]

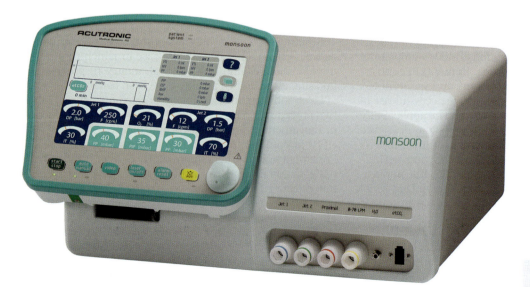

Figure 13-2 The Acutronic Monsoon 3 Universal Ventilator.

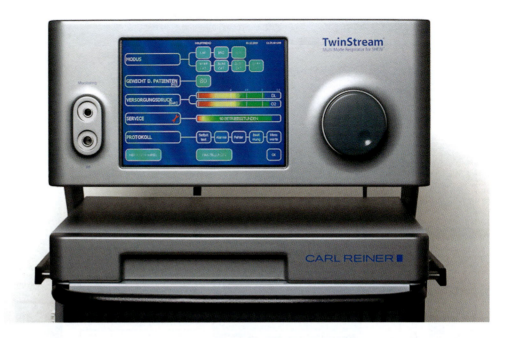

Figure 13-3 Carl Reiner Twin-Stream ventilator.

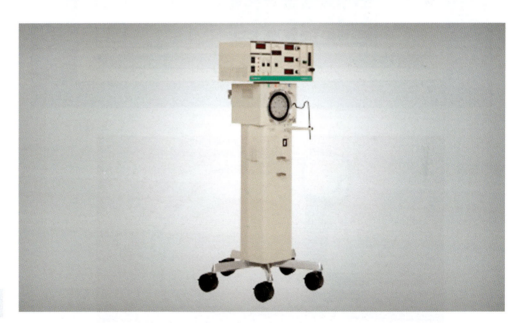

Figure 13-4 Sensormedics 3100B ventilator.

5. *Negative-pressure high-frequency oscillators.* These ventilators use an external shell with an oscillating pressure imposed into the space surrounding the patient's chest, as was done with the "iron lung" but at high frequencies. The Hayek RTX oscillator is an example of this class of ventilator.

The initial focus of HFV was in care of patients with acute respiratory distress syndrome (ARDS), and devices such as the Percussionaire that are well suited to alveolar recruitment may be ill-suited to respiratory immobilization because they impose slow phasic changes in lung volume. Another early application was in tubeless ventilation during laryngotracheal surgery. Devices employing modalities such as superimposed HFJV to improve the efficiency of carbon dioxide elimination produce tidal oscillations in lung volume. Respiratory immobilization exists to minimize changes in lung volume, thus discussion of HFV will focus on the most commonly employed modality for lung immobilization—HFJV.

The following types of jet ventilators have been developed:

1. *Manually operated pneumatic devices.* The Sanders injector is a manually operated valve with pressure reduction that is connected to a high-pressure source such as wall oxygen or an oxygen cylinder. VBM Medical manufactures the Manuject III (Noblesville, Ind.) (Figure 13-6), which is approved for "transtracheal ventilation in specific emergency situations of upper airway obstruction, used in conjunction with a transtracheal catheter, or a cricothyrotomy needle, which is inserted through the

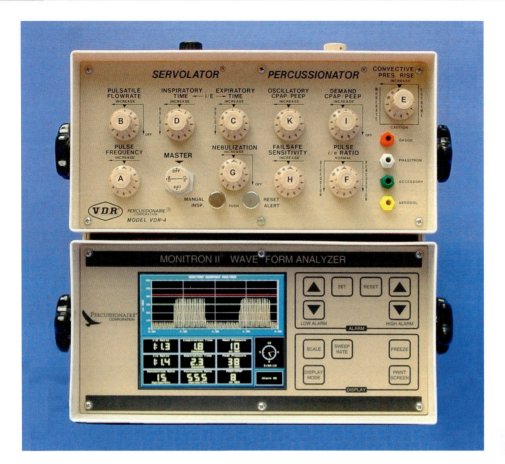

Figure 13-5 The Percussionaire VBR-4 ventilator.

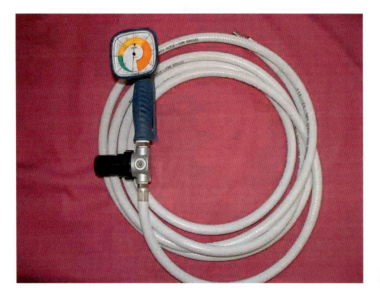

Figure 13-6 The VBM Manuject III.

cricothyroid membrane."* Although it is possible to use a Sanders injector as a high-frequency device, use beyond a few minutes is challenging, and producing stable lung volumes is difficult.

2. *Fluidic valve devices.* Fluidic valves were used in early ventilators such as the Bird Mark II, now produced by JD Medical (Phoenix, Arizona), shown in Figure 13-7.

All that is necessary is a source of compressed gas. The ventilator consists of two parallel channels, with one output channel of each valve being connected to the switching channel of the other. This creates a bistable oscillator. Tuning is achieved by adjusting three valves that control overall flow and the flow through the two switching channels. Achieving consistent results with fluidic valved devices can be challenging, but the portability and low cost of the device may be a compelling factor.

*See http://www.accessdata.fda.gov/cdrh_docs/pdf11/K112783.pdf. Accessed April 21, 2013.

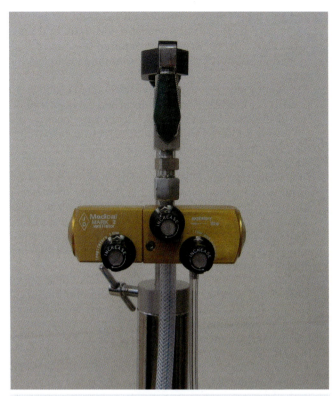

Figure 13-7 The JD Medical Mark 2 ventilator.

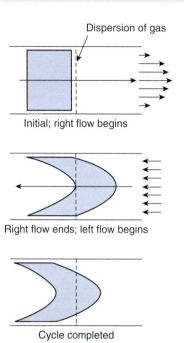

Figure 13-8 Axial dispersion of gas in an airway. An initial plug of gas in the airway *(upper panel)* is carried to the right by a high-velocity jet, resulting in a parabolic profile *(center panel)*. Exhalation carries gas to the left in a plug flow pattern *(bottom panel)*, resulting in opposing flow within a single airway. (Redrawn from Chang HK. Mechanisms of gas transport during ventilation by high-frequency oscillation. *J Appl Physiol.* 1984;56[3]:553-563.)

3. *Electronically controlled devices.* Electronically controlled devices, such as the Acutronic Monsoon Universal Ventilator (see Figure 13-2), use a microprocessor-controlled solenoid valve. The device has built-in safety features to prevent barotrauma and has the capacity to add humidity to the inspired gas.

Physics of High-Frequency Jet Ventilation

The attraction of HFJV is its ability to eliminate carbon dioxide with lung excursions that are close to the anatomical dead space. Carbon dioxide is eliminated by the following combination of effects[21]:

1. *Convection.* Convection is simple bulk flow of gas back and forth down the large airways. It is responsible for the majority of carbon dioxide elimination in frequencies employed clinically.
2. *Axial dispersion.* Axial dispersion is the result of different flow profiles during inspiration and expiration that permit net flow to occur in opposite directions within the airway, as illustrated in Figure 13-8. These effects make the actual dead space smaller than the anatomical dead space.
3. *Pendelluft.* Pendelluft is the to-and-fro movement of gas between adjacent lung segments of different time constants. It brings carbon dioxide closer to the large airways, where convection can remove it, as illustrated in Figure 13-9.
4. *Diffusion.* Diffusion is the result of Brownian motion of gas and will also bring carbon dioxide closer to the large airways where convection can remove it.

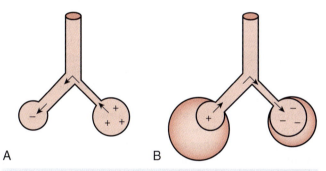

Figure 13-9 When two adjacent lung units are ventilated at high rates, flow is dominated by resistance. **A** represents early inspiration, and the unit on the left has emptied more completely because of its larger bronchiole and is filled partially by the unit on the right. **B** represents end inspiration, and the unit on the left has completely filled and now empties into the smaller unit on the left. (Redrawn from Chang HK. Mechanisms of gas transport during ventilation by high-frequency oscillation. *J Appl Physiol.* 1984;56[3]:553-563.)

These effects operate in different areas of the lung, with convection dominating the large airways and diffusion most prominent in the alveoli. Carbon dioxide is eluted from the lung by the combination of these effects, albeit less efficiently than with conventional ventilation.

Entrainment

Entrainment of side stream gas is commonly seen during HFJV. This phenomenon has been erroneously labeled the Venturi effect,[22] which is depicted in Figure 13-10. Entrainment is simply the effect of friction of the fast-moving jet stream acting to accelerate adjacent gas. It requires no

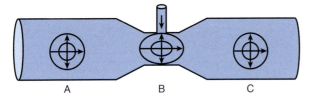

Figure 13-10 The Venturi effect. Gas moving down a tube at point *A* encounters a constriction at point *B*. The forward velocity increases, but because mean velocity in all directions is proportional to temperature, velocity in the direction of the wall decreases. Transmural pressure is proportional to velocity of gas hitting the wall, so as transmural pressure drops, a pressure gradient allows inflow from the side channel.

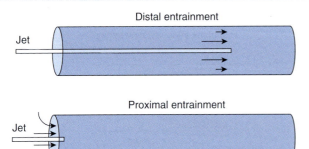

Figure 13-11 Entrainment. In the *upper panel,* the tip of the jet cannula is placed distally. Frictional forces along the wall of the tube limit entrainment. In the *lower panel,* the tip is in the proximal position and frictional forces do not limit entrainment.

special geometry and thus is not correctly described as the Venturi effect. When entrainment occurs in a tube, this increase in velocity down the tube will result in a decrease in transmural pressure because of the same laws of physics responsible for the Venturi effect. The amount of gas entrained is highly dependent on the site of entrainment and is significantly greater at the entrance to the tube than within the tube (Figure 13-11).

Entrainment is also affected by airway resistance and lung compliance. Although entrainment of volatile agents into the jet stream has been described,[23] the efficiency of agent delivery is low, can be expected to vary as conditions change, and thus has not been pursued. Entrainment can be from ambient air, an open blow-by system, or a semi-closed circle system. The latter permits conservation of inspiratory humidity, as will be discussed later, and offers the ability to add positive end-expiratory pressure (PEEP) and rapidly convert to conventional ventilation. These features are useful despite the increased dead space such systems impose.

Carbon Dioxide Elimination

Elimination of carbon dioxide from the lung is the result of total minute ventilation (the sum of delivered and entrained volume) and respiratory efficiency. It is not possible to precisely predict the arterial carbon dioxide that will result from a particular set of conditions, but it is possible for carbon dioxide to change over time. Several factors influence the rate of carbon dioxide elimination, as follows:

1. *Driving pressure.* Driving pressure affects the amount of gas delivered by the ventilator, the entrained volume,

and the lung volume. Driving pressures of 20 pounds per square inch (psi) are typically adequate, and pressures above 30 psi are rarely required to achieve normocarbia but may be useful in expanding an atelectatic lung.

2. *Respiratory rate.* As respiratory rates increase above 30 breaths per minute, efficiency of carbon dioxide elimination decreases.[24] Rates above 120 breaths per minute are rarely required to eliminate perceived respiratory motion, and carbon dioxide elimination is generally adequate at this frequency.

3. *Inspiratory fraction.* Efficiency tends to be highest at an inspiratory fraction of 0.4. Higher fractions favor larger lung volume, and lower fractions favor lower volume. Although desaturation during HFJV for respiratory immobilization is only rarely noted, reasons do exist for why a large lung would be particularly advantageous during radiation therapy.

4. *Catheter position.* Catheter position affects efficiency; a more distal position yields more efficient elimination.[25] With distal injection, the ventilator must work against a higher resistance in the delivery system and thus a lower tidal volume will be achieved for a given ventilator setting.

5. *Mechanical load.* Respiratory mechanical load affects efficiency, principally by reducing the entrained volume.[26] Both changes in airway resistance, as is seen with bronchospasm, and changes in lung compliance, as seen with pulmonary edema or externally applied pressure, can affect entrainment.

Breath Stacking

The other concern during HFJV is that of breath stacking, which may result in pulmonary barotrauma. Expiration is usually passive during mechanical ventilation, consisting of exponentially decreasing flow governed by the airway resistance and lung compliance. As expiratory time drops, the volume remaining in the lung at the start is increasing. Inspiration is active and less sensitive to resistance and compliance, and lung volume will thus increase until the increased volume produces an expiratory flow equal to the inspiratory flow. This phenomenon is termed breath stacking, or auto-PEEP. It should be noted that this is a normal physiological process and atelectasis would ensue without it. Auto-PEEP can be seen in conventional ventilation but is more associated with HFJV,[27] because it is more easily employed in cases of tracheal stenosis. Breath stacking during conventional and HFJV can be seen in Figure 13-12, with lung volumes measured by respiratory inductance plethysmography.

Breath stacking is influenced by both extrinsic and intrinsic factors. Much of our understanding of the extrinsic factors comes from simple mechanical analogs and may not adequately represent actual patients. The most important factor is airway diameter; with endotracheal tube sizes above 4.5 mm internal diameter, driving pressures in excess of 30 psi are typically required to obtain significant breath stacking.[28] Use of endotracheal tubes of 7 mm internal diameter or greater may largely avoid significant breath stacking. The larger diameter of the LMA

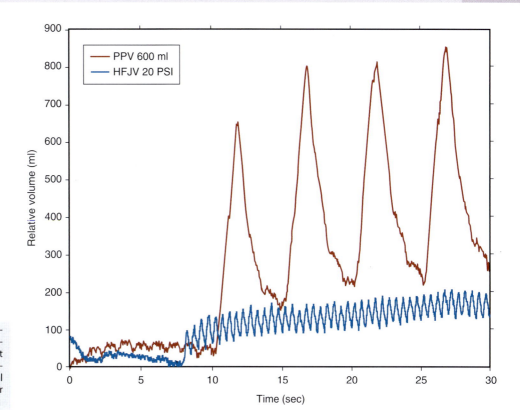

Figure 13-12 Thoracic volume measured by respiratory inductance plethysmography under high-frequency jet ventilation at 20 psi *(blue)* and positive-pressure ventilation at 600 mL tidal volume *(red)*, each producing similar carbon dioxide elimination.

may further reduce the potential for breath stacking. The position of the jet catheter also affects breath stacking. The proximal position may result in twice the effect of the distal position[29] because of greater entrainment, as depicted in Figure 13-11.

Intrinsic factors include tracheal stenosis and high lung compliance. The location of the catheter influences breath stacking in stenosis. Caution should be exercised when placing the jet catheter close to the stenosis,[30] although jet ventilation distal to the site of obstruction can be employed[31] with appropriate caution. Lung compliance is increased with severe emphysema, and breath stacking is more likely. Again, HFJV can be safely employed with an abundance of caution.[32]

When setting the jet ventilator, it is preferable to pursue strategies that result in more breath stacking rather than more efficient removal of carbon dioxide and to favor hypercarbia over atelectasis. Although it may comfort the clinician to unwaveringly maintain the arterial carbon dioxide at 40 mm Hg, evidence demonstrates that transient hypercarbia is not deleterious and may be beneficial.[33] Atelectasis and hypoxia, however, are generally bad. Thus the author favors a proximal location for the jet catheter and uses a semi-closed circle system for entrainment.

Monitoring of High-Frequency Jet Ventilation

During HFJV, an undiluted alveolar sample is not available between breaths. In most situations, it is possible to interrupt jet ventilation, deliver three tidal breaths, and measure the end tidal carbon dioxide on the third breath. Transcutaneous carbon dioxide measurement has been demonstrated

to have a correlation of 0.94 when measured by arterial blood gas.[34] Newer units that employ lower temperature on the earlobe have simplified transcutaneous measurement.[35] In settings such as the electrophysiology laboratory, arterial access is commonly available. Monitoring of carbon dioxide may be useful in identifying the minority of patients in whom hypercarbia is unanticipated, approximately 10% of patients in the author's experience.[36] It is unknown whether correcting hypercarbia alters outcome.

Monitoring airway pressure during HFJV can be accomplished in several ways. A useful feature of the Acutronic Monsoon is the pause pressure, the pressure in the jet tubing 100 ms after the solenoid valve has closed. Under conditions typically employed in respiratory immobilization, this pressure has good correlation with changes in functional residual capacity (FRC) assessed with respiratory inductance plethysmography.[37] Pressure can also be measured via a second lumen of a catheter such as the Biro catheter.[38] A limitation of measuring pressure in the central airway is that as respiratory frequency increases, the gradient between central airway pressure and alveolar pressure increases,[39] and thus central airway pressures do not precisely measure auto-PEEP.

Several methods have been described in a research context but have not yet been developed as commercial products. Respiratory inductance plethysmography employs elastic bands that contain wires through which a magnetic field is induced. The magnetic inductance reflects the encircled cross section, which is related to tidal volume. Our group has demonstrated that respiratory inductance plethysmography can accurately detect HFJV.[40] Measurement of gas flow during HFJV is complicated, because any detector placed within the jet stream will disrupt flow, and measurements made in the expiratory path are affected by entrained volume. This problem can be addressed by excluding this flow from the calculation of volume.[41]

Although transcutaneous monitoring may be worth pursuing in some settings, capnometry is readily available in anesthetizing locations and suffices for most applications.

Humidification of Inspired Gas

During open HFJV, humidification is necessary for all but the shortest of durations, because the high volume of dry gas will rapidly desiccate the airway.[42] Various approaches to humidification of the jet stream have been described.[43,44] Nebulization of water into the jet stream was the approach taken with the Monsoon 2, whereas the Monsoon 3 uses steam generation to provide humidification. When using a semi-closed circle system, some humidification is provided by entrainment of moist gas from the circuit, and water from the jet ventilator may accumulate in heat-moisture exchange filters and rain out along the anesthesia circuit. When higher levels of humidification are desired, such as in patients with chronic bronchitis, use of an open system with blow-by entrainment may be warranted, but for normal patients, circuit entrainment is generally well tolerated.

Hemodynamic Effects of High-Frequency Jet Ventilation

Much of the information on hemodynamic effects of HFV was gleaned from patients with ARDS, in whom HFV was employed to reduce intrapulmonary pressure. The principal benefit of HFJV is to permit the FRC to be maintained with lower mean intrathoracic pressure, which reduces the pulmonary vascular resistance.[45] This is less of an issue in patients who do not have ARDS.

The Physiology of Apnea

The intent of respiratory immobilization is to eliminate tidal breathing. Although administration of neuromuscular blocking agents to awake patients can certainly do this, it is unlikely that this elimination would be embraced. HFV can sustain normocarbia, but it alone is not sufficient to produce prolonged apnea in most awake patients.[46] Chemical drive is only one component of respiratory drive; the action of HFV may be mostly exerted through activation of pulmonary stretch receptors.[47] Lung volume and respiratory frequency have been shown to independently modulate the apneic threshold.[48] The state of consciousness is also central to the ability to produce sustained apnea, with quiet wakefulness and non–rapid eye movement (REM) sleep far more susceptible than REM sleep.[49] Opioids will certainly raise the apneic threshold. Apnea thus seems to be the norm in anesthetized patients who are normocarbic and receiving significant doses of opioids, and in the author's experience with several thousand cases, muscle relaxants are not required to ablate spontaneous ventilation.

Anesthetic Management

As previously noted, volatile agents can be entrained during HFJV but would be wasteful and unreliable. The author can attest to the difficulty of this approach from efforts to use HFJV for extracorporeal shockwave lithotripsy before the introduction of propofol, although Warner et al[3] reported use of entrained isoflurane with a ventilator driven by an oxygen and nitrous oxide blender.[3] With the advent of reliable intravenous agents such as propofol and remifentanil, there seems little motivation to pursue volatile agents.

Anesthetic requirements during these procedures may be fairly low, because of the minimally invasive nature of the procedures. During pulmonary vein isolation for atrial fibrillation, we often maintain patients on propofol 50 mcg/kg/min and remifentanil 0.1 mcg/kg/min. Over 95% of our patients require phenylephrine infusions to maintain normotension.[36]

Muscle relaxants are rarely required in maintenance of anesthesia for respiratory immobilization, particularly during pulmonary vein isolation, in which identification of the course of the phrenic nerve by high-output pacing is often required.[50]

During these procedures, patients are typically placed on fluoroscopy tables intended for brief procedures. Patients unsurprisingly develop back and neck pain after several hours immobilized on a rigid surface. It is advisable to provide analgesia, including ketorolac and longer-acting opioids, before emergence.

Future Directions

As previously mentioned, the production of prolonged apnea requires more than normocarbia. Conversely, HFJV can be applied via the natural airway in awake patients. Advances in the understanding of respiratory neurobiology may someday provide drugs that permit awake patients undergoing peroral HFJV to sustain apnea during minimally invasive procedures such as diagnostic imaging and radiation therapy. Anesthesiologists are uniquely qualified to perform such respiratory maneuvers safely. The time to master these techniques is upon us, for if we do not, others surely will.

References

1. Carlson CA, Roysen PG, Banner MJ, Gravenstein JS. Conventional vs high frequency jet ventilation for extracorporeal shock-wave lithotripsy. *Anesthesiology*. 1985;63:A530.
2. Schulte AM, Esch J, Kochs E, Meyer WH. Improved efficiency of extracorporal shock wave lithotripsy during high frequency jet ventilation. *Anesthesiology*. 1985;63(6):A177.
3. Warner MA, Warner ME, Buck CF, Segura JW. Clinical efficacy of high frequency jet ventilation during extracorporeal shock wave lithotripsy of renal and ureteral calculi: a comparison with conventional mechanical ventilation. *J Urol*. 1988;139(3):486–487.
4. Cormack JR, Hui R, Olive D, Said S. Comparison of two ventilation techniques during general anesthesia for extracorporeal shock wave lithotripsy: high-frequency jet ventilation versus spontaneous ventilation with a laryngeal mask airway. *Urology*. 2007;70(3):7–10.
5. Canty DJ, Dhara SS. High frequency jet ventilation through a supraglottic airway device: a case series of patients undergoing extra-corporeal shock wave lithotripsy. *Anaesthesia*. 2009;64(12):1295–1298.
6. Mucksavage P, Mayer WA, Mandel JE, Van Arsdalen KN. High-frequency jet ventilation is beneficial during shock wave lithotripsy utilizing a newer unit with a narrower focal zone. *Can Urol Assoc J*. 2010;4(5):333–335.

7. Clark DL, Connors BA, Evan AP, Handa RK, Gao S. Effect of shock wave number on renal oxidative stress and inflammation. *BJU Int.* 2011;107(2):318–322.

8. Goode JS, Taylor RL, Buffington CW, Klain MM, Schwartzman D. High-frequency jet ventilation: utility in posterior left atrial catheter ablation. *Heart Rhythm.* 2006;3(1):13–19.

9. Hutchinson MD, Garcia FC, Mandel JE, et al. Efforts to enhance catheter stability improve atrial fibrillation ablation outcome. *Heart Rhythm.* 2012;10(3):347–353.

10. Mandel JE, Perry I, Boonn WW, Litt H. Use of high-frequency jet ventilation for respiratory immobilization during coronary artery CT angiography. *J Clin Anesth.* 2009;21(8):599–601.

11. Chen JX, Gottschalk A, Kathuria S, Gandhi D. Undulating microcatheter tip motion with respiratory cycle during intracranial aneurysm embolization: description of a case and strategy for its mitigation. *J Neurointerv Surg.* 2012;4(3):e8.

12. Yin F, Kim JG, Haughton C, et al. Extracranial radiosurgery: immobilizing liver motion in dogs using high-frequency jet ventilation and total intravenous anesthesia. *Int J Radiat Oncol Biol Phys.* 2001;49(1):211–216.

13. Fritz P, Kraus HJ, Dölken W, et al. Technical note: gold marker implants and high-frequency jet ventilation for stereotactic, single-dose irradiation of liver tumors. *Technol Cancer Res Treat.* 2006;5(1):9–14.

14. Biro P, Spahn DR, Pfammatter T. High-frequency jet ventilation for minimizing breathing-related liver motion during percutaneous radiofrequency ablation of multiple hepatic tumours. *Br J Anaesth.* 2009;102(5):650–653.

15. Abderhalden S, Biro P, Hechelhammer L, Pfiffner R, Pfammatter T. CT-guided navigation of percutaneous hepatic and renal radiofrequency ablation under high-frequency jet ventilation: feasibility study. *J Vasc Interv Radiol.* 2011;22(9):1275–1278.

16. Lara-Guerra H, Kalloger SE, Powell T, et al. Tomographic comparison of ventilation techniques for CT-guided thoracoscopic staple excision of subcentimeter lung nodules. *J Invest Surg.* 2006;19(3):185–191.

17. Fritz P, Kraus HJ, Mühlnickel W, et al. High-frequency jet ventilation for complete target immobilization and reduction of planning target volume in stereotactic high single-dose irradiation of stage I non-small cell lung cancer and lung metastases. *Int J Radiat Oncol Biol Phys.* 2010;78(1):136–142.

18. Sjöstrand UH, Smith RB. Overview of high frequency ventilation. *Int Anesthesiol Clin.* 1983;21(3):1–10.

19. Kraincuk P, Kepka A, Ihra G, Schabernig C, Aloy A. A new prototype of an electronic jet-ventilator and its humidification system. *Crit Care.* 1999;3(4):101–110.

20. Allan PF, Osborn EC, Chung KK, Wanek SM. High-frequency percussive ventilation revisited. *J Burn Care Res.* 2010;31(4):510–520.

21. Chang HK. Mechanisms of gas transport during ventilation by high-frequency oscillation. *J Appl Physiol.* 1984;56(3):553–563.

22. Ihra G, Aloy A. On the use of Venturi's principle to describe entrainment during jet ventilation. *J Clin Anesth.* 2000;12(5):417–419.

23. Gravenstein N, Weber W, Banner MJ. Entrainment of anesthetic agents from the circle system during high frequency jet ventilation and anesthesia. *Anesthesiology.* 1986;65:A148.

24. Fletcher R, Malmkvist G, Lührs C, et al. Isocapnic high frequency jet ventilation: dead space depends on frequency, inspiratory time and entrainment. *Acta Anaesthesiol Scand.* 1991;35(2):153–158.

25. Benhamou D, Ecoffey C, Rouby JJ, Spielvogel C, Viars P. High frequency jet ventilation: the influence of different methods of injection on respiratory parameters. *Br J Anaesth.* 1987;59(10):1257–1264.

26. Berdine GG, Strollo PJ. Effect of mechanical load on tidal volume during high-frequency jet ventilation. *J Appl Physiol.* 1988;64(3):1217–1222.

27. Beamer WC, Prough DS, Royster RL, Johnston WE, Johnson JC. High-frequency jet ventilation produces auto-PEEP. *Crit Care Med.* 1984;12(9):734–737.

28. Dworkin R, Benumof JL, Benumof R, Karagianes TG. The effective tracheal diameter that causes air trapping during jet ventilation. *J Cardiothorac Anesth.* 1990;4(6):731–736.

29. Spackman DR, Kellow N, White SA, Seed PT, Feneck RO. High frequency jet ventilation and gas trapping. *Br J Anaesth.* 1999;83(5):708–714.

30. Ihra GC, Heid A, Pernerstorfer T. Airway stenosis-related increase of pulmonary pressure during high-frequency jet ventilation depends on injectors position. *Anesth Analg.* 2009;109(2):461.

31. Atkins JH, Mirza N, Mandel JE. Case report: respiratory inductance plethysmography as a monitor of ventilation during laser ablation and balloon dilatation of subglottic tracheal stenosis. *J Otorhinolaryngol Relat Spec.* 2009;71(5):289–291.

32. Myles PS, Evans AB, Madder H, Weeks AM. Dynamic hyperinflation: comparison of jet ventilation versus conventional ventilation in patients with severe end-stage obstructive lung disease. *Anaesth Intensive Care.* 1997;25(5):471–475.

33. Kregenow A, Swenson R. The lung and carbon dioxide: implications for permissive and therapeutic hypercapnia. *Eur Respir J.* 2002;20(1):6–11.

34. Simon M, Gottschall R, Gugel M, et al. Comparison of transcutaneous and end-tidal CO_2-monitoring for rigid bronchoscopy during high-frequency jet ventilation. *Acta Anaesthesiol Scand.* 2003;47(7):861–867.

35. Eberhard P. The design, use, and results of transcutaneous carbon dioxide analysis: current and future directions. *Anesth Analg.* 2007;105(6 Suppl):S48–S52.

36. Elkassabany N, Garcia F, Tschabrunn C, et al. Anesthetic management of patients undergoing pulmonary vein isolation for treatment of atrial fibrillation using high-frequency jet ventilation. *J Cardiothorac Vasc Anesth.* 2012;26(3):433–438.

37. Bourgain JL, Desruennes E, Cosset MF, et al. Measurement of end-expiratory pressure during transtracheal high frequency jet ventilation for laryngoscopy. *Br J Anaesth.* 1990;65(6):737–743.

38. Biro P. Jet ventilation for surgical interventions in the upper airway. *Anesthesiol Clin.* 2010;28(3):397–409.

39. Simon BA, Weinmann GG, Mitzner W. Mean airway pressure and alveolar pressure during high-frequency ventilation. *J Appl Physiol.* 1984;57(4):1069–1078.

40. Atkins JH, Mandel JE, Weinstein GS, Mirza N. A pilot study of respiratory inductance plethysmography as a safe, noninvasive detector of jet ventilation under general anesthesia. *Anesth Analg.* 2010;111(5):1168–1175.

41. Young JD, Sykes MK. A method for measuring tidal volume during high frequency jet ventilation. *Br J Anaesth.* 1988;61(5):601–605.

42. Circeo LE, Heard SO, Griffiths E, Nash G. Overwhelming necrotizing tracheobronchitis due to inadequate humidification during high-frequency jet ventilation. *Chest.* 1991;100(1):268–269.

43. Kan AF, Gin T, Lin ES, Oh TE. Factors influencing humidification in high-frequency jet ventilation. *Crit Care Med.* 1990;18(5):537–539.

44. Zandstra DF, Stoutenbeek CP, Miranda DR. Efficacy of a heat and moisture exchange device during high-frequency jet ventilation. *Intensive Care Med.* 1987;13(5):355–557.

45. Kawahito S, Kitahata H, Tanaka K, Nozaki J, Oshita S. Transesophageal echocardiographic assessment of pulmonary arterial and venous flow during high-frequency jet ventilation. *J Clin Anesth.* 2000;12(4):308–314.

46. George RJ, Winter RJ, Johnson MA, Slee IP, Geddes DM. Effect of oral high frequency ventilation by jet or oscillator on minute ventilation in normal subjects. *Thorax.* 1985;40(10):749–755.

47. Kohl J, Koller EA. Blockade of pulmonary stretch receptors reinforces diaphragmatic activity during high-frequency oscillatory ventilation. *Pflugers Arch.* 1988;411(1):42–46.

48. van Vught AJ, Versprille A, Jansen JR. Suppression of spontaneous breathing during high-frequency jet ventilation: separate effects of lung volume and jet frequency. *Intensive Care Med.* 1987;13(5):315–322.

49. Dempsey JA. Crossing the apnoeic threshold: causes and consequences. *Exp Physiol.* 2005;90(1):13–24.

50. Fan R, Cano O, Ho SY, et al. Characterization of the phrenic nerve course within the epicardial substrate of patients with nonischemic cardiomyopathy and ventricular tachycardia. *Heart Rhythm.* 2009;6(1):59–64.

14 *Anesthesia for Upper Gastrointestinal Endoscopy*

BASAVANA G. GOUDRA, JONATHAN W. TANNER, PREET MOHINDER SINGH, and GREGORY G. GINSBERG

Gastrointestinal (GI) endoscopies are among the most common non–operating room procedures requiring anesthesia. This chapter reviews considerations and challenges related to anesthesia for upper GI endoscopy procedures. These include esophagogastroduodenoscopy (EGD), endoscopic ultrasound (a variation on EGD employing a specialized endoscope with a miniature ultrasound transducer affixed to its distal tip), and endoscopic retrograde cholangiopancreatography (ERCP). The biggest challenge for the anesthesia provider is that because these procedures involve insertion of an endoscope into the patient's mouth, the patient's airway must be shared with the gastroenterologist.

Anesthesia is not required for all GI endoscopy procedures. In fact, gastroenterologists can successfully complete endoscopies in most patients (frequently with no or minimal comorbidities) with moderate sedation such as midazolam and fentanyl. Propofol may have advantages over midazolam in terms of efficiency (i.e., faster sedation and recovery) and patient satisfaction, but it cannot be administered by gastroenterologists in many venues, and involving an anesthesiologist is expensive. For sicker patients or more complex procedures, most gastroenterologists prefer to have an anesthesiologist provide sedation and care to ensure patient safety and comfort and to allow the gastroenterologist to concentrate on the procedure. Insurance companies may question reimbursement for the expense of an anesthesiologist for a relatively healthy patient having a diagnostic EGD. However, they probably will not question the need for an anesthesiologist for a more complicated situation such as a therapeutic intervention or a patient with American Society of Anesthesiologists physical status 3 or greater, for which there are clear indications.

Patient Populations Presenting for Upper Gastrointestinal Endoscopic Procedures

Gastroesophageal reflux disease and its potential sequelae, including Barrett's esophagus and esophageal cancer, are common indications for EGD. The incidences of Barrett's esophagus and esophageal cancer are increasing. Barrett's esophagus is a precursor of esophageal cancer. Fortunately, effective endoscopic therapeutic interventions are available that can decrease the need for a debilitating esophagectomy. However, the endoscopic interventions can be lengthy and uncomfortable. Many patients who undergo esophagectomy enjoy long-term survival, but they frequently present to the gastroenterologist for repeated dilations.

Conditions for which surgery was seen as the only curative option, such as tracheoesophageal fistula, are now treated endoscopically with a high degree of success. Bariatric surgery is gaining popularity in developed nations, and EGD is often performed for assessment before or after the surgery. Placement of stents, cautery of bleeding arteriovenous malformations, and banding of esophageal varices are other growing areas of endoscopic practice.

The most frequent indication for ERCP is common bile duct stones. Gallstone disease is estimated to affect more than 20 million adults in the United States, at an annual cost of $6.2 billion.[1] Of patients undergoing laparoscopic cholecystectomy for symptomatic cholelithiasis and patients with acute biliary pancreatitis, 5% to 10% and 18% to 33%, respectively, also will have choledocholithiasis.[2]

Patients with pancreatic cancer often need endoscopic ultrasound or ERCP for staging or palliation. The pancreas is the 10th most common site of new cancer and the 4th-leading cause of cancer death in the United States and worldwide. In 2010 an estimated 43,140 new cases of pancreatic cancer were diagnosed in the United States; this accounts for 2.8% of all cancers.[3]

Although many advanced endoscopic procedures are currently the privilege of tertiary gastroenterology centers, they are likely to be performed more widely in the future.

Preprocedure Evaluation

In general, patients presenting for an inpatient EGD or ERCP are likely to be far sicker than their outpatient counterparts. The comorbidities discussed in the following paragraphs should be kept in mind while conducting a preoperative evaluation. The time available for a comprehensive evaluation in a busy endoscopy unit may be limited; the anesthesiologist should triage and allocate appropriate time for a given patient.

Hypertension and coronary artery disease are extremely common in this patient population. The procedure in a patient presenting for surveillance EGD who has undergone recent coronary stent placement, with either a bare metal or drug-eluting stent, may be postponed if issues concerning ongoing anticoagulation are not addressed.[4] If the patient presents for cancer staging or for a therapeutic ERCP, however, the risks of postponement might exceed the risks of the procedure. The risk-to-benefit ratio for fine-needle aspiration cytology and any other potential instigation of bleeding should be discussed in advance with the gastroenterologist. A cardiologist should also be consulted for guidance in these situations.

Cardiac rhythm disorders are not uncommon. Chronic atrial fibrillation with anticoagulation is less frequent, with wider availability and success of antiarrhythmic medications and ablation procedures. Patients with a pacemaker or automatic implantable cardioverter-defibrillator are increasingly encountered. Therapeutic EGD or ERCP might involve use of electrocautery close to these devices. It is prudent to have a magnet available, although prophylactic use is unnecessary. When applied, the magnet may activate the backup mode (fixed-rate pacing); in such an event, pacemaker evaluation and resetting are recommended.

Ventricular assist devices (VADs) are more commonly used. In our hospital, these patients are managed by noncardiac anesthesiologists for noncardiac procedures. In the absence of pulsatile flow, pulse oximeter and noninvasive blood pressure readings may be unreliable. Communication with the VAD coordinator nurse regarding physiological parameters such as volume and vasodilation status is important.

Patients with chronic obstructive airway disease who require supplemental oxygen at baseline may occasionally present for EGD or ERCP. These patients usually can be anesthetized for endoscopy without endotracheal intubation and sent home on the same day.

Obstructive sleep apnea is present in approximately 70% of patients with morbid obesity presenting for bariatric surgery.[5] An accurate airway assessment is important. Intubation is rarely necessary in these patients for EGD, although elective intubation may be considered for prolonged ERCP.

Considering the frequency of diabetes mellitus in the population, it is impossible to schedule all such patients as the first case of the day. Most of these patients can be fed almost immediately after the procedure and return to their insulin or oral treatment regimen. Holding the morning dose of hypoglycemic agent and insulin may be all that is necessary.

Patients on chronic opioid therapy require significantly higher than average doses of intravenous anesthetic agents and opioids. Gastroenterologists will often request anesthesia for these patients.

Endoscopic procedures have low cardiac risk. Therefore, according to recent guidelines,[6] preprocedural electrocardiograms (ECGs) are not indicated in asymptomatic patients, even if they are older than 60 years of age or have known cardiovascular disease. Likewise, laboratory testing is not usually needed before endoscopy, with rare exceptions such as coagulation studies and platelet count in patients with liver disease undergoing therapeutic endoscopic procedures.

Anesthetic Drugs for Gastrointestinal Endoscopy

Propofol is the cornerstone when anesthesia services are provided for EGD and ERCP.[7] Smooth intravenous induction and maintenance, quick and clear-headed recovery, and low incidence of postprocedure nausea and vomiting make it an attractive anesthetic agent in this setting. The anesthesia provider should, however, be mindful of the fact that patients are often under general anesthesia during some or most of an endoscopy procedure with propofol;

this has attendant risks, especially loss of airway control. The anesthesia provider must also appreciate the pharmacokinetic and pharmacodynamic variability of propofol, especially when used in combination with other drugs (such as short-acting opioids). As a result, a patient with a seemingly adequate dose can be still awake, and a patient with a smaller dose can be apneic, be unresponsive, and require airway support. Additionally, instrumentation of an inadequately sedated patient can cause reflex coughing and laryngospasm despite the fact that propofol does not increase airway irritability.

Although propofol is not absolutely contraindicated in patients with a mild egg allergy,[8] patients occasionally present with a history of severe egg allergy or propofol allergy. One alternative to propofol is etomidate. Etomidate is advantageous because of its minimal cardiorespiratory depression but disadvantageous because of the increased incidence of nausea or vomiting and tonic or clonic movements in contrast to propofol. Both etomidate and propofol may produce a burning sensation when injected intravenously; this unpleasant effect can be mitigated by pretreatment with intravenous lidocaine, which may also have some general anesthetic properties and suppress coughing from endoscope insertion.

Another alternative to propofol is the combination of a benzodiazepine and an opioid such as midazolam and remifentanil. Remifentanil is an ultra–short-acting opioid. Its pharmacodynamic properties are similar to those of the other commonly used opioids, but its pharmacokinetic properties are unique. Unlike all other opioids, remifentanil is metabolized by esterases, because of the presence of an ester moiety at the active site, and esterases are ubiquitous, being present in many tissues, including plasma and red blood cells. Its fixed context-sensitive half-time stems from this unique metabolism. As a result of rapid elimination, its context-sensitive half-time is approximately 2 to 4 minutes. It is important to administer it as a small bolus (1 to 2 mcg/kg) infused over a period of at least 2 minutes. This is followed by an infusion at 0.06 to 0.2 mcg/kg/min. Administration of 0.5 to 2 mg midazolam 2 or 3 minutes before is useful for amnesia, although remifentanil itself has amnestic properties.[9] Midazolam can be repeated again in small doses during the procedure. After 4 to 5 minutes of remifentanil infusion, patients tolerate GI endoscopy quite well. It is important not to be tempted to increase the remifentanil infusion, because apnea and rigidity can ensue. Frequently, patients receiving remifentanil can stop breathing, although they are conscious and cooperative, and they need to be reminded to take deep breaths. Supplemental oxygen should be administered. The patients usually tolerate endoscopy well and often have no recollection of the procedure.

Limited data exist regarding the use of ketamine for endoscopy.[10] Ketamine produces a less familiar state of anesthesia: the patient might give an impression of staring, with eyeballs rolling, and he or she might even move. The mere mention of ketamine may conjure up concern about psychomimetic reactions, but the incidence of those can be greatly reduced by coadministration of midazolam, propofol, or both.[11] Although ketamine's cardiovascular stimulation may be undesirable in some patients (such as those prone to myocardial ischemia), it may be advantageous in some hemodynamically unstable (e.g., septic or bleeding) patients. In most patients, ketamine will offset hypotension caused by propofol. One potential problem with ketamine for endoscopy is that it promotes salivation, which can be mitigated by preprocedure anticholinergic administration but that is associated with further tachycardia and postprocedural dry mouth. Ketamine's lack of respiratory depression is attractive for upper GI endoscopy, particularly in patients with obstructive sleep apnea. Ketamine may also be particularly advantageous in patients with asthma because of its bronchodilating properties. Ketamine is an analgesic as well, so additional analgesics may not be needed in patients undergoing endoscopy.

Dexmedetomidine, a selective α_2-adrenergic receptor agonist,[12] has properties unlike those of other commonly used anesthetic drugs. Its action is similar to that of clonidine, another α_2 agonist, but it is six times more selective. The drug is now approved for sedation[13] in nonintubated patients, so its inclusion in the GI endoscopy armory is relevant. Almost all studies agree that patients receiving dexmedetomidine maintain spontaneous ventilation with almost no assistance, apart from an occasional chin lift. A few studies have been conducted on the role of dexmedetomidine in GI endoscopy.[14-17] Coadministration of midazolam and a short-acting opioid will help achieve a higher success rate. Dexmedetomidine is administered with a loading dose over 10 minutes, and its effects of sedation and hypotension tend to linger longer than those of propofol. Thus, although dexmedetomidine may be appropriate for certain patients, such as those particularly prone or sensitive to respiratory depression from other agents, it is not as practical for routine, rapid turnover cases.

In summary (Table 14-1), for most patients, propofol is the basis of anesthesia for upper GI endoscopy although in particular patients alternative drugs may be more attractive. The details of intravenous administration, especially target-controlled infusion (TCI) versus traditional intravenous infusion, are discussed in a separate chapter, so discussion here is limited to their application for endoscopy. Depending on which side of the Atlantic Ocean one is practicing, the tools for intravenous anesthetic delivery will vary. Use of TCI pumps will definitely reduce the variability, and that reduction might be especially useful for endoscopy. They are known to reduce the number of changes to the infusion settings necessary for surgical anesthesia. In the setting of endoscopy, however, in which the change of stimulation is less frequent than in surgical procedures, such a luxury may not be necessary.

Airway Management

Anesthetizing in any location needs to be taken as seriously as in an operating room. Preoperative evaluation with special attention to airway and aspiration risk factors must be thorough. An anesthesia machine is not required, but a breathing circuit capable of positive-pressure ventilation (such as Mapleson C), laryngoscope, face masks, oral and nasal airways, laryngeal mask airways, various sizes of endotracheal tubes, and emergency drugs should be readily available. Because of its remote location, it is also important to have additional airway adjuncts such as Bougies, stylets, video laryngoscopes, and carbon dioxide detectors. It is important to check the availability and functionality of these before the start of every procedure. Airway emergencies such as laryngospasm and other airway obstruction often occur with little notice during upper GI endoscopy. Being ready for any airway situation (or not) could be the difference between apnea-related cardiac arrest and a safe discharge home.

Options for airway management for upper GI endoscopic procedures range from natural (with supplemental oxygen by nasal cannula) to endotracheal intubation.[18] In fact, a study of ERCPs with laryngeal mask airways has been published.[19] Another choice used in our practice is insertion of a nasal trumpet. Insertion of a nasal airway may provoke epistaxis, so use of a vasoconstrictor nasal spray or oral insertion of the nasal trumpet should be considered, particularly in patients who have received anticoagulation therapy. Even for advanced endoscopic procedures, including complicated ERCPs, endotracheal intubation is rarely used in our practice, with the exception of patients with a stomach full of food or blood. It should be noted that gastric contents can be suctioned by the endoscopist under direct vision.

The experience of the anesthesiologist in providing anesthesia for endoscopy procedures seems to play a major part in this decision; anesthesiologists unfamiliar with this area of practice seem to intubate more frequently.[18] It is a tightrope walk to keep the patients unresponsive and comfortable while spontaneously breathing. Avoiding endotracheal intubation is beneficial in the rapid turnover, outpatient endoscopy setting. In this population, irrespective of the drugs chosen and the tool used to administer them, the central aim of anesthesia is to have an unresponsive patient who is spontaneously ventilating and maintaining the airway with little or no support. Airway manipulations such as chin lift, jaw thrust, and neck extension and various devices help maintain a patent airway, and their use should not be seen as failure of the technique. Having a dedicated team of

Table 14-1   Comparison of Drugs for Anesthesia for Upper Gastrointestinal Endoscopy

Drug	Site of Action	Time of Onset (min)	Notable Clinical Effects	Notable Drawbacks	Time for Recovery (min)
Propofol	GABA receptor	½-1	Amnesia, hypnosis	PK/PD variability, apnea, hypotension	5-7 (for a 30- to 45-min procedure)
Remifentanil	μ Receptor	1-2	Analgesia	Bradycardia, hypoxemia, rigidity	2-3
Ketamine	NMDA receptor	1-2	Dissociative anesthesia	Tachycardia, salivation	5-10
Dexmedetomidine	α_2 Receptor	8-10	Sedation	Slow loading and offset, bradycardia	15-20
Remimazolam	GABA receptor	3-5	Sedation	None so far	10-15

GABA, γ-aminobutyric acid; *NMDA*, N-methyl-D-aspartate; *PK/PD*, pharmacokinetics/pharmacodynamics.

providers with experience in anesthesia for endoscopy and an appreciation of pharmacokinetic and pharmacodynamic variability will help master this technique and greatly facilitate efficiency without compromising safety. The gastroenterologist must be aware that scope removal during the procedure may be needed urgently for airway management. Not every situation, procedure, and patient factor can be addressed, but the following items can be used as broad principles for airway management in upper GI endoscopy.[20]

1. Most patients with normal airway anatomy and physiology presenting for a short diagnostic upper GI endoscopy do not need any special airway apart from nasal cannula for supplemental oxygen administration.

2. Most ERCPs in our hospital are done without an endotracheal tube. Anesthesia is induced after prone positioning. A nasal trumpet can be inserted soon after induction and connected to a breathing system, as seen in Figure 14-1. Apnea lasting 30 to 45 seconds after induction is not uncommon, but the stimulation of gastroscope insertion helps restart spontaneous ventilation. The nasal trumpet allows some degree of controlled ventilation, if necessary. More importantly, it allows delivery of 100% oxygen at the laryngeal inlet. High-frequency jet ventilation is also useful in this setting. Endotracheal intubation is the airway of choice for endoscopic drainage of a pancreatic pseudocyst.

3. Most therapeutic upper GI endoscopies such as endoscopic mucosal resection, Barrett's eradication, application of variceal banding, and resection of larger gastroduodenal polyps are managed similarly to ERCPs. These procedures may involve frequent scope withdrawal and reinsertion, so it is important to maintain or increase the depth of anesthesia to prevent coughing. Patients undergoing treatment for tracheoesophageal fistula, especially with a history of aspiration, should be considered for endotracheal intubation.

4. Morbidly obese patients often present for upper GI endoscopy before weight reduction surgery. Obstructive sleep apnea is very common in this group. We use nasal trumpets after induction, occasionally supplemented with supraglottic jet ventilation. Use of supraglottic jets provides ventilation and also probably prevents the upper airway from collapsing. This is a technique that requires experience and maintenance of adequate depth of anesthesia at all times. If in doubt, these patients are better handled with endotracheal intubation. In any event, equipment for difficult intubation should be at hand.

5. Patients who had previous esophagectomy for cancer or achalasia frequently present for esophageal dilation. In the absence of gastric motility issues, these patients can be handled safely with supplemental nasal oxygen or a nasal trumpet connected to breathing system. Stretching with a balloon or a Bougie can be stimulating, and deepening of anesthesia in anticipation is important.

6. Patients with a documented pharyngeal pouch are anesthetized after awake endotracheal intubation. Application of cricoid pressure may not be useful in this scenario.

7. Patients with limited mouth opening or neck extension as a result of radiation treatment for oropharyngeal cancer often present for repeated esophageal dilations of radiation-induced stricture. In the absence of any nasopharyngeal airway obstruction and if ventilation by mask is not expected to be difficult, these patients can be safely managed with nasal cannula or nasal trumpet.

8. Patients who had prior weight loss surgery sometimes present for endoscopic evaluation. Insufficient evidence exists to recommend endotracheal intubation in this subgroup.[21] Each individual patient needs to be evaluated with regard to potential for aspiration and accordingly managed.

9. GI bleeding is common in patients with ventricular assist devices. Although it is recommended[22] to treat them as having a full stomach because of the position of the devices, in our practice oxygen is delivered with nasal cannula or nasal trumpet for EGD. The potential risks of rapid sequence induction and intubation in these very sick patients outweigh any benefits.

Conduct of Anesthesia for Upper Gastrointestinal Endoscopy

As with all anesthetics, an understanding of the procedure makes administration of the anesthetic smoother. Common indications for upper GI endoscopy can be found in Box 14-1. Advanced endoscopic procedures are technically challenging for endoscopists and anesthesia providers alike. The patients are often elderly and ill; they are not usually supine; the room is often darkened; equipment such as fluoroscopy machine, ultrasound machine, and/or video display extends over the patient; and there is competition for space around the patient's mouth and airway. For EGD, gastroenterologists usually prefer the patient to assume the left lateral position, whereas for ERCP, they usually prefer the patient to be prone, with head turned to the side. A bite block is usually inserted by the gastroenterology team; it is easiest to get the patient in position, with the bite block in place, before induction of anesthesia, unless the anesthesiologist plans to intubate the patient's trachea. As indicated earlier, insertion of the endoscope is usually the most stimulating part of the procedure, except if dilation is performed. Topical pharyngeal anesthesia may improve tolerance of endoscopy.[23] A simple EGD may

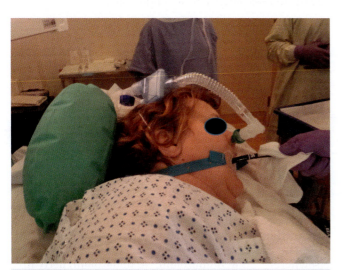

Figure 14-1 Mapleson C breathing circuit connected to nasal trumpet via endotracheal tube connector.

Box 14-1   Common Indications for Upper Gastrointestinal Endoscopy Procedures

Diagnostic

Isolated dysphagia, odynophagia, Barrett's esophagus
Persistent vomiting, gastroesophageal reflux disease
Chronic anemia, melena
Acute upper gastrointestinal bleed
Peptic ulcer, duodenal biopsy
Portal hypertension
Small bowel enteroscopy
Evaluation before bariatric surgery

Therapeutic

Common bile duct stones
Biliary, pancreatic stenting, dilatation
Variceal bleed
Foreign body extraction
Esophageal stricture dilatation
Esophageal stenting
Percutaneous endoscopic gastrostomy
Endoscopic mucosal resection (for neoplasms)

Box 14-2   Complications Related to Sedation for Upper Gastrointestinal Endoscopy

Airway Obstruction

Apnea
Failed airway management under deep sedation

Inadequate or Excessive Sedation

Desaturation
Laryngospasm
Aspiration

---

take a few minutes, although a complicated ERCP can take over an hour. Antibiotics are not usually indicated, even in patients with valvular heart disease.

In our practice, induction is typically with propofol. The dose is variable—it depends on the patient's age, weight, height, comorbidity, and medication history, all of which influence the pharmacokinetics and pharmacodynamics. We typically start with approximately 1 to 1.5 mg/kg, although less in elderly patients. Propofol may be preceded (1 to 2 minutes before) with fentanyl 25 to 50 mcg for an antitussive effect. At the peak clinical effect of propofol, signaled by loss of eyelash reflex, unresponsiveness, and sometimes apnea, a nasal trumpet can be inserted and connected to a Mapleson C breathing system (see Figure 14-1). The gastroscope is introduced at the same time to provide sufficient stimulation to initiate (if patient was apneic) and sustain spontaneous ventilation.

The gastroenterologist may request glucagon for GI relaxation. Glucagon is usually supplied as a vial with 1 mg powder and a vial with 1 mL solvent; the usual initial dose is between 0.2 and 0.5 mg intravenously. It may affect blood glucose, so it should be used with caution in patients with diabetes or insulinoma.

Postprocedure pain is rare except for mild throat irritation, so more than 100 mcg or so of fentanyl is excessive except in the patient on chronic opioid therapy. Postprocedure abdominal pain could be a sign of visceral perforation, and approximately 5% of patients will have pancreatitis after ERCP, so make sure the gastroenterologist is aware of this symptom.

Monitoring

Routine monitoring via pulse oximetry, blood pressure at least every 5 minutes, and continuous ECG during anesthesia are among the standards of the American Society of Anesthesiologists. Those standards were recently revised to

state that exhaled carbon dioxide should also be monitored, unless precluded or invalidated by the nature of the patient, procedure, or equipment. Obtaining accurate capnography during upper gastrointestinal endoscopy can be difficult, but it is important for recognizing apneic periods that might otherwise go unnoticed during the procedure. Artifacts can be produced if the endoscopist uses carbon dioxide for insufflation. Other techniques of respiratory monitoring are emerging based on acoustics or pulse plethysmograph analysis.[24] Transcutaneous carbon dioxide monitoring has been attempted, but its use in this setting is of questionable value.

Complications

Providing anesthesia at remote locations carries significant risk for morbidity and mortality.[25-27] Inadequate oxygenation and ventilation seem to be the most common problems. Approximately half of all deaths reported in closed claim studies in the GI endoscopy suite are the result of airway mismanagement. Titration to appropriate levels at which patients are appropriately sedated yet adequately ventilating is not always easy because of pharmacokinetic and pharmacodynamic variability of sedative medications.[28] Apnea, laryngospasm, and aspiration are more specific to EGD and ERCP (Box 14-2). As mentioned, preparedness for any airway eventuality is the key for a successful and safe anesthetic for endoscopy.

Future

The future of anesthesia for EGD and ERCP will depend on the development of new drugs that can potentially replace propofol. Although pain on injection can be unpleasant (sometimes the only unpleasant experience of the whole anesthetic), its major drawback is its propensity to cause hypotension and apnea, which sometimes requires airway support and, rarely, even endotracheal intubation. The additional cost of anesthesiologist involvement inevitably calls for a suitable replacement that also can be used safely by the gastroenterologist, particularly in subsets of low-risk patients. SEDASYS is a computer-based system with built-in safety features that can be safely used to sedate low-risk colonoscopy patients and is discussed elsewhere.[29,30] Remimazolam, a midazolam derivative metabolized by ester hydrolysis, is a newer drug undergoing clinical trials. It is unlikely to fill this void because of apnea and more importantly long induction and recovery times. The drugs in sight at various stages of development are unlikely to replace propofol in the near future. Even if an intravenous anesthetic can be designed with rapid elimination and thereby quick recovery, the doses required are likely to be higher and thus increase the cost. In any event, with the trends of older, sicker patient populations and more complex procedures, the role of anesthesia providers for upper GI endoscopies seems currently secure and likely to expand in both the inpatient and outpatient settings.

References

1. Everhart JE, Ruhl CE. Burden of digestive diseases in the United States. I. Overall and upper gastrointestinal diseases. *Gastroenterology.* 2009;136(2):376–386.
2. American Society of Gastrointestinal Endoscopy Standards of Practice Committee, Maple JT, Ben-Menachem T, Anderson MA, et al. The role of endoscopy in the evaluation of suspected choledocholithiasis. *Gastrointest Endosc.* 2010;71(1):1–9.
3. Vincent A, Herman J, Schulick R, Hruban RH, Goggins M. Pancreatic cancer. *Lancet.* 2011;378(9791):607–620.
4. American Society of Anesthesiologists Committee on Standards and Practice Parameters. Practice alert for the perioperative management of patients with coronary artery stents: a report by the American Society of Anesthesiologists Committee on Standards and Practice Parameters. *Anesthesiology.* 2009;110(1):22–23.
5. Frey WC, Pilcher J. Obstructive sleep-related breathing disorders in patients evaluated for bariatric surgery. *Obes Surg.* 2003;13(5):676–683.
6. American College of Cardiology, American Heart Association Task Force on Practice Guidelines (Writing Committee to Revise the 2002 Guidelines on Perioperative Cardiovascular Evaluation for Noncardiac Surgery), American Society of Echocardiography, American Society of Nuclear Cardiology, Heart Rhythm Society, Society of Cardiovascular Anesthesiologists, Society for Cardiovascular Angiography and Interventions, et al. ACC/AHA 2007 guidelines on perioperative cardiovascular evaluation and care for noncardiac surgery: executive summary. *Anesth Analg.* 2008;106(3):685–712.
7. Goudra BG, Mandel JE. Target-controlled infusions/patient-controlled sedation. *Tech Gastrointest Endosc.* 2009;11(4):181–187.
8. Baombe JP, Parvez K. Towards evidence-based emergency medicine: best BETs from the Manchester Royal Infirmary. BET 1: is propofol safe in patients with egg anaphylaxis? *Emerg Med J.* 2013;30(1):79–80.
9. Vennila R, Hall A, Ali M, et al. Remifentanil as single agent to facilitate awake fibreoptic intubation in the absence of premedication. *Anaesthesia.* 2011;66(5):368–372.
10. Varadarajulu S, Eloubeidi MA, Tamhane A, Wilcox CM. Prospective randomized trial evaluating ketamine for advanced endoscopic procedures in difficult to sedate patients. *Aliment Pharmacol Ther.* 2007;25(8):987–997.
11. Badrinath S, Avramov MN, Shadrick M, Witt TR, Ivankovich AD. The use of a ketamine-propofol combination during monitored anesthesia care. *Anesth Analg.* 2000;90(4):858–862.
12. Kaur M, Singh P. Current role of dexmedetomidine in clinical anesthesia and intensive care. *Anesth Essays Res.* 2011;5(2):128–133.
13. Iirola T, Ihmsen H, Laitio R, et al. Population pharmacokinetics of dexmedetomidine during long-term sedation in intensive care patients. *Br J Anaesth.* 2012;108(3):460–468.
14. Muller S, Borowics SM, Fortis EAF, et al. Clinical efficacy of dexmedetomidine alone is less than propofol for conscious sedation during ERCP. *Gastrointest Endosc.* 2008;67(4):651–659.
15. Dere K, Sucullu I, Budak ET, et al. A comparison of dexmedetomidine versus midazolam for sedation, pain and hemodynamic control, during colonoscopy under conscious sedation. *Eur J Anaesthesiol.* 2010;27(7):648–652.
16. Jalowiecki P, Rudner R, Gonciarz M, et al. Sole use of dexmedetomidine has limited utility for conscious sedation during outpatient colonoscopy. *Anesthesiology.* 2005;103(2):269–273.
17. Demiraran Y, Korkut E, Tamer A, et al. The comparison of dexmedetomidine and midazolam used for sedation of patients during upper endoscopy: a prospective, randomized study. *Can J Gastroenterol J.* 2007;21(1):25–29.
18. Goudra BG, Singh PM, Sinha AC. Anesthesia for ERCP: impact of anesthesiologist's experience on outcome and cost. *Anesthiol Res Pract.* 2013. [Internet]. May 28, 2013 [cited June 7, 2013]. http://www.hindawi.com/journals/arp/2013/570518/abs/.
19. Osborn IP, Cohen J, Soper RJ, Roth LA. Laryngeal mask airway: a novel method of airway protection during ERCP—comparison with endotracheal intubation. *Gastrointest Endosc.* 2002;56(1):122–128.
20. Goudra BG, Singh PM, Sinha A. Outpatient endoscopic retrograde cholangiopancreatography: safety and efficacy of anesthetic management with a natural airway in 653 consecutive procedures. *Saudi J Anaesth.* 2013;7(3):259–265.
21. Herbella FAM, Vicentine FPP, Del Grande JC, Patti MG, Arasaki CH. Postprandial proximal gastric acid pocket in patients after Roux-en-Y gastric bypass. *J Gastrointest Surg.* 2010;14(11):1742–1745.
22. Stone ME, Soong W, Krol M, Reich DL. The anesthetic considerations in patients with ventricular assist devices presenting for noncardiac surgery: a review of eight cases. *Anesth Analg.* 2002;95(1):42–49.
23. Evans LT, Saberi S, Kim HM, Elta GH, Schoenfeld P. Pharyngeal anesthesia during sedated EGDs: is "the spray" beneficial? A meta-analysis and systematic review. *Gastrointest Endosc.* 2006;63(6):761–766.
24. Goudra BG, Penugonda LC, Speck RM, Sinha AC. Comparison of acoustic respiration rate, impedance pneumography and capnometry monitors for respiration rate accuracy and apnea detection during GI endoscopy anesthesia. *Open J Anesth.* 2013;03(02):74–79.
25. Metzner J, Posner KL, Domino KB. The risk and safety of anesthesia at remote locations: the US closed claims analysis. *Curr Opin Anaesthesiol.* 2009;22(4):502–508.
26. Bhananker SM, Posner KL, Cheney FW, et al. Injury and liability associated with monitored anesthesia care: a closed claims analysis. *Anesthesiology.* 2006;104(2):228–234.
27. Hug Jr CC. MAC should stand for maximum anesthesia caution, not minimal anesthesiology care. *Anesthesiology.* 2006;104(2):221–223.
28. Gan TJ. Pharmacokinetic and pharmacodynamic characteristics of medications used for moderate sedation. *Clin Pharmacokinet.* 2006;45(9):855–869.
29. Pambianco DJ, Vargo JJ, Pruitt RE, Hardi R, Martin JF. Computer-assisted personalized sedation for upper endoscopy and colonoscopy: a comparative, multicenter randomized study. *Gastrointest Endosc.* 2011;73(4):765–772.
30. Martin JF, Bridenbaugh P, Gustafson M. The SEDASYS System is not intended for the sedation of high-risk patients. *Gastrointest Endosc.* 2011;74(3):723.

15 Anesthesia for Colonoscopy

ESTHER D. GARAZI, CHRISTOPHER D. PRESS, and PEDRO P. TANAKA

History of Anesthesia for Gastrointestinal Endoscopic Procedures

Sedation and analgesia are common components to most upper and lower endoscopic procedures. Although diagnostic upper and lower endoscopy can be performed without sedation, the use of sedative medications improves patient comfort and the quality of the procedure.[1,2] The use of sedation in part depends on the country and reflects local practices. The decision to include an anesthesiologist in the care of a patient with a gastrointestinal (GI) issue also may depend on the location of the procedure and ready availability of trained anesthesia staff. Anesthesiologists tend to be more involved in sedation when procedures are being performed in an ambulatory surgery center instead of an office-based setting, where resources are limited.[3]

Since the U.S. Preventive Services Task Force mandated screening colonoscopies for all patients between the ages of 50 and 75 years, colonoscopies have become one of the most common medical procedures in the United States.[4] In 2002 it was estimated that more than 14 million colonoscopies were performed.[5] Although diagnostic colonoscopies can be done without sedation, the use of sedative medications improves overall outcomes — patients describe improved comfort, and proceduralists note that sedating the patient improves the diagnostic quality of the procedure.[6,7] Sedation for endoscopy has traditionally been administered by a nurse or endoscopist; however, as the number and complexity of cases have increased, participation by a trained anesthesiologist has become more commonplace in the endoscopy suite. Anesthesiologists tend to be more involved in sedation when procedures are performed in an ambulatory surgery center as compared with an office based–setting, where there are limited resources.[8]

General Considerations

GENERAL REASONS TO REQUEST AN ANESTHESIA PROVIDER

Several factors can contribute to the decision to use anesthesiology-based sedation for an endoscopic procedure. Certain patients commonly warrant anesthesiology-based care, including those with multiple or problematic comorbidities or airway concerns and pediatric patients. In addition, highly complex, long, or high-risk procedures are performed most safely under general anesthesia to prevent patient movement interfering with the procedure. Finally, patients with a history of failed gastroenterologist-administered sedation will benefit from the skills of a trained anesthesia provider (Box 15-1).[9]

The majority of patients can tolerate endoscopic procedures without general anesthesia by titrating the level of sedation to achieve a safe balance between patient comfort and optimal procedure conditions. Most endoscopic procedures are performed with the patient under moderate sedation.[10] Table 15-1 lists the criteria for varying levels of sedation.[11]

PREOPERATIVE EVALUATION

Patients must be evaluated for each procedure, with safety a top priority. Empty-stomach status must be confirmed with patients before proceeding with an elective procedure such as a colonoscopy. Preoperatively the anesthesiologist should always perform an airway examination. This includes evaluation for characteristics of difficult mask ventilation (Box 15-2).[12] Discuss with the patient all possible comorbidities associated with the sedation and anesthesia that will be used during the procedure. Ask the patient about previous experience with anesthetics, to identify patients who could be difficult to sedate or who could react poorly to sedation. Discuss what the patient expects from the procedure. Remember that patient comfort is an important factor in patient satisfaction for colonoscopies.[7]

Communication between the proceduralist and anesthesiologist is key to understanding how long the procedure will take and for ensuring that the patient will be able to tolerate sedation for the entirety of the colonoscopy. Older age in women, body mass index greater than 25 kg/m², diverticular disease in women, and history of constipation in men are predictors of increased time to complete an outpatient colonoscopy.[13] The anesthesia plan should

---

Box 15-1 Guidelines for Anesthesiology Assistance During Gastrointestinal Endoscopy

Prolonged procedure requiring deep sedation or general anesthesia
Anticipated intolerance to standard sedation regimens
Increased risk because of comorbidity (ASA 3 to 5)
Increased risk for airway obstruction (e.g., severe obstructive sleep apnea, stridor)
Dysmorphic facial features (e.g., Pierre-Robin, trisomy 21)
Oral abnormalities (e.g., macroglossia, small mouth opening, trismus)
Neck abnormalities (e.g., cervical stenosis, thick neck, trauma)
Uncooperative or pediatric patient

Modified from American Association for Study of Liver Diseases; American College of Gastroenterology; American Gastroenterological Association Institute; American Society for Gastrointestinal Endoscopy; Society for Gastroenterology Nurses and Associates; Vargo JJ, DeLegge MH, Feld AD, et al. Multisociety sedation curriculum for gastrointestinal endoscopy. Gastrointest Endosc. 2012;76:e1-e25.

Table 15-1   Continuum of Depth of Sedation

Signs	Minimal Sedation Anxiolysis	Moderate Sedation/ Analgesia	Deep Sedation/ Analgesia	General Anesthesia
Responsiveness	Normal response to verbal stimulation	Purposeful response to verbal or tactile stimulation	Purposeful response after repeated or painful stimulation	Unarousable even with painful stimulation
Airway	Unaffected	No intervention required	Intervention may be required	Intervention often required
Spontaneous ventilation	Unaffected	Adequate	May be inadequate	Frequently inadequate
Cardiovascular function	Unaffected	Usually maintained	Usually maintained	May be impaired

Modified from Gross J, Bailey PL, Connis R, et al. Practice guidelines for sedation and analgesia by nonanesthesiologists. *Anesthesiology.* 2002;6(4):1004-1017.[33]

Box 15-2   Predictors of Difficult Mask Ventilation and Difficult Intubation

Increased body mass index (>30 kg/m^2)
History of snoring or sleep apnea
Presence of beard
Lack of teeth
Age greater than 55 years
Mallampati class III or IV
Limited mandibular protrusion
Male gender
Airway masses or tumors

Modified from El-Orbany M, Woehlck HJ. Difficult mask ventilation. Anesth Analg. *2009;109(6);1870-1880.*

---

be adjusted accordingly and always contain alternative options in the event the initial plan does not work.

MONITORING

The recent advancements in safety for patients undergoing anesthesia are due in part to improved monitoring. In the past several decades, key monitors have increased anesthesia safety. The basic monitors now mandated by the American Society of Anesthesiologists (ASA) to be used during all procedures requiring anesthesia, are electrocardiogram, blood pressure (noninvasive or invasive), end-tidal capnography, oxygen saturation, and temperature.[14]

Additional monitors might be necessary on a patient-to-patient basis. For example, electroencephalographic (EEG) monitoring can be used to identify the depth of anesthesia to avoid awareness during general anesthesia, although the efficacy of EEG monitors for this indication is still debated. Continuous physical examination is the typical means of monitoring the depth of anesthesia for patients undergoing a colonoscopy. Ideally, patients should be able to verbally communicate with the anesthesia provider if provoked.

POSITIONING

Patient position is a particularly important consideration because many endoscopic procedures require the patient to be in the lateral or prone position, making it difficult if not impossible to access the airway if airway management techniques must be implemented. Therefore careful preoperative airway evaluation is paramount. If concern exists about airway management, the safest plan is to proceed with general anesthesia with endotracheal intubation, depending on the patient's associated comorbidities.

Once the patient has been positioned for the procedure, all monitors should be checked to ensure they are working properly. In addition, functional intravenous access should be confirmed before the patient is handed over to the proceduralist.

ANESTHETIC CHOICES

Anesthesia providers have the ability to vary the amount of sedation necessary to ensure the patient gets through the procedure safely and comfortably. In devising the anesthetic plan, focus should be on the level of sedation necessary to achieve this goal (see Table 15-1).[9] Monitored anesthesia care can be provided with the myriad medications listed in Table 15-2.

In the outpatient setting, which is where most diagnostic colonoscopies are performed, the goal of care is to provide a safe and effective anesthetic, with minimal side effects and quick recovery. Combinations of anesthetic agents are often the best means of achieving this goal. For example, medications such as propofol, when used in addition to a short-acting opiate such as fentanyl, provide the ideal level of amnesia, anxiolysis, and analgesia.[7] Combining propofol with other sedative medications can help reduce the amount of any one administered medication, thereby preventing propofol's negative cardiovascular effects.[15] In the preoperative period, take note of a patient's anesthetic history to identify patients at risk for bad reactions or side effects with these medications. One effect of note is the patient who becomes extremely nauseous with opiates. In patients with a history of difficult sedation, ketamine has shown to be an effective adjunct in moderate sedation.[16] In the inpatient setting, in which colonoscopies are in contrast to the outpatient setting, anesthesiologists are not limited by the expectation that the patient will be going home that day, so medications that have a longer-lasting effect, such as ketamine, are more readily used.

It is essential to maintain the airway of patients identified preoperatively as presenting with a potentially problematic airway. For these patients, the safest way to do the procedure might be general anesthesia with a protected airway. It is important to have this discussion preoperatively with the proceduralist and the patient.

Level of Sedation

The necessary levels of sedation to achieve safe and successful endoscopic procedures, ranging from no sedation to

Table 15-2   Favorable Sedative Effect Profile of Common Sedative Agents

Effect	Midazolam	Fentanyl	Propofol	Ketamine	Dexmedetomidine
Amnesia	+		+ >30mcg/kg/m	+ dissociative	
Analgesia		+		+	+
Anxiolysis	+	+/−			+

general anesthesia, are determined by patient-related and procedure-related factors. Patient-related factors include comorbidities, airway concerns, medication tolerance, and amount of pain or anxiety. Important procedure-related factors include patient position, type of procedure, duration, and complexity of procedure.

Patient position is a particularly important consideration, because many endoscopic procedures require the patient to be in the lateral or prone position, in which access to the airway becomes difficult, if not impossible, if airway management techniques must be implemented. Airway accessibility consideration increases during upper endoscopic procedures when the endoscope is advanced through the oral cavity. When concern for airway management exists, the safest plan is to proceed with general anesthesia with endotracheal intubation, often with a rapid sequence induction.

The majority of patients can tolerate endoscopic procedures without general anesthesia by titrating the level of sedation to achieve a safe balance between patient comfort and optimal procedure conditions. Most endoscopic procedures are performed with the patient under moderate sedation. Table 15-1 lists the criteria for varying levels of sedation.[17] In the United States; interest is growing on the part of the insurers to have clear indications for the use of an anesthesiologist.

Pharmacology: Common Sedative Medications

The choice of sedative medication depends on the provider and should be based on a combination of the procedure being performed and the individual patient. Traditional sedation for endoscopies typically entails a combination of opioids and benzodiazepines, usually midazolam and fentanyl, respectively, administered under the supervision of the endoscopist. The diverse array of sedative medications can allow sedation to be tailored according to each individual patient's needs based on the side effect profile of each medication (see Table 15-2).

Midazolam. Benzodiazepines have historically been the sedative agents favored by gastroenterologists. Along with their sedative effects, benzodiazepines have the added benefit of providing anxiolysis. Midazolam (Versed), in particular, is preferred because of its amnesic effects, fast onset, and short duration of action. When used alone, benzodiazepines have only modest hemodynamic effects.[18] Initial dosing of 1 to 2 mg is standard for young, healthy adults and provides significant anxiolysis. Additional doses of 1 mg every 2 to 5 minutes can then be administered as needed throughout the procedure to achieve adequate levels of sedation. When midazolam is given in conjunction with an opioid, such as fentanyl, synergism reduces the amount of midazolam needed for sedation. Patients older than 60 years of age or classified as having ASA 3 or

greater status often require smaller doses of midazolam for the same effect. Because the liver metabolizes midazolam, dose adjustments are also indicated in patients with significant liver disease.

The major disadvantage of midazolam is its respiratory depression, especially when given in combination with an opioid. The respiratory depressant effect can last up to 2 hours.[19] However, benzodiazepines can be reversed with flumazenil, which competitively antagonizes the central effects on gamma-aminobutyric acid (GABA) receptors. In addition, paradoxical reactions to midazolam, including disinhibition and aggression, have been reported.[20]

Fentanyl. Fentanyl is a short-acting synthetic opioid that is frequently given as an analgesic during endoscopic procedures. Its fast onset and short duration of action make it a better choice than other opioid analgesics, such as morphine or meperidine[21]. Fentanyl in combination with midazolam is considered part of the "traditional" sedation approach used by endoscopists without the supervision of an anesthesiologist. Initial doses of 50 to 100 mcg can be supplemented with boluses of 25 to 100 mcg, based on the individual patient. As with benzodiazepines, the dose should be reduced for elderly and critically ill patients and with hepatic impairment. Fentanyl is also safe to use in the pediatric population, with an initial dose of 0.5 mcg/kg, up to a maximum initial dose of 50 mcg.

Common side effects of fentanyl are similar to the side effects of all opioid narcotics and include bradycardia and respiratory depression. The respiratory depressant effects can be reversed with naloxone if needed.

Propofol. Propofol has come into favor for use by endoscopists as a replacement for traditional sedation because it increases patient comfort and decreases recovery times. It also improves the diagnostic quality of the procedure.[22,23] Propofol can be administered as an infusion or as intermittent boluses to achieve the desired sedation levels. Continuous infusions allow for easy titration to the desired level of sedation with relatively fast recovery after the infusion is terminated.[24] Propofol may have significant advantages during more complex procedures, such as endoscopic retrograde cholangiopancreatography (ERCP), in which deep sedation is needed.[25] Infusion rates for moderate sedation are 25 to 75 mcg/kg/min, but may be considerably less in elderly or critically ill patients. Propofol infusions for sedation may also cause some degree of amnesia, which can be beneficial to patient satisfaction.[26] Finally, the antiemetic properties of propofol may be especially useful when providing sedation for upper endoscopic procedures. In the pediatric population, propofol is an effective regimen alone or in combination with other sedative agents.[27]

The common side effects of propofol include hypoventilation, decreased muscle tone, cardiac depression, and hypotension. Therefore caution must be used when administering propofol as a sole means of sedation in patients who have significant cardiopulmonary disease or airway abnormalities.

Dexmedetomidine. Dexmedetomidine has more recently gained favor among anesthesiologists as an agent for inducing mild to moderate levels of sedation. As a nonselective alpha-2 receptor agonist, dexmedetomidine provides sedation, anxiolysis, and analgesia.[28] Although its high cost can make it prohibitively expensive, it still may be a favorable sedative in patients with hypoventilation concerns because it has minimal effect on respiratory drive. It is not very effective as a sole agent for colonoscopy, but can be very effective when supplemented with fentanyl or other agents.[29] Dexmedetomidine is given as an optional initial bolus of 0.5 to 1 mg/kg over 10 minutes, followed by an infusion of 0.2 to 0.7 mcg/kg/hr.

The main concern with dexmedetomidine is that its sympatholytic effects can trigger significant hypotension and bradycardia. However, for endoscopic procedures, it can be used in conjunction with ketamine to blunt some of the hemodynamic consequences of sympatholysis.

Ketamine. Ketamine is unique in that is has both sedative and analgesic properties without impairing respiratory drive or cardiovascular tone. It is a useful sedation adjunct for complex procedures, such as ERCP or endoscopic ultrasound (EUS), or for difficult-to-sedate patients undergoing colonoscopy.[16] Ketamine is frequently administered in combination with low-dose midazolam to prevent some of the hallucinogenic effects associated with ketamine administration. Ketamine boluses are also useful adjuncts to propofol or dexmedetomidine infusions because its stimulant effect on the respiratory and cardiovascular systems can counteract the cardiac and respiratory depressant effects of these agents. Bolus dosing of 0.1 to 0.3 mg/kg every 2 to 5 minutes, titrating to the desired effect, is a reasonable dose in a healthy adult, with a maximum dose of 1 mg/kg. Intramuscular or intravenous ketamine also can be useful in the pediatric population for sedation during endoscopic procedures.[30,31]

Complications

Preoperatively, it is important to identify and discuss with patients the complications associated with sedation. Patients should be aware that aspiration is a possible complication of sedation and monitored anesthesia care. In particular, the increased use of propofol for colonoscopies has raised the concern of the increased incidence of aspiration. The rate of aspiration events during sedation for colonoscopy is approximately 0.10% to 0.14%.[32]

Anesthesia providers should be ready to treat any of the complications associated with the procedure, such as a vagal response with insufflation, colonic laceration, and bleeding. Anesthesia providers usually can overcome these complications by having atropine or glycopyrrolate readily available in advance and ensuring adequate access.

Conclusion

Colonoscopies are better tolerated when analgesia and sedation are provided. Although proceduralists provide sedation during many colonoscopies, anesthesiologists are often consulted for care in complex cases and for critically ill patients or patients who have failed traditional sedation. Propofol has now become a popular alternative to the traditional benzodiazepine and opioid regimens of the past; however, a combination of multiple sedative agents tailored to individual patient needs is always warranted. The most complex endoscopic procedures, especially upper endoscopies, may require general anesthesia for the safety of the patient.

References

1. Dumonceau J, Riphaus A, Aparicio, et al. European Society of Gastrointestinal Endoscopy; European Society of Gastroenterology and Endoscopy Nurses and Associates. European Society of Anaesthesiology guideline: non-anaesthesiologist administration of propofol for GI endoscopy. *Eur J Anaesthesiol*. 2010;27(11):960–974.
2. McQuaid K, Laine L. A systematic review and meta-analysis of randomized, controlled trials of moderate sedation for routine endoscopic procedures. *Gastrointest Endosc*. 2008;67(6):910–923.
3. Liu H, Waxman D, Main R, Mattke S. Utilization of anesthesia services during outpatient endoscopies and colonoscopies and associated spending in 2003-2009. *JAMA*. 2012;307(11):1178–1184.
4. U.S. Preventive Services Task Force. Screening for colorectal cancer: U.S. Preventive Services Task Force recommendation statement. *Ann Intern Med*. 2008;149(9):627–637.
5. Seeff LC, Richards TB, Shapiro JA, et al. How many endoscopies are performed for colorectal cancer screening? Results from CDC's survey of endoscopic capacity. *Gastroenterology*. 2004;127(6):1670–1677.
6. Dumonceau JM, Riphaus A, Aparicio JR, et al. European Society of Gastrointestinal Endoscopy; European Society of Gastroenterology and Endoscopy Nurses and Associates. European Society of Anaesthesiology guideline: non-anesthesiologist administration of propofol for GI endoscopy. *Endoscopy*. 2010;42:960–974.
7. McQuaid KR, Laine LA. Systematic review and meta-analysis of randomized, controlled trials of moderate sedation for routine endoscopic procedures. *Gastrointestinal Endoscopy*. 2008;67:910–923.
8. Liu H, Waxman DA, Main R, Mattke S. Utilization of anesthesia services during outpatient endoscopies and colonoscopies and associated spending in 2003–2009. *JAMA*. 2012;307:1178–1184.
9. American Association for Study of Liver Diseases, American College of Gastroenterology, American Gastroenterological Association Institute, American Society for Gastrointestinal Endoscopy, Society for Gastroenterology Nurses and Associates, Vargo JJ, DeLegge MH, Feld AD, et al. Multisociety sedation curriculum for gastrointestinal endoscopy. *Gastrointest Endosc*. 2012;76:e1–e25.
10. Heuss LT, Schnieper P, Drewe J, et al. Risk stratification and safe administration of propofol by registered nurses supervised by the gastroenterologist: a prospective observational study of more than 2000 cases. *Gastrointest Endosc*. 2003;57(6):664–671.
11. American Society of Anesthesiologists Task Force on Sedation and Analgesia by Non-Anesthesiologists. Practice guidelines for sedation and analgesia by non-anesthesiologists. *Anesthesiology*. 2002;96(4):1004–1017.
12. El-Orbany M, Woehlck HJ. Difficult mask ventilation. *Anesth Analg*. 2009;109(6):1870–1880.
13. Anderson JC, Messina CR, Cohn W, et al. Factors predictive of difficult colonoscopy. *Gastrointest Endosc*. 2001;54(5):558–562.
14. Eichhorn JH. Prevention of intraoperative anesthesia accidents and related severe injury through safety monitoring. *Anesthesiology*. 1989;70(4):572–577.
15. Wang D, Wang S, Chen J, et al. Propofol combined with traditional sedative agents versus propofol-alone sedation for gastrointestinal endoscopy: a meta-analysis. *Scand J Gastroenterol*. 2013;48(1):101–110.
16. Varadarajulu S, Eloubeidi MA, Tamhane A, Wilcox CM. Prospective randomized trial evaluating ketamine for advanced endoscopic procedures in difficult to sedate patients. *Aliment Pharmacol Ther*. 2007;25(8):987–997.

17. Heuss LT, Schnieper P, Drewe J, Pflimlin E, Beglinger C. Risk stratification and safe administration of propofol by registered nurses supervised by the gastroenterologist: a prospective observational study of more than 2000 cases. *Gastroint Endosc.* 2003;57:664–671.

18. Wong RC. The menu of endoscopic sedation: all-you-can-eat, combination set, á la carte, alternative cuisine, or go hungry. *Gastrointest Endosc.* 2001;54(1):122–126.

19. Cole SG, Brozinsky S, Isenberg JI. Midazolam, a new more potent benzodiazepine, compared with diazepam: a randomized, double-blind study of preendoscopic sedatives. *Gastrointest Endosc.* 1983;29(3):219–222.

20. Robin C, Trieger N. Paradoxical reactions to benzodiazepines in intravenous sedation: a report of 2 cases and review of the literature. *Anesth Prog.* 2002;49(4):128–132.

21. Triantafillidis JK, Merikas E, Nikolakis D, Papalois AE. Sedation in gastrointestinal endoscopy: current issues. *World J Gastroenterol.* 2013 Jan 28;19(4):463–481.

22. Qadeer MA, Vargo JJ, Khandwala F, et al. Propofol versus traditional sedative agents for gastrointestinal endoscopy: a meta-analysis. *Clin Gastroenterol Hepatol.* 2005;3(11):1049–1056.

23. Singh H, Poluha W, Cheung M, et al. Propofol for sedation during colonoscopy. *Cochrane Database Syst Rev.* 2008;(4). CD006268.

24. Wilson E, Mackenzie N, Grant IS. A comparison of propofol and midazolam by infusion to provide sedation in patients who receive spinal anaesthesia. *Anaesthesia.* 1988;43(Suppl):91–94.

25. Jung M, Hofmann C, Kiesslich R, Brackertz A. Improved sedation in diagnostic and therapeutic ERCP: propofol is an alternative to midazolam. *Endoscopy.* 2000;32(3):233–238.

26. Grounds RM, Lalor JM, Lumley J, Royston D, Morgan M. Propofol infusion for sedation in the intensive care unit: preliminary report. *Br Med J (Clin Res Ed).* 1987;294:397–400.

27. Van Beek EJ, Leroy PL. Safe and effective procedural sedation for gastrointestinal endoscopy in children. *J Pediatr Gastroenterol Nutr.* 2012;54(2):171–185.

28. Kamibayashi T, Maze M. Clinical uses of alpha2-adrenergic agonists. *Anesthesiology.* 2005;93:1345–1349.

29. Jalowiecki P, Rudner R, Gonciarz M, et al. Sole use of dexmedetomidine has limited utility for conscious sedation during outpatient colonoscopy. *Anesthesiology.* 2005;103(2):269–273.

30. Law AK, Ng DK, Chan K-K. Use of intramuscular ketamine for endoscopy sedation in children. *Pediatr Int.* 2003;45(2):180–185.

31. Green SM, Klooster M, Harris T, Lynch EL, Rothrock SG. Ketamine sedation for pediatric gastroenterology procedures. *J Pediatr Gastroenterol Nutr.* 2001;32(1):26–33.

32. Cooper GS, Kou TD, Rex DK. Complications following colonoscopy with anesthesia assistance: a population-based analysis. *JAMA Intern Med.* 2013;173(7):551–556.

33. Gross J, Bailey PL, Connis R, et al. Practice guidelines for sedation and analgesia by nonanesthesiologists. *Anesthesiology.* 2002;96(4):1004–1017.

16 Anesthesia in the Bronchoscopy Suite

MARK A. LEIBEL, W. KIRKE ROGERS, and RICHARD E. GALGON

An increasing number of pulmonary disorders are amenable to flexible or rigid bronchoscopic diagnostic or therapeutic intervention. New techniques such as endobronchial ultrasound, electromagnetic navigational bronchoscopy, and treatment of central airway obstruction, including tumor debulking and placement of airway stents, require specialized equipment and the physical space to store and use it. The increase in variety and volume of procedures led to the development of dedicated procedural space in many hospitals—interventional pulmonology or bronchoscopy suites.

Many bronchoscopic procedures can be performed with minimal sedation. Thus the continual presence of a trained anesthesia provider is not always necessary. However, because of procedural or patient complexity, anesthesia providers are being increasingly consulted to provide care in these settings. For several reasons, the pulmonology suite can be an intimidating location for the anesthesiologist or nurse anesthetist. Familiarity with the physical space and ancillary staff may be limited as a result of the intermittent request for anesthesia services. Patients often have multiple baseline comorbidities with tenuous respiratory or cardiac status. Procedures are typically short, with rapid patient turnover and limited time for preprocedural evaluation. The airway must be shared with the bronchoscopist, and the patient's head is often turned away from the anesthesiologist. Anesthesia providers who do not frequently perform in these cases may be somewhat unfamiliar with the specialized ventilatory and intravenous anesthetic techniques used for these procedures. Finally, the procedure suite may be located distant from the main operating rooms, limiting the availability of assistance in an emergency.

The goal of this chapter is to provide an overview of the procedures and accompanying airway and ventilation choices, anesthetic management issues, and complications unique to the adult interventional bronchoscopy suite.

Interventional Bronchoscopic Techniques

Modern interventional bronchoscopy encompasses a variety of diagnostic and therapeutic procedures. An in-depth discussion of all techniques exceeds the scope of this chapter; therefore we have chosen to briefly examine a few important procedures that are either becoming widespread or show great potential for transforming interventional bronchoscopic practice over the next decade. Common anesthetic techniques and airway choices for each procedure are detailed in Table 16-1.

ENDOBRONCHIAL ULTRASOUND WITH TRANSBRONCHIAL NEEDLE ASPIRATION

Endobronchial ultrasound with transbronchial needle aspiration (EBUS-TBNA) is a less invasive procedure than traditional mediastinoscopy; both are intended to yield tissue for diagnostic purposes. For EBUS, an ultrasound transducer integrated into a dedicated bronchoscope is placed either directly in contact with the tracheal or bronchial wall or indirectly via a saline-inflated balloon, displaying real-time ultrasound images. Fine needle aspiration of lymph nodes can then be performed under ultrasound visualization. Procedural indications include staging of non–small cell lung cancer, diagnosis of suspected lung cancer without endobronchial lesions, and evaluation of unexplained mediastinal lymphadenopathy. EBUS-TBNA may be diagnostically superior to computed tomography (CT) and positron emission tomography (PET)[1,2] and has overall accuracy similar to that of mediastinoscopy but with less invasiveness and the ability to sample hilar lymph nodes.[3] As the required technology is maturing and becoming more widely available, EBUS-TBNA is quickly becoming the standard of care.

EBUS with or without biopsies is usually only minimally stimulating, and most procedures can be completed under conscious sedation; however, general anesthesia may be requested in several instances. First, sampling adequacy is improved with sampling a higher number of lymph node stations.[4] When extensive staging is performed, particularly when lymph nodes are less than 1 cm in their largest dimension, procedures can become quite prolonged. Patient intolerance may necessitate general anesthesia. Further, some pulmonologists prefer general anesthesia when a large number of stations are sampled, believing it improves diagnostic yield. Finally, the saline-filled balloon can occasionally completely obstruct the airway; cases have been reported in which coughing against the obstruction led to negative-pressure pulmonary edema,[5] a problem obviated by general anesthesia with muscle relaxation.

ELECTROMAGNETIC NAVIGATIONAL BRONCHOSCOPY

Electromagnetic navigational bronchoscopy (ENB) was developed as a guidance system to assist the bronchoscopist

Table 16-1 Anesthesia for Interventional Bronchoscopic Techniques

Bronchoscopic Technique	Recommended Anesthetic Technique	Recommended Airway
DIAGNOSTIC		
Endobronchial ultrasound with transbronchial needle aspiration (EBUS-TBNA)	Conscious sedation versus less commonly general anesthesia	None versus SGA
Electromagnetic navigational bronchoscopy (ENB)	Conscious sedation versus less commonly general anesthesia	None versus SGA
THERAPEUTIC		
Treatment of central airway obstruction	TIVA with rigid bronchoscopy versus awake fiberoptic intubation; reduced FiO_2; consider Heliox and maintenance of spontaneous ventilation even with rigid bronchoscopy	ETT versus rigid bronchoscopy
Airway stents	General anesthesia, often TIVA with rigid bronchoscopy	ETT versus rigid bronchoscopy
Bronchoscopic balloon dilation	TIVA with paralysis; jet ventilation versus bag-mask ventilation between balloon inflations	Rigid bronchoscopy
Bronchoscopic lung volume reduction (BLVR)	Conscious sedation versus general anesthesia	None versus SGA
Radiofrequency ablation	Conscious sedation versus general anesthesia if lung isolation is necessary; reduced FiO_2	None versus double-lumen endotracheal tube if lung isolation is necessary
Bronchial thermoplasty	Conscious sedation	None versus SGA

ETT, Endotracheal tube; *SGA*, supraglottic airway; *TIVA*, total intravenous anesthesia.

in performing a biopsy of difficult-to-access peripheral, pulmonary nodules. The technology combines multidirectional CT (MDCT) imaging, magnetic field localization, and a steerable probe with a magnetized tip. During the procedure, the bronchoscope is guided into the area of interest and the tip location is displayed on the MDCT image. Diagnostic yield of biopsies for small peripheral lung nodules is much improved over previous techniques.[6,7] Other potential uses include placement of fiducial markers for stereotactic radiotherapy and marking of nodules for surgical wedge resection. Sedation and anesthetic needs are similar to those of EBUS and dictated by patient comorbidities, needs of the bronchoscopist, and anticipated procedure duration.

TREATMENT OF CENTRAL AIRWAY OBSTRUCTION

In modern practice, relief of obstruction of the central airways (trachea, mainstem bronchi, and bronchus intermedius) remains the main indication for therapeutic bronchoscopy.

Obstruction can result from intraluminal malignancy, external compression by mediastinal mass, massive hemoptysis with clot, or benign causes such as foreign body, postintubation tracheal stenosis, or tracheobronchomalacia. A variety of therapeutic approaches exist, with selection depending on cause, urgency, and availability. Laser ablation, electrocautery, argon plasma coagulation (APC), mechanical debridement, and airway stents can provide immediate relief of obstruction. In contrast, cryotherapy, brachytherapy, and photodynamic therapy produce delayed effects. If intervention is urgent because of severe or progressive obstruction, effort should be made to stabilize the patient to enable completion of diagnostic studies (such as CT imaging) to aid in developing an optimal treatment strategy. In this situation, heliox, given its lower density than air or 100% oxygen, can improve gas flow across highly narrowed areas of the airway and reduce turbulent flow conditions. If heliox is ineffective or not available, consideration must be given for intubation distal to the obstruction, typically accomplished with fiberoptic bronchoscopy. Alternatively, rigid bronchoscopy in expert hands can be lifesaving.

The neodymium-doped yttrium aluminum garnet (Nd:YAG) laser and other "hot" therapies, such as electrocautery and APC, are designed to vaporize tissue and achieve superior coagulation and thus are often chosen to treat obstructing central airway lesions. Unfortunately, these thermal techniques also carry an increased risk for airway and procedure room fires. Microdebriders, which mechanically debulk airway tumors, were developed as "cold" therapies that still can rapidly open an airway. Although inferior to thermal techniques in controlling bleeding, microdebriders also avoid some of their potential complications.

APC is based on gas flow, and many lasers have a gas-cooled fiber that is used to apply the energy. Case reports have documented intravascular gas during use of the Nd:YAG laser and even cardiac arrest secondary to gas embolism during bronchoscopic APC.[8,9] In animal studies, gas emboli were more frequent with higher laser coolant flow and longer laser pulse generation,[10] a finding the authors speculatively ascribed to positive-pressure ventilation forcing air through small bronchovascular defects. Therefore current procedural recommendations include using the lowest possible setting for laser coolant flow, using noncontact mode, and applying thermal ablation only during apnea or spontaneous breathing.

AIRWAY STENTS

Indications for airway stenting include extrinsic airway compression, mixed extrinsic and endoluminal lesions, recurrence of airway compromise after treatment of intraluminal lesions, inoperable nonmalignant disease, and treatment of airway fistulas.[11,12] Stents can be made of silicone, expandable metal, or a combination of both, such as a covered metal stent. Metal stents resist migration because they become embedded in airway tissue and tend to generate a proliferative granulation response. Unfortunately, this also means that metal stents can be difficult and potentially dangerous to remove if in place for more than a few weeks. Expandable metal stents can be placed via flexible or rigid bronchoscope. Fluoroscopy is often used to guide placement. Because silicone stents do not collapse, a rigid bronchoscope must be used for placement.

Complications are common with all stent types. Granulation tissue formed after metal stent placement may occasionally cause airway obstruction and necessitate reintervention, often by Nd:YAG laser ablation. Removal of metal stents is best accomplished with a rigid bronchoscope and jet ventilation. Silicone stents are much easier to remove but are prone to migration, mucous obstruction, and infection.

BRONCHOSCOPIC BALLOON DILATATION

Bronchoscopic balloon dilatation is commonly used to treat nontraumatic subglottic stenosis, often in conjunction with injection of corticosteroids or the anti-neoplastic drug mitomycin-C in an attempt to reduce the rate of restenosis. Total intravenous anesthesia (TIVA) with paralysis is often used in combination with intermittent bag-mask ventilation or jet ventilation before and after balloon dilatation, which typically lasts 1 to 3 minutes and can be performed repeatedly during a single procedure. During balloon dilatation, it is important to maintain adequate muscle relaxation and monitor for diaphragmatic firing to prevent respiratory effort against the occluded airway and the subsequent development of negative-pressure pulmonary edema. Further, improvement in stenosis is often delayed, so the anesthesia provider must be particularly vigilant in monitoring for airway obstruction and adequate ventilation both immediately after the procedure and in the postanesthesia care unit (PACU).

RADIOFREQUENCY ABLATION

Radiofrequency ablation (RFA) is a minimally invasive treatment modality that has previously been used to treat patients with hepatic, renal, and breast tumors. After the RFA electrode is inserted into the target lesion, alternating radiofrequency currents are generated, leading to frictional heating and ultimately coagulative necrosis and cell death. The procedure tends to be well tolerated and is often done under conscious sedation. However, achieving effective targeting of pulmonary neoplastic lesions and protecting nontargeted tissues can be challenging. Deflating the target lung can be helpful but may move the lesion too close to central structures. A technique to obtain improved tumor positioning has been described using lung isolation with a double-lumen endotracheal tube (DLT) with static inflation of the target lung by either clamping the DLT lumen supplying the target lung or applying CPAP to maintain target lung inflation.[13] Although not reported with RFA of pulmonary lesions, the use of high oxygen concentrations may pose a fire risk.

BRONCHIAL THERMOPLASTY

In poorly controlled chronic asthma, airway smooth muscle hypertrophy is a component of airway remodeling, which contributes to ongoing symptoms. Bronchial thermoplasty, which uses heat generated by radiofrequency energy to destroy bronchial smooth muscle, has been shown in at least two trials to (1) improve prebronchodilator forced expiratory volume in 1 second (FEV_1), (2) reduce severe exacerbations, (3) decrease rescue medication use, and (4) improve reported quality of life for patients with severe asthma.[14,15] Current guidelines, however, limit bronchial thermoplasty as a treatment option to selected patients with severe persistent asthma already on maximal medical therapy.[16] Bronchial thermoplasty is generally well tolerated and can usually be accomplished under conscious sedation. However, if the anesthesiologist is involved, he or she must be aware of the increased risk for respiratory complications in the first 24 hours after the procedure, primarily acute bronchospasm or increased mucous plugging, occasionally resulting in lobar collapse.

BRONCHOSCOPIC LUNG VOLUME REDUCTION

The National Emphysema Treatment Trial was published in 2003, demonstrating that in a carefully selected patient population with severe heterogeneous emphysema, lung volume reduction surgery (LVRS) reduced mortality, improved exercise tolerance, and improved quality of life.[17] However, LVRS was associated with considerable morbidity and mortality, causing investigators to speculate that less invasive bronchoscopic interventions might achieve similar benefits while minimizing perioperative risk. Multiple techniques are currently under study, including intrabronchial valves, lung volume reduction coils, lung sealant, and bronchoscopic thermal vapor ablation. The goal for any of these procedures is to achieve segmental or lobar collapse to effectively reduce lung volume, thus reducing air trapping and improving elastic recoil and expiratory flows. Although results for many of these modalities are somewhat promising, none are ready for widespread adoption, and optimal anesthetic techniques have not yet been described.

Preoperative Evaluation

HISTORY AND REVIEW OF SYSTEMS

The majority of patients presenting for interventional bronchoscopic procedures are classified as American Society of Anesthesiologists physical status 3 or higher.[18] Tobacco abuse is a common risk factor for the majority of upper airway and pulmonary pathological conditions necessitating bronchoscopic intervention. Unsurprisingly, smoking-related diseases such as obstructive or less commonly restrictive pulmonary disease, coronary artery disease, congestive heart failure, peripheral vascular disease, cerebral ischemic disease, hypertension, malnutrition, and malignancies outside the lungs and airway are extremely common in this population. Heavy alcohol use, type 2 diabetes mellitus, and obesity are also common. Sequelae of the aforementioned pathological conditions that can affect anesthetic management include chronic kidney disease, obstructive sleep apnea, gastroparesis and gastroesophageal reflux disease, and limited neck mobility. The review of systems should further focus on the patient's functional status, symptom control of baseline pulmonary or cardiac disease and any environmental triggers, presence of orthopnea, specific triggers for cough, and the severity of reflux disease.

Rigid bronchoscopy requires neck hyperextension, so patients presenting for this procedure should be assessed for risk factors for cervical spine subluxation such as trisomy 21 (Down syndrome) cervical ankylosis, or rheumatoid or other inflammatory arthritis with cervical involvement.[19] Inquiring about previous chemotherapy is important, particularly the use of bleomycin and its associated risks for pulmonary fibrosis and acute oxygen toxicity, as well as doxorubicin and its potential for causing cardiomyopathy. Patients with previous lung transplantation or cystic fibrosis require increased sedative dosing during flexible bronchoscopy.[20] Interestingly, advanced age alone does not confer an increased risk for complications from either flexible or rigid bronchoscopy.[21,22]

PREPROCEDURE STUDIES

Patients with suspected chronic obstructive pulmonary disease (COPD) should undergo spirometry and also should have a baseline arterial blood gas sample drawn if COPD is determined to be severe (FEV_1 <40% predicted and/or room air oxygen saturation [SaO_2] <93%).[23] If biopsies are to be performed, coagulation tests, including international normalized ratio, partial thromboplastin time, and platelet count, may be considered.[24] Other laboratory studies such as a complete blood count or metabolic panel should not be routinely ordered unless prompted by the history and review of systems. Radiographic images must be reviewed, particularly when central airway obstruction is present or suspected, allowing the anesthesiologist to assess the potential for clinical airway compromise. Large bullae typical of severe emphysema suggest an increased risk for pneumothorax or other barotrauma with jet ventilation or even conventional positive-pressure ventilation.

Management of Anesthesia: Pharmacology

PREMEDICATION

Anticholinergics

In a consensus statement on the use of sedation and topical anesthesia during flexible bronchoscopy, the American College of Chest Physicians advised against the routine use of anticholinergic medication as a bronchodilator or antisialagogue.[25] However, glycopyrrolate 0.005 mg/kg (approximately 0.2 to 0.4 mg for an average-size adult) is not unreasonable in selected cases, such as when aerosolized local anesthetic is to be used, and is generally better tolerated and more effective than atropine in decreasing secretions.[25]

Sedatives

Oral clonidine, at a dose of 150 mcg or up to 3 mcg/kg, has been suggested as a premedicant because it has some sedative effect and can blunt the hemodynamic response to bronchoscopy or laryngoscopy,[26] though additional sedative medicines are likely to be needed during awake fiberoptic bronchoscopy.[27] Other preprocedure sedatives and anxiolytics such as midazolam (0.25 to 2 mg intravenously) or diazepam (2.5 to 10 mg intravenously) should be minimized because of the risk for respiratory depression in an undermonitored patient. Oversedation with benzodiazepines also can lead to disinhibition, complicating a bronchoscopic procedure that could otherwise be performed in a lightly sedated and cooperative

patient. Supplemental oxygen should be routinely provided before administering any sedatives, and anxiolytics should be used in only extremely anxious patients.

Steroids

Multiple studies have suggested that a 24-hour course of dexamethasone or other corticosteroid can reduce laryngeal edema and decrease the risk for postextubation stridor or obstruction in a critical care setting,[28] but there is no solid evidence that the routine use of corticosteroids has any benefit in most bronchoscopic procedures. Nonetheless, many practitioners administer dexamethasone 0.2 to 0.5 mg/kg (up to 10 mg) intravenously to prevent airway swelling in cases of longer duration or when extensive inflammation of vocal cords or airway mucosa is expected. This may not be an unreasonable approach, because at least two small studies have suggested that a prophylactic dose of dexamethasone 0.2 mg/kg can at least decrease the incidence of postoperative sore throat and hoarseness in patients intubated for relatively short procedures.[29,30] Although high-dose steroids have many potential adverse effects, the risk for significant complications after a single prophylactic dose of dexamethasone is likely negligible.[31]

Antiemetics

Published guidelines on postoperative nausea and vomiting (PONV) prophylaxis do not recommend routine antiemetic administration.[32] However, the risk for aspiration during and after bronchoscopic interventions may be higher than that for other procedures. Given that many of the patients undergoing such procedures have limited pulmonary reserve, aggressive PONV prophylaxis may be warranted. Because multiple drug classes have similar efficacy, medication selection is based on side effect profile, patient factors, physician preference, availability, and cost. Dexamethasone given preprocedurally is an effective antiemetic and is often given for other reasons, as discussed earlier.

Antacids and Gastrokinetics

Reducing gastric acidity may decrease the risk for chemical pneumonitis in patients who aspirate, although no evidence supports the routine use of acid-reducing drugs in patients undergoing bronchoscopic procedures. Although protein pump inhibitors are the most potent class, they may take more than 24 hours for full effect and thus have a limited role as preoperative medications.[33] In contrast, histamine-2 (H_2) antagonists may produce a clinically significant increase in gastric pH and reduction in gastric volume 30 to 60 minutes after an intravenous dose or 2 to 3 hours after an oral dose. Metoclopramide is often used as a prokinetic in patients with gastroparesis. Less effective in increasing gastric pH than H_2 blockers, metoclopramide also has more potential side effects and drug and disease interactions, making it a less attractive option. In patients with high aspiration risk presenting without sufficient time for other medications to take effect, a nonparticulate antacid such as 0.3 M sodium citrate can be administered with a resultant immediate increase in gastric pH.

Bronchodilators

Many authorities recommend that patients with asthma or COPD with a reversible component routinely receive a short-acting bronchodilator preprocedurally,[34] although such premedication may not produce any benefit in COPD.[35] Atropine has been long suggested to have protective bronchodilatory properties when given before bronchoscopic procedures.[36] However, more recent studies failed to show meaningful improvement in lung function or sustained benefit postprocedurally.[25]

LOCAL ANESTHETICS AND AIRWAY REFLEX SUPPRESSION

Successful bronchoscopy in a patient not receiving general anesthesia requires adequate suppression of airway reflexes to facilitate the procedure. The degree and location of necessary reflex suppression depend on the planned airway management and route of bronchoscopy. Perineural injections, topicalization with local anesthetics, or a combination of these techniques may be used. In either case, lidocaine is the preferred local anesthetic because of its rapid onset, appropriately short duration of action, and relative safety.[25] The total cumulative dose of lidocaine used through all procedures described in the following section should absolutely not exceed 8.2 mg/kg [37]; most practitioners are more conservative and limit maximum lidocaine administration to 5 mg/kg.

Nasal Anesthesia

Adequate nasal anesthesia usually can be achieved using a combination of a vasoconstricting nasal spray, such as oxymetazoline or phenylephrine, followed by application of viscous lidocaine jelly. This process usually provides adequate sensory blockade and lubrication to allow passage of a nasal trumpet, bronchoscope, or endotracheal tube (ETT). Alternatively, the pterygopalatine ganglion (providing sensory input to the anterior third of the nasal septum and posterior nasal cavity) can be blocked by soaking a cotton ball or cotton-tipped applicator in 2% to 4% lidocaine with epinephrine (1:200,000) or phenylephrine (1:20,000), passing it slowly to the posterior wall of the nasopharynx, and leaving it in place for 5 to 10 minutes.[38]

Anesthesia of the Posterior Oropharynx and Upper Airway

For an awake patient to tolerate either nasotracheal or orotracheal bronchoscopy or intubation, sequential blockade of the superior laryngeal nerve and recurrent laryngeal nerve is required, via either perineural injections or less invasive mucosal saturation. Direct regional blockade of the superior laryngeal nerve is performed bilaterally at the level of the thyrohyoid membrane, just inferior to the cornu of the hyoid bone. A small-bore needle is directed anteroinferomedially until the greater cornu is contacted; the needle is then withdrawn slightly, and after negative aspiration is confirmed, 2 mL of 2% to 4% lidocaine with epinephrine 1:200,000 is injected. The block is repeated in the same fashion on the contralateral side.[38] Recurrent laryngeal nerve blockade is necessary to suppress coughing when the bronchoscope is passed through the vocal cords and into the trachea and can be readily achieved by translaryngeal block. A 20- or 22-gauge needle on a syringe under constant negative pressure is advanced through the cricothyroid membrane until air is aspirated, and then 4 mL of 2% to 4% lidocaine with epinephrine is injected. Patients invariably cough with the

delivery of the local anesthetic solution, which helps disperse the local anesthetic but increases the risk for puncturing the back wall of the trachea with the needle.[38] To minimize this risk, some practitioners prefer to use a 20- or 22-gauge peripheral intravenous catheter-over-needle to access the trachea. After aspiration of air, the needle is removed, air aspiration is repeated to confirm catheter location in the airway, and the local anesthetic solution is delivered. Ultrasound guidance has recently been used to facilitate this procedure.[39] Remember that the induction of coughing potentially could be life-threatening in patients with severe central airway obstruction,[40] and another approach to airway management may be required.

Although direct regional blockade of the superior and recurrent laryngeal nerves is possible, adequate anesthesia usually can be achieved less invasively with topical local anesthetic application and mucosal saturation. After administration of a drying agent such as glycopyrrolate to reduce oropharyngeal secretions and improve local anesthetic absorption, 5 mL of 4% lidocaine or another local anesthetic can be aerosolized via a standard nebulizer attached to a face mask or mouthpiece and is well tolerated in nearly all patients. With enough time, aerosolized local anesthetic usually provides adequate initial anesthesia of the oropharynx and upper airway. Denser anesthesia of more distal structures can then be achieved through a combination of gargled, swallowed, or sprayed liquid or viscous local anesthetic. Benzocaine spray can be used, but excessive administration can cause methemoglobinemia.[41] Finally, the working channel of a flexible bronchoscope can be used to sequentially inject 1 to 2 mL of 2% to 4% lidocaine over the epiglottis, just above the vocal cords, just below the cords, and at the carina. Systemic lidocaine levels are generally negligible even when administered to mucosa using a combination of methods.[42]

MODERATE SEDATION

Standard flexible bronchoscopy in an otherwise healthy patient usually requires little more than moderate conscious sedation with adequate airway reflex suppression via any of the previously described techniques. Intravenous fentanyl 2 to 2.5 mcg/kg titrated over the duration of the procedure in 12.5- to 50-mcg aliquots and midazolam 0.5 to 2 mg usually provide adequate sedation, anxiolysis, and some degree of cough suppression. Higher doses of benzodiazepines tend to cause disinhibition and may actually lead to increased coughing. Between 500 to 1000 mcg of alfentanil was used more commonly in the past as an alternative to fentanyl to achieve adequate sedation for flexible bronchoscopy.[43,44] Adding midazolam to alfentanil may increase the risk for hypoxia without improving sedation or decreasing discomfort.[43]

When anesthesiologists are consulted, the most common choice for moderate sedation is propofol, administered either by intermittent boluses (10 to 20 mg)[18] or as a low-dose infusion (10 to 50 mcg/kg/min). In contrast to the combination of midazolam and fentanyl, propofol offers more rapid recovery and easier titration in bronchoscopic cases lasting more than 20 minutes.[45-47]

Remifentanil by infusion can be used as a sole agent for moderate sedation or as an infusion after 0.5 to 2 mg of midazolam for particularly anxious patients. The initial infusion rate should be 0.1 mcg/kg/min started 5 minutes before beginning bronchoscopy, with the infusion then weaned to approximately 0.05 mcg/kg/min as tolerated during the procedure. This regimen usually provides adequate sedation and cough suppression for bronchoscopy and has even been used for more stimulating procedures, such as tracheoplasty using combined laser and balloon dilation,[48] although providers may find that patients need to be "coached" to breathe. Remifentanil offers an advantage as a sole agent over other opioids because patients predictably awaken within 4 to 5 minutes of discontinuation of its infusion, regardless of infusion duration.

Dexmedetomidine has been studied as a sedative for bronchoscopic procedures[49] but has the disadvantage of requiring a loading infusion, typically 0.5 to 1 mcg/kg over 10 to 20 minutes, before the initiation of a maintenance infusion of 0.2 to 0.7 mcg/kg/hr. Given the relatively short duration and fast turnover of most procedures performed in a bronchoscopy suite, this relatively long loading time may result in significant inconvenience and cost ineffectiveness. Nonetheless, the use of dexmedetomidine is appealing because of its lack of blunting of respiratory drive while providing analgesia. Dexmedetomidine can be associated with clinically significant bradycardia and hypotension at any point during its use, as well as occasional hypertension during the initial load.

General Anesthesia

INDUCTION

General anesthesia may be necessary for long cases, procedures in which immobility is necessary, or when significant stimulation is anticipated. Induction of general anesthesia should be relatively rapid and without coughing while maintaining hemodynamic stability.

Inhaled sevoflurane can be used to gently induce general anesthesia and may be the preferred choice of induction in cases of critical airway stenosis because spontaneous ventilation is maintained. A single-breath vital capacity technique in which the patient, beginning from maximal exhalation, deeply inhales 8% sevoflurane and then holds the breath is reported to be most effective in healthy volunteers.[50] Although a single-breath induction has been successfully reported in patients with airway stenosis,[51] patients with pulmonary disease tend to do better with a tidal volume technique in which the concentration of sevoflurane is slowly titrated up, with the patient taking regular normal tidal volume breaths, because many cannot take large breaths and hold them without coughing.

As in general operating rooms, propofol at 1 to 2 mg/kg is the most commonly used primary induction medication in the bronchoscopy suite. Ketamine is an attractive induction agent because of its unique characteristics; as an indirect sympathomimetic, it is a potent bronchodilator with relative preservation of respiratory drive and cardiac function. At an induction dose of 1 to 2 mg/kg, psychotropic side effects are rarely encountered after benzodiazepine premedication (e.g., midazolam 1 to 2 mg). Etomidate 0.2 to 0.3 mg/kg is an alternative induction agent for patients with impaired left ventricular function. Complete opioid-based or benzodiazepine-based induction regimens are rarely appropriate for bronchoscopic procedures because the doses required to achieve adequate anesthetic depth do not allow emergence in a timely manner.

MAINTENANCE

Either TIVA or inhalational anesthetic can be employed for maintenance of general anesthesia, although TIVA is often preferred for bronchoscopic procedures because of its multiple advantages. Most notably, recurrent insertion and removal of the bronchoscope, as well as frequent airway suctioning, cause inconsistent delivery of volatile agents. TIVA ensures uninterrupted delivery of anesthetic separate from ventilation and avoids exposing procedural room personnel to leaked inhalational agent. Other advantages of TIVA when propofol-based include less PONV, decreased cough at emergence,[52] and less depression of bronchial mucous transport velocity.[53] Inhalational anesthetics may predispose patients to increased bleeding at the site of needle puncture during biopsies, perhaps because volatile agents cause local vasodilation in the bronchial mucosa.[5] Finally, jet ventilation and other specialized modes of ventilation may be technically incompatible with the delivery of volatile anesthetic.

Propofol can be used as a sole agent for maintenance of anesthesia for flexible bronchoscopy at a dose of 75 to 250 mcg/kg/min, but it is usually necessary to add an opioid to suppress coughing in nonparalyzed patients or to blunt the hemodynamic response to more stimulating procedures, such as rigid bronchoscopy. Either intermittent low-dose fentanyl (12.5- to 50-mcg aliquots to a total of <2 to 2.5 mcg/kg for the duration of a typical case) or a remifentanil infusion (0.1 to 0.3 mcg/kg/min) are commonly used.[5] A higher dose of remifentanil (0.5 mcg/kg/min) together with propofol more effectively attenuates the hemodynamic response to insertion of a rigid bronchoscope,[54] but more frequently causes hypotension. Remifentanil has a reliably short duration of action, with 3 to 10 minutes to arousal after its discontinuation regardless of the duration or dose of infusion, allowing predictable emergence. Arousal from propofol is short and fairly predictable after short cases typical of bronchoscopic procedures. Prolonged use, however, may lead to unpredictably prolonged emergence. If a target-controlled infusion, currently not available in the United States, is administered, appropriate induction and maintenance plasma concentration targets for propofol are 7 mcg/mL and less than 5 to 6 mcg/mL, respectively, if a remifentanil infusion or intermittent fentanyl boluses are used concurrently. The most commonly reported initial effect-site target concentration for remifentanil infusions in bronchoscopic procedures is 2 to 5 ng/mL.

MUSCLE RELAXATION

It is worth remembering that most procedures performed in the bronchoscopy suite do not absolutely require pharmacological muscle relaxation if quiescent conditions can be achieved by other means. Even procedures requiring rigid bronchoscopy, jet ventilation, laser therapy, and stent placement have been safely performed without paralysis.[55,56] Potential advantages of avoiding neuromuscular blockade include shortened emergence and no chance of residual paralysis or recurarization of patients with baseline or anticipated limited pulmonary reserve after the procedure. Despite this, many proceduralists and anesthesia providers prefer muscle relaxation for procedures with a high risk for airway injury or hemorrhage or the potential for spontaneous respiratory effort against an obstructed or occluded airway, which can lead to negative-pressure pulmonary edema.

Management of Anesthesia: Airway Choice

Appropriate airway choice depends on a variety of patient-related and procedure-related factors, as well as the preferences and experience of the interventional bronchoscopist and anesthesiologist. Many patients undergoing interventional bronchoscopic procedures have significant baseline comorbidities and limited cardiopulmonary reserve. These patients often do not tolerate the transient hypoxia associated with bronchoscopy and may require high-flow oxygen supplementation or positive-pressure ventilation. Supraglottic airways (SGAs) are now used more often than endotracheal tubes (ETTs) as a conduit for the flexible fiberoptic bronchoscope but may not achieve adequate seal pressures for controlled ventilation and are contraindicated in patients at high risk for aspiration. Treatment of central airway obstruction or hemoptysis, foreign body removal, and silicone stent placement generally require rigid bronchoscopy.

NO AIRWAY

Many short, minimally stimulating procedures may be safely completed with intravenous sedation without the need for airway device placement. In these cases, good topicalization with local anesthetics is necessary to minimize sedation and its associated risks. If procedurally acceptable, maintaining the patient in an upright or sitting position improves respiratory mechanics and may reduce aspiration risk. Typical monitoring with pulse oximetry is mandatory; if available, capnography is helpful to monitor ventilation.

SUPRAGLOTTIC AIRWAYS

SGAs are increasingly popular for many types of surgery, including those necessitating positive-pressure ventilation, and may have special advantages during fiberoptic bronchoscopic procedures. For example, use of an SGA allows fiberoptic bronchoscopic examination of the vocal cords or proximal infraglottic masses. During endoscopic ultrasound, use of an SGA may allow closer approximation of the ultrasound transducer to the tracheal or bronchial mucosa to obtain better ultrasound images, whereas use of an ETT can force the bronchoscope into the middle of the trachea, increasing transducer and tissue impedance mismatching. In addition, higher lymph node stations, which would be blocked by an ETT, can be imaged and sampled, if appropriate.

For patients receiving general anesthesia, SGAs have been shown to reduce the risk for airway-related complications, including laryngospasm during emergence, postoperative hoarse voice, PONV, and coughing, in contrast to ETTs,[57] although this has not been specifically validated in patients undergoing bronchoscopy. SGAs, particularly designs lacking a gastric vent port, do not protect against aspiration and should generally be avoided in patients with increased aspiration risks.

The choice of any particular SGA over another is often based on availability and physician preference; however, patient and procedural factors combined with known device performance characteristics, such as airway seal pressure and air tube internal diameter, length, and shape, should be considered. Preferable SGA characteristics are summarized in Box 16-1 and include an airway seal pressure of 18 cm H_2O or greater, a built-in bite block, a relatively small periglottic cuff that minimizes glottic distortion and facilitates examination of supraglottic structures, a short and relatively flexible air tube with a larger inner diameter, and proved potential for use as intubating conduit during an emergency. Several SGAs, including the widely used LMA Classic (LMA, San Diego, Calif.), have epiglottic aperture bars designed to prevent the epiglottis from

---

Box 16-1 Desirable Qualities for Supraglottic Airways To Be Used During Flexible Bronchoscopy

Built-in bite block: *Examples:* Air-Q sp (Mercury Medical, Clearwater, Fla.), iGel (Intersurgical, Liverpool, NY)

Relatively small pharyngeal cuff: May negatively affect seal pressure but decreases distortion of periglottic anatomy. *Examples:* iGel (Intersurgical), Portex (Smiths Medical, Dublin, Ohio), Soft Seal Laryngeal Mask (Smiths Medical)

Short air tube: Eases manipulation of the bronchoscope and facilitates use of SGA as an intubating conduit, allowing ETT to reach vocal cords. *Examples:* Ambu (Ambu, Glen Burnie, Md.) Aura-i (Ambu), Air-Q sp (Mercury Medical)

Large inner diameter: Allows use of larger bronchoscopes and facilitates ventilation around the bronchoscope

Semi-rigid air tube: Provides countertraction, easing manipulation of the bronchoscope.

Gastric access port: Allows drainage of stomach, reducing risk for aspiration during positive-pressure ventilation. *Examples:* LMA Supreme (LMA, San Diego, Calif.), iGel (Intersurgical)

Proven potential for use as an ETT intubating conduit in an emergency: *Examples:* Air-Q sp (Mercury Medical), iGel (Intersurgical)

Proven potential for use during positive-pressure ventilation: Most newer-generation SGAs

ETT, Endotracheal tube; *SGA,* supraglottic airway.

Box 16-2 Undesirable Qualities for Supraglottic Airways To Be Used During Flexible Bronchoscopy

Epiglottic aperture bars: Designed to reduce risk of the epiglottis obstructing airflow but prohibits or hinders insertion of bronchoscope. *Example:* LMA Classic (LMA, San Diego, Calif.)

Flexible air tube: Airway tube can be positioned away from the surgical field but is counterproductive in bronchoscopic procedures; also, flexible air tubes tend to have a smaller diameter than the air tubes on similarly sized standard SGAs. *Example:* LMA Flexible (LMA)

Gastric port that extends into lumen of the air tube: Allows placement of a larger nasogastric tube but interferes with movement of bronchoscope. *Example:* LMA ProSeal (LMA)

Acute anterior curve in air tube: May facilitate initial placement and seating of SGA but can make passage of a bronchoscope more difficult. *Examples:* LMA Supreme; Ambu and Aura-i (Ambu, Glen Burnie, Md.)

SGA, Supraglottic airway.

Once fire is noted, it should be clearly announced, the procedure should be halted, and any flammable objects should be immediately removed from the airway, including sponges and the ETT if one was used. The flow of all gases must be stopped and the flames doused with saline. Some authorities recommend keeping a 50-mL syringe of 0.9% saline immediately available during laser surgery.[80] If fire persists, a carbon dioxide fire extinguisher can be used.[62] Once the fire is out, ventilation must be reestablished with the anesthesia circuit or a self-inflating resuscitation bag, preferably with room air. If a volatile anesthetic is being administered, this should be changed to a TIVA in anticipation of rigid bronchoscopy being performed to assess airway injury and remove any debris.[62] Routine corticosteroids or antibiotics have not been proved beneficial after an airway fire.

TRACHEAL LACERATION OR RUPTURE

Traumatic intubation, balloon dilatation of a stricture, or airway stent removal all can result in tracheobronchial rupture or laceration. Unfortunately, such a complication is often not diagnosed until after the procedure. Head and neck emphysema, hemoptysis, dry cough, and dyspnea should raise suspicion for tracheal disruption in the appropriate clinical setting. Chest imaging may show pneumomediastinum; bronchoscopy or CT scan can confirm the diagnosis.[81]

Traumatic intubation most commonly lacerates the membranous portion of the trachea, often a few centimeters above the carina.[82] Rupture related to balloon dilation is usually at the site of balloon inflation, again on the posterior tracheal wall.[83] Minor lacerations usually can be managed conservatively,[81] but immediate thoracic surgery consultation is recommended for tracheal rupture.[82,84] Passing an endotracheal tube under bronchoscopic guidance beyond the rupture and then inflating the cuff distal to the injury is sometimes recommended.[85]

LOSS OF AIRWAY

Creation of a percutaneous airway is a rarely performed but potentially lifesaving procedure of last resort in the patient with a failed airway. Associated conditions possibly encountered in a bronchoscopy suite include massive postprocedure hemorrhage or emesis, airway edema, and obstructing masses. Anesthesia providers as a group are understandably reluctant to perform emergency surgical procedures, and studies have suggested that anesthesiologists are very poor at correctly identifying the cricothyroid membrane, especially in obese patients.[86] Nonetheless, a surgical airway is a potentially lifesaving procedure, and we believe that cricothyroidotomy should be considered a core skill for anyone providing anesthesia in a bronchoscopy suite.

Emergency tracheotomy is generally beyond the scope of anesthesia providers. Needle or Seldinger cricothyroidotomies are commonly described in anesthesia textbooks but require special kink-resistant cannulas and equipment to administer high-pressure ventilation. A simple technique for surgical cricothyroidotomy has been described that relies only on equipment that is immediately available in standard anesthesia carts—a no. 11 scalpel blade, an elastic bougie such as an Eschmann stylet, and a 6.0 endotracheal tube.[87] This procedure is detailed in Box 16-3.

Box 16-3   Emergency Cricothyroidotomy

1. **Skin incision**
- Cleanse neck with an alcohol-based solution.
- Grasp larynx with the nondominant hand.
- Identify the thyroid cartilage, cricothyroid membrane, and cricoid ring.
- Use dominant hand to make a vertical incision with a no. 11 blade knife over the cricothyroid membrane.
- Place the nondominant index finger into the vertical incision and move it side to side to clearly feel the cricothyroid membrane.
2. **Incision of cricothyroid membrane**
- Make a 5-mm horizontal incision through the cricothyroid membrane.
- Place an elastic bougie into the defect, and advance until resistance is felt.
- If immediately available, insert a tracheal hook into the hole and retract the larynx upward.
3. **Endotracheal tube placement**
- Advance a cuffed 6.0 endotracheal tube over the elastic bougie, up to the cricothyroid membrane.
- Align the bevel of the endotracheal tube with the horizontal incision of the cricothyroid membrane, and then gently advance the ETT through the divided cricothyroid membrane.
- Stop advancing once the cuff of the ETT has passed into the trachea, and inflate the ETT cuff.

Modified from MacIntyre A, Markarian MK, Carrison D, et al. Three-step emergency cricothyroidotomy. Mil Med. 2007;172(12):1228-1230.
ETT, Endotracheal tube.

Conclusion

The interventional bronchoscopy suite can be a challenging environment in which to provide anesthesia. Performance of a safe anesthesia requires thorough consideration of environmental factors, patient factors, the surgical or bronchoscopic technique to be employed, and the relative merits of various airway devices, ventilatory techniques, and pharmacological regimens.

References

1. Yasufuku K, Pierre A, Darling G, et al. A prospective controlled trial of endobronchial ultrasound-guided transbronchial needle aspiration compared with mediastinoscopy for mediastinal lymph node staging of lung cancer. *J Thorac Cardiovasc Surg.* 2011;142(6):1393–1400. e1.
2. Hwangbo B, Kim SK, Lee H-S, et al. Application of endobronchial ultrasound-guided transbronchial needle aspiration following integrated PET/CT in mediastinal staging of potentially operable non-small cell lung cancer. *Chest.* 2008;135(5):1280–1287.
3. Ernst A, Eberhardt R, Krasnik M, Herth FJF. Efficacy of endobronchial ultrasound-guided transbronchial needle aspiration of hilar lymph nodes for diagnosing and staging cancer. *J Thorac Oncol.* 2009;4(8):947–950.
4. Depew ZS, Edell ES, Midthun DE, et al. Endobronchial ultrasound-guided transbronchial needle aspiration: determinants of sampling adequacy. *J Bronchol Interventional Pulmonol.* 2012;19(4):271–276.
5. Sarkiss M, Kennedy M, Riedel B, et al. Anesthesia technique for endobronchial ultrasound-guided fine needle aspiration of mediastinal lymph node. *J Cardiothorac Vasc Anesth.* 2007;21(6):892–896.
6. Gildea TR, Mazzone PJ, Karnak D, Meziane M, Mehta AC. Electromagnetic navigation diagnostic bronchoscopy: a prospective study. *Am J Respir Crit Care Med.* 2006;174(9):982–989.

7. Eberhardt R, Anantham D, Herth F, Feller-Kopman D, Ernst A. Electromagnetic navigation diagnostic bronchoscopy in peripheral lung lesions. *Chest*. 2007;131(6):1800–1805.

8. Tellides G, Ugurlu BS, Kim RW, Hammond GL. Pathogenesis of systemic air embolism during bronchoscopic Nd:YAG laser operations. *Ann Thorac Surg*. 1998;65(4):930–934.

9. Reddy C, Majid A, Michaud G, et al. Gas embolism following bronchoscopic argon plasma coagulation: a case series. *Chest*. 2008;134(5):1066–1069.

10. Feller-Kopman D, Lukanich JM, Shapira G, et al. Gas flow during bronchoscopic ablation therapy causes gas emboli to the heart: a comparative animal study. *Chest*. 2008;133(4):892–896.

11. Makris D, Marquette C-H. Tracheobronchial stenting and central airway replacement. *Curr Opin Pulmon Med*. 2007;13(4):278–283.

12. Lund ME, Garland R, Ernst A. Airway stenting: applications and practice management considerations. *Chest*. 2007;131(2):579–587.

13. Elliott BA, Curry TB, Atwell TD, Brown MJ, Rose SH. Lung isolation, one-lung ventilation, and continuous positive airway pressure with air for radiofrequency ablation of neoplastic pulmonary lesions. *Anesth Analg*. 2006;103(2):463–464.

14. Pavord ID, Cox G, Thomson NC, et al. Safety and efficacy of bronchial thermoplasty in symptomatic, severe asthma. *Am J Respir Crit Care Med*. 2007;176(12):1185–1191.

15. Thomson NC, Chaudhuri R, Spears M. Emerging therapies for severe asthma. *BMC Med*. 2011;6(9):102.

16. Du Rand IA, Barber PV, Goldring J, et al. British Thoracic Society guideline for advanced diagnostic and therapeutic flexible bronchoscopy in adults. *Thorax*. 2011;66(suppl 3):iii1–21.

17. Ramsey SD, Berry K, Etzioni R, et al. Cost effectiveness of lung-volume-reduction surgery for patients with severe emphysema. *New Engl J Med*. 2003;348(21):2092–2102.

18. Grendelmeier P, Kurer G, Pflimlin E, Tamm M, Stolz D. Feasibility and safety of propofol sedation in flexible bronchoscopy. *Swiss Med Wkly*. 2011;141(Aug):w13248.

19. Wain JC. Rigid bronchoscopy: the value of a venerable procedure. *Chest Surg Clin North Am*. 2001;11(4):691–699.

20. Chhajed PN, Glanville AR. Management of hypoxemia during flexible bronchoscopy. *Clin Chest Med*. 2003;24(3):511–516.

21. Hehn BT, Haponik E, Rubin HR, Lechtzin N, Diette GB. The relationship between age and process of care and patient tolerance of bronchoscopy. *J Am Geriatr Soc*. 2003;51(7):917–922.

22. Davoudi M, Shakkottai S, Colt HG. Safety of therapeutic rigid bronchoscopy in people aged 80 and older: a retrospective cohort analysis. *J Am Geriatr Soc*. 2008;56(5):943–944.

23. Global Strategy for Diagnosis, Management, and Prevention of COPD. Global Initiative for Chronic Obstructive Lung Disease (GOLD), 2011. http://www.goldcopd.org.

24. Brickey DA, Lawlor DP. Transbronchial biopsy in the presence of profound elevation of the international normalized ratio. *Chest*. 1999;115(6):1667–1671.

25. Wahidi MM, Jain P, Jantz M, et al. American College of Chest Physicians consensus statement on the use of topical anesthesia, analgesia, and sedation during flexible bronchoscopy in adult patients. *Chest*. 2011;140(5):1342–1350.

26. Matot I, Kuras Y, Kramer MR. Effect of clonidine premedication on haemodynamic responses to fibreoptic bronchoscopy. *Anaesthesia*. 2000;55(3):269–274.

27. De Padua AI, De Castro M, Schmidt A, et al. Clonidine as a pre-anesthetic agent for flexible bronchoscopy. *Respir Med*. 2004;98(8):746–751.

28. Fan T, Wang G, Mao B, et al. Prophylactic administration of parenteral steroids for preventing airway complications after extubation in adults: meta-analysis of randomised placebo controlled trials. *BMJ*. 2008;337(1):a1841.

29. Park S-H, Han S-H, Do S-H, et al. Prophylactic dexamethasone decreases the incidence of sore throat and hoarseness after tracheal extubation with a double-lumen endobronchial tube. *Anesth Analg*. 2008;107(6):1814–1818.

30. Thomas S, Beevi S. Dexamethasone reduces the severity of postoperative sore throat. *Can J Anaesth Can J Anesth*. 2007;54(11):897–901.

31. Hawkins DB, Crockett DM, Shum TK. Corticosteroids in airway management. *Otolaryngol Head Neck Surg*. 1983;91(6):593–596.

32. Gan TJ, Meyer T, Apfel CC, et al. Consensus guidelines for managing postoperative nausea and vomiting. *Anesth Analg*. 2003;97(1):62–71.

33. Ng A, Smith G. Gastroesophageal reflux and aspiration of gastric contents in anesthetic practice. *Anesth Analg*. 2001;93(2):494–513.

34. British Thoracic Society Bronchoscopy Committee. British Thoracic Society guidelines on diagnostic flexible bronchoscopy. *Thorax*. 2001;56(suppl 1):i1–21.

35. Stolz D, Pollak V, Chhajed PN, et al. A randomized, placebo-controlled trial of bronchodilators for bronchoscopy in patients with COPD. *Chest*. 2007;131(3):765–772.

36. Neuhaus A, Markowitz D, Rotman HH, Weg JG. The effects of fiberoptic bronchoscopy with and without atropine premedication on pulmonary function in humans. *Ann Thorac Surg*. 1978;25(5):393–398.

37. Langmack EL, Martin RJ, Pak J, Kraft M. Serum lidocaine concentrations in asthmatics undergoing research bronchoscopy. *Chest*. 2000;117(4):1055–1060.

38. Kundra P, Kutralam S, Ravishankar M. Local anaesthesia for awake fibreoptic nasotracheal intubation. *Acta Anaesthesiol Scand*. 2000;44(5):511–516.

39. De Oliveira GS, Fitzgerald P, Kendall M. Ultrasound-assisted translaryngeal block for awake fibreoptic intubation. *Can J Anaesth*. 2011;58(7):664–665.

40. Conacher ID. Anaesthesia and tracheobronchial stenting for central airway obstruction in adults. *Br J Anaesth*. 2003;90(3):367–374.

41. Wright RO, Lewander WJ, Woolf AD. Methemoglobinemia: etiology, pharmacology, and clinical management. *Ann Emerg Med*. 1999;34(5):646–656.

42. Vloka J, Hadzic A, Kitain E. A simple adaptation to the Olympus LF1 and LF2 flexible fiberoptic bronchoscopes for instillation of local anesthetic. *Anesthesiology*. 1995;82(3):792.

43. Greig JH, Cooper SM, Kasimbazi HJ, et al. Sedation for fibre optic bronchoscopy. *Respir Med*. 1995;89(1):53–56.

44. Houghton CM, Raghuram A, Sullivan PJ, O'Driscoll R. Pre-medication for bronchoscopy: a randomised double blind trial comparing alfentanil with midazolam. *Respir Med*. 2004;98(11):1102–1107.

45. Crawford M, Pollock J, Anderson K. Comparison of midazolam with propofol for sedation in outpatient bronchoscopy. *Br J Anaesth*. 1993;70:419–422.

46. Clarkson K, Power CK, O'Connell F, Pathmakanthan S, Burke CM. A comparative evaluation of propofol and midazolam as sedative agents in fiberoptic bronchoscopy. *Chest*. 1993;104(4):1029–1031.

47. Stolz D, Kurer G, Meyer A, et al. Propofol versus combined sedation in flexible bronchoscopy: a randomised non-inferiority trial. *Eur Respir J*. 2009;34(5):1024–1030.

48. Andrews BT, Graham SM, Ross AF, et al. Technique, utility, and safety of awake tracheoplasty using combined laser and balloon dilation. *Laryngoscope*. 2007;117(12):2159–2162.

49. Liao W, Ma G, Su Q, et al. Dexmedetomidine versus midazolam for conscious sedation in postoperative patients undergoing flexible bronchoscopy: a randomized study. *J Int Med Res*. 2012;40:1371–1380.

50. Yurino M, Kimura H. A comparison of vital capacity breath and tidal breathing techniques for induction of anaesthesia with high sevoflurane concentrations in nitrous oxide and oxygen. *Anaesthesia*. 1995;50(4):308–311.

51. Baraka AS, Siddik SS, Taha SK, Jalbout MI, Massouh FM. Low frequency jet ventilation for stent insertion in a patient with tracheal stenosis. *Can J Anaesth*. 2001;48(7):701–704.

52. Hohlrieder M, Tiefenthaler W, Klaus H, et al. Effect of total intravenous anaesthesia and balanced anaesthesia on the frequency of coughing during emergence from the anaesthesia. *Br J Anaesth*. 2007;99(4):587–591.

53. Ledowski T, Paech MJ, Patel B, Schug SA. Bronchial mucus transport velocity in patients receiving propofol and remifentanil versus sevoflurane and remifentanil anesthesia. *Anesth Analg*. 2006;102(5):1427–1430.

54. Prakash N, McLeod T, Gao Smith F. The effects of remifentanil on haemodynamic stability during rigid bronchoscopy. *Anaesthesia*. 2001;56(6):576–580.

55. Perrin G, Colt HG, Martin C, et al. Safety of interventional rigid bronchoscopy using intravenous anesthesia and spontaneous assisted ventilation: a prospective study. *Chest*. 1992;102(5):1526–1530.

56. Raiten J, Elkassabany N, Mandel JE. The use of high-frequency jet ventilation for out of operating room anesthesia. *Curr Opin Anaesthesiol*. 2012;25(4):482–485.

57. Yu SH, Beirne OR. Laryngeal mask airways have a lower risk of airway complications compared with endotracheal intubation: a systematic review. *J Oral Maxillofac Surg*. 2010;68(10):2359–2376.

58. Lawson RW, Peters JI, Shelledy DC. Effects of fiberoptic bronchoscopy during mechanical ventilation in a lung model. *Chest*. 2000;118(3):824–831.

59. Ernst A, Silvestri GA, Johnstone D. Interventional pulmonary procedures: guidelines from the American College of Chest Physicians. *Chest*. 2003;123(5):1693–1717.

60. Baumann HJ, Klose H, Simon M, et al. Fiber optic bronchoscopy in patients with acute hypoxemic respiratory failure requiring noninvasive ventilation: a feasibility study. *Crit Care*. 2011;15(4):R179.

61. Murgu SD, Pecson J, Colt HG. Bronchoscopy during noninvasive ventilation: indications and technique. *Respir Care*. 2010;55(5):595–600.

62. Caplan RA, Barker SJ, Connis RT, et al. Practice advisory for the prevention and management of operating room fires. *Anesthesiology*. 2008;108(5):786–801. quiz 971–972.

63. Orr JB. Helium-oxygen gas mixtures in the management of patients with airway obstruction. *Ear Nose Throat J*. 1988;67(12): 866, 868–869.

64. Milner QJ, Abdy S, Allen JG. Management of severe tracheal obstruction with helium/oxygen and a laryngeal mask airway. *Anaesthesia*. 1997;52(11):1087–1089.

65. Reuben AD. Heliox for asthma in the emergency department: a review of the literature. *Emerg Med J*. 2004;21(2):131–135.

66. Linck SL. Use of heliox for intraoperative bronchospasm: a case report. *AANA J*. 2007;75(3):189–192.

67. Nakstad ER, Opdahl H, Skjønsberg OH, Borchsenius F. Intrabronchial airway pressures in intubated patients during bronchoscopy under volume controlled and pressure controlled ventilation. *Anaesth Intensive Care*. 2011;39(3):431–439.

68. Searl CP, Perrino A. Fluid management in thoracic surgery. *Anesthesiol Clin*. 2012;30(4):641–655.

69. Bolliger CT, Mathur PN, Beamis JF, et al. ERS/ATS statement on interventional pulmonology. European Respiratory Society/American Thoracic Society. *Eur Respir J*. 2002;19(2):356–373.

70. Hautmann H, Gamarra F, Henke M, Diehm S, Huber RM. High frequency jet ventilation in interventional fiberoptic bronchoscopy. *Anesth Analg*. 2000;90(6):1436–1440.

71. Bruhn J, Myles PS, Sneyd R, Struys MMRF. Depth of anaesthesia monitoring: what's available, what's validated and what's next? *Br J Anaesth*. 2006;97(1):85–94.

72. Cooper RM. The use of an endotracheal ventilation catheter in the management of difficult extubations. *Can J Anaesth*. 1996;43(1):90–93.

73. Izbicki G. Is routine chest radiography after transbronchial biopsy necessary? A prospective study of 350 cases. *Chest*. 2006;129(6):1561–1564.

74. Wong DH, Weber EC, Schell MJ, et al. Factors associated with postoperative pulmonary complications in patients with severe chronic obstructive pulmonary disease. *Anesth Analg*. 1995;80:276–284.

75. Lee P, Mehta AC, Mathur PN. Management of complications from diagnostic and interventional bronchoscopy. *Respirology*. 2009;14(7):940–953.

76. Carr IM, Koegelenberg CFN, Von Groote-Bidlingmaier F, et al. Blood loss during flexible bronchoscopy: a prospective observational study. *Respiration*. 2012;84(4):312–318.

77. Goldman JM, Currie DC, Morgan AD, Collins JV. Arterial oxygen saturation during bronchography via the fibreoptic bronchoscope. *Thorax*. 1987;42(9):694–695.

78. Haynes D, Baumann MH. Management of pneumothorax. *Semin Respir Crit Care Med*. 2010;31(6):769–780.

79. Ho AM-H, Wan S, Karmakar MK. Flooding with carbon dioxide prevents airway fire induced by diathermy during open tracheostomy. *J Trauma*. 2007;63(1):228–231.

80. English J. Anaesthesia for airway surgery. *Contin Educ Anaesth Crit Care Pain*. 2006;6(1):28–31.

81. Kim JH, Shin JH, Song H-Y, et al. Tracheobronchial laceration after balloon dilation for benign strictures: incidence and clinical significance. *Chest*. 2007;131(4):1114–1117.

82. Carbognani P, Bobbio A, Cattelani L, et al. Management of postintubation membranous tracheal rupture. *Ann Thorac Surg*. 2004;77(2):406–409.

83. Kim JH, Kim YH, Shin JH, et al. Deep tracheal laceration after balloon dilation for benign tracheobronchial stenosis: case reports of two patients. *Br J Radiol*. 2006;79(942):529–535.

84. Mussi A, Ambrogi MC, Menconi G, Ribechini A, Angeletti CA. Surgical approaches to membranous tracheal wall lacerations. *J Thorac Cardiovasc Surg*. 2000;120(1):115–118.

85. Miñambres E, Burón J, Ballesteros MA, et al. Tracheal rupture after endotracheal intubation: a literature systematic review. *Eur J Cardiothorac Surg*. 2009;35(6):1056–1062.

86. Aslani A, Ng S-C, Hurley M, et al. Accuracy of identification of the cricothyroid membrane in female subjects using palpation: an observational study. *Anesth Analg*. 2012;114(5):987–992.

87. MacIntyre A, Markarian MK, Carrison D, et al. Three-step emergency cricothyroidotomy. *Mil Med*. 2007;172(12):1228–1230.

17 Adult Anesthesia in the Radiology Suite

DANIEL RUBIN and THOMAS CUTTER

One of the driving forces in the genesis of the field of interventional radiology was its minimally invasive nature. As catheters and stents replaced the physiologically taxing "open" procedure, patients were able to have an intervention they may not otherwise have survived. Initially, local anesthesia and light sedation were usually sufficient to provide a comfortable experience for the patient with minimal risk, but continued improvements in imaging and device technology have made more complex procedures possible in sicker patients. This has made "local with sedation" a more challenging proposition for the interventionalist. The increasing need for an anesthesiologist seems like a natural progression since the line between the radiology suite and the operating room continues to be blurred. The knowledge and skill of an anesthesiologist play an undeniable role in providing appropriate anesthetic and physiological support for patients undergoing these procedures. The anesthesiologist's understanding of the procedure and the proper application of pharmacology and other interventions is becoming necessary to decrease morbidity and improve patient care.

It is beyond the scope of this chapter to discuss and detail all of the various procedures performed in the radiology suite. Our goal is to discuss the fundamental issues that exist in the radiology suite, with an emphasis on the more common and more challenging procedures performed there. As the field of interventional radiology continues to expand the number and complexity of procedures performed, the need for presence of an anesthesiologist will continue to expand with it.

Radiopaque Contrast

Intravenous contrast is commonly used in interventional radiology procedures. The overall incidence of adverse reactions using high-osmolar contrast agents is 5% to 8%, with severe reactions occurring in 1 in 1000 to 2000 examinations.[1] Moderate reactions are those requiring therapeutic measures without hospitalization. Development of nonionic and lower osmolality contrast agents has decreased the incidence and severity of contrast reactions to 1% to 4%. Severe, life-threatening reactions in low-osmolality contrast agents continue to be rare and are reported to be less than 0.2%.[2] Contrast reactions are classified as either anaphylactoid or chemotoxic, with anaphylactoid being more common and chemotoxic typically more severe (Box 17-1).

Anaphylactoid reactions can manifest as nausea, vomiting, urticaria, pruritus, bronchospasm, and cardiovascular collapse. The exact mechanism is still unclear but likely involves the direct release of histamine from basophils and mast cells, which directly or indirectly activates the complement, coagulation, fibrinolytic, and kinin systems.[1] It does not appear to be mediated by an antibody-antigen interaction, despite resembling the typical symptoms of an allergic reaction. The magnitude of the reaction is not dependent on the dose or concentration of the contrast agent, and as with true allergic reactions, symptoms are typically seen within 1 hour after administration of contrast. Preexisting activation of these systems in critically ill patients may increase the severity and activation of the contrast reaction. Currently no evidence suggests that shellfish allergy predisposes patients to a contrast reaction, but patients with a history of significant allergies, asthma, or anxiety have an increased risk for anaphylactoid reactions, and premedication should be considered.[2] Patients with previous anaphylactoid reactions may benefit from premedication with corticosteroids and histamine-1 blockers. A commonly used regimen is to give prednisone 50 mg 13 hours, 7 hours, and 1 hour before contrast administration and diphenhydramine 50 mg 1 hour before contrast administration.[3]

Chemotoxic reactions to intravascular contrast are due to the inherent chemical properties of the contrast agent on specific organ systems. Because the contrast itself causes the reaction, the severity is directly proportional to its dose and concentration. Important factors are (hyper) osmolality, calcium binding, and the nature and concentration of its cations (sodium or meglumine). Critically ill patients who are already sensitive to significant volume shifts, arrhythmias, and renal insufficiency are at greater risk for chemotoxic reactions.

Treatment of acute contrast reactions is largely supportive. Once an adverse reaction has manifested, the injection of further contrast material should be immediately stopped. An urticarial rash may be self-limited or the harbinger of

---

Box 17-1 Classification of Severity of Reactions to Contrast Media

Minor: Nausea, vomiting (limited), urticarial (limited), pruritus, diaphoresis
Moderate: Faintness, vomiting (severe), urticaria (profound), facial edema, laryngeal edema, bronchospasm (mild)
Severe: Hypotensive shock, pulmonary edema, respiratory arrest, cardiac arrest, seizures

From Bush WH, Swanson DP. Acute reactions to intravascular contrast media: types, risk factors, recognition, and specific treatment. AJR Am J Roentgenol. 1991;157(6):1154.

a worsening anaphylactoid reaction. The anesthesiologist should be vigilant for the development of bronchospasm, angioedema, hypotension, bradycardia, and sudden cardiovascular collapse. Beta-agonists, intravenous fluids, epinephrine, atropine, and the ability to secure the airway should be readily available in any location where intravenous contrast is administered.

Contrast-induced nephrotoxicity (CIN) is thought to result from the chemotoxic effects of the contrast on the renal tubules or by direct vasoconstriction. It is described as a sudden deterioration in renal function after the intravascular administration of iodinated contrast material that cannot be explained by another nephrotoxic event.[3] It is rare in patients without preexisting renal dysfunction or critical illness, but studies suggest an increased risk is also seen in patients with diabetes mellitus, heart failure, older age, hypertension, and anemia.[4] A dose-dependent correlation exists between the severity of injury and the dose of contrast, so the risks for worsening renal injury must be weighed against the benefits of the study or intervention planned. Strategies to help prevent CIN in patients with renal dysfunction are hydration with crystalloid and the administration of N-acetylcysteine and sodium bicarbonate. N-acetylcysteine 600 mg given 24 hours and 12 hours before and 12 hours and 24 hours after administration of contrast coupled with prehydration before administration of nonionic, low-osmolality contrast decreased the incidence of CIN in patients with preexisting renal disease as assessed by serum creatinine.[5] Sodium bicarbonate also decreased the incidence of CIN in patients with preexisting renal dysfunction with the administration of 154 mEq/L of sodium bicarbonate as a bolus of 3 mL/kg/hr for 1 hour before contrast administration, followed by an infusion of 1 mL/kg/hr for 6 hours after the procedure.[6]

Patients with diabetes and preexisting renal dysfunction who take metformin have developed severe lactic acidosis after an iodinated contrast study. If possible, metformin should be discontinued at the time of or before the procedure, withheld for 48 hours subsequent to the procedure, and reinstituted only after renal function has been reevaluated and found to be normal.[7]

Radiation Safety

The primary safety concern for the anesthesiologist in the interventional radiology suite is ionizing radiation. Computed tomography and simple x-rays carry little risk, and fluoroscopy poses the greatest. The three primary sources are scatter radiation from the patient, direct radiation from the beam, and leakage from the radiation source, with scatter radiation from the patient providing the greatest risk.

A typical fluoroscope comprises a radiation source and an image intensifier. The orientation of the fluoroscopy beam in the anterior–posterior plane places the radiation source below the patient and the image intensifier above the patient. This minimizes scatter radiation by deflecting it down to the floor, away from medical personnel. Biplane machines employ an additional laterally facing fluoroscope to improve visualization, decrease contrast dose, and shorten procedure time. The lateral scope's radiation source is classically positioned on the opposite side of the

interventionalist to decrease his radiation exposure. Anesthesia personnel are frequently located on the same side as the radiation source and can be exposed to four times greater radiation levels than the interventionalist.[8] The anesthesia team should communicate to the interventionalist when they need to access the patient, during which fluoroscopy should not be used, to decrease unnecessary radiation exposure. Anesthesia providers should avoid placing their hands into the x-ray beam unless absolutely necessary for patient safety (Figure 17-1).

The two primary methods to decrease overall radiation exposure are distancing oneself from the source of radiation and shielding. Standard lead aprons with thyroid collars decrease the radiation from fluoroscopy by a factor of 10 and should be worn by all anesthesia personnel while in the radiology suite.[9] Providers wearing aprons that do not provide adequate shielding in the back should avoid turning away from the beam while it is in use. When possible, transparent leaded acrylic shielding also should be placed between anesthesia providers and the patient to further decrease x-ray exposure. Anastasian et al[8] showed that anesthesiologists' eyes are exposed to a significant amount of radiation that could lead to cataracts and recommend that providers who spend considerable time in interventional radiology should consider using the lightweight leaded glasses that are commonly worn by interventionalists.

In addition to lead shielding, anesthesia providers should distance themselves as far as safely possible from the patient. The dose of radiation to which a provider is exposed is inversely proportional to the square of the distance from the source of radiation. Interventions such as administering a bolus of medication, adjusting ventilator settings, or checking neuromuscular blockade all increase radiation

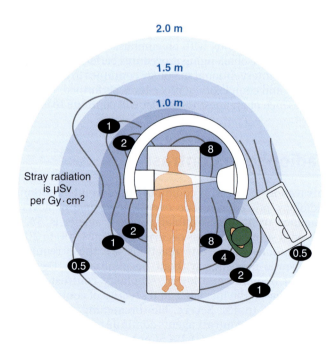

Figure 17-1 Distribution of scatter radiation from a lateral C-arm with the radiation source on the same side as the anesthesiologist. (From Anastasian ZH, Strozyk D, Meyers PM, Wang S, Berman MF. Radiation exposure of the anesthesiologist in the neurointerventional suite. *Anesthesiology*. 2011;114[3]:517.)

exposure.[8] Even small distances can decrease radiation exposure significantly; therefore "remote" access using intravenous extension tubing or ventilator extension tubing may allow the anesthesia provider to be positioned farther away.

Digital subtraction angiography (DSA) and road-mapping are two techniques that aid the interventionalist during complex vascular procedures. These image acquisition techniques are highly sensitive to patient movement and breathing, and image quality is degraded easily. Patients are required to remain motionless and apneic for periods of up to 15 seconds to acquire adequate images. Because of the high levels of radiation, the anesthesiologist may choose to leave the immediate area, which is still within the standards for basic anesthetic monitoring endorsed by the American Society of Anesthesiologists (ASA) if the patient can be monitored remotely.[10]

General Considerations

CHOICE OF ANESTHETIC

The diversity and complexity of interventional radiology procedures have dramatically expanded over the past two decades. Although the vast majority of procedures are performed under light or moderate sedation by a nurse and supervised by the interventionalist, an anesthesiologist is indicated if the patient has significant comorbidities or other issues that will make moderate sedation challenging or the procedure requires a general anesthetic.[11] Procedures performed in the United States are typically performed with more sedation than those performed in Europe, but general anesthesia is employed more often in Europe. The reason for this is unclear, but patient expectations and patient anxiety may play a role.[12,13] A discussion with the interventionalist before every procedure should include the expected procedure length, procedural stimulation, positioning, and need for patient cooperation. Biliary and percutaneous urological procedures that are particularly stimulating have been performed successfully under neuraxial blockade, obviating the need for general anesthesia or deep sedation.[14,15]

PATIENT POSITIONING

Just as in the operating room, procedures performed in the radiology suite may last from 10 minutes to several hours. It is imperative for patients undergoing long procedures under moderate or deep sedation to be positioned as comfortably as possible. Foam padding, lumbar support, and a comfortable pillow all help ensure patient comfort during the procedure and may decrease the amount of sedation necessary. During femoral cannulation the patient must be completely supine, but a pillow may be placed under the knees for added support once the femoral sheath is in place. Some patients may not be able to lie supine for extended periods because of comorbid conditions, such as arthritis, chronic obstructive pulmonary disease, obstructive sleep apnea, pleural effusions, or congestive heart failure, and these should be discussed with the radiologist. Some procedures may allow for or require patients to be in the semirecumbent position. Extra care should be taken in patients undergoing placement of venous-access devices, because the patient position will increase the risk for venous air embolism during cannulation, especially in the spontaneously breathing patient. Some procedures (e.g., placement of percutaneous nephrostomy tubes and kyphoplasty) require the patient to be placed in the prone position, and specialized equipment and materials should be employed—just as they are in the surgical suite.

PATIENT ACCESS

Depending on the type of procedure, access to the patient may be severely limited. The traditional arrangement with the anesthesiologist at the head of the bed is altered by the presence of fluoroscopy equipment and the radiologist. Certain procedures that focus around the head and neck, such as interventional neuroradiology procedures and transjugular intrahepatic portosystemic shunting (TIPS), make it especially difficult to access and secure the airway in an emergency situation. The patient's arms are typically tucked and secured to allow for free movement of the fluoroscopy machine, which will require intravenous access and monitoring equipment, such as arterial lines, to be placed before the procedure starts (Figure 17-2).

TEMPERATURE

Maintaining normothermia during a procedure can be challenging in interventional radiology suites because the temperature is typically at or below 68° F because of the sensitivity of the radiology equipment.[16] Strategies that actively warm the patient, such as forced-air warming

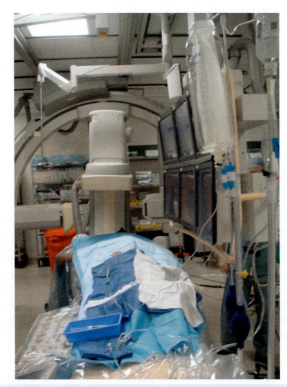

Figure 17-2 Interventional neurology suite. Anesthesia providers are located behind the imaging monitors on the right and the interventional neuroradiologist is located on the left.

blankets and fluid warmers, and those that minimize heat loss, such as humidifiers on the ventilator circuit and low-flow anesthesia, should be employed for long procedures. Applying the usual forced-air warming blankets can be difficult because of the need for access by the radiologist.

ANESTHESIA EQUIPMENT

Because anesthesia is required for only a small number of cases, the anesthesiologist typically uses space "borrowed" from the interventionalist. Important considerations include positioning the anesthesia machine a sufficient distance from the patient to allow the fluoroscopy machine adequate travel for imaging. Extensions on intravenous tubing, arterial pressure tubing, and ventilator tubing are usually required to allow adequate distance from the patient. Neurointerventional radiology typically employs a biplane fluoroscopy machine to help minimize radiation. The rotation of this device requires that all tubing, monitors, and ventilator circuits travel inferior to the patient. The ASA standards should be followed for equipment in all off-site cases and include adequate oxygen supply and backup, suction, a waste scavenging system, electrical outlets with backup power supply, emergency equipment for cardiopulmonary resuscitation, trained support staff and two-way communication for assistance, and a rehearsed plan.[17] Nitrous oxide should not be used with anesthesia machines that rely on activated charcoal filters (F/AIR filter canisters, Harvard Apparatus, Holliston, Mass.) because it cannot be effectively removed by these systems.

PATIENT MOTION

A discussion with the radiologist should take place before the start of the procedure about the importance of patient movement with regard to its impact on image acquisition and quality. For example, DSA and road-mapping require the patient to be completely motionless and apneic to acquire sufficient image quality.

MONITORING

The standards for basic anesthetic monitoring should apply to all patients having anything more than light sedation. Access to the patient may make ventilation assessment difficult for some procedures. The ASA recommends that during moderate or deep sedation the adequacy of ventilation should be evaluated by continual observation of qualitative clinical signs and monitoring for the presence of exhaled carbon dioxide unless precluded or invalidated by the nature of the patient, procedure, or equipment.[10] More invasive monitoring such as arterial lines and central venous pressure monitoring may be necessary for certain interventional neuroradiology procedures such as acute stroke or the coiling of arteriovenous malformations. If arterial pressure monitoring is required only during the procedure, it may be possible to measure it from the arterial sheath placed by the interventionalist, thereby obviating the need for a specific radial artery cannula. It should be noted that the arterial pressure waveform may be dampened by the coaxial catheter in the arterial sheath. Fluids administered by the interventionalist should be monitored throughout the procedure because large volumes of fluid may be given during lengthy procedures. Foley catheterization should be considered in patients undergoing lengthy procedures so that urine output can help guide fluid management decisions.

It must be stressed that the location of the radiology suite is often a fair distance from the general operating rooms. Adequate rescue equipment, particularly airway devices, should be brought to, or located near, the radiology suite in case of emergency. In the patient with a difficult airway undergoing a general anesthetic, it may be safer to induce anesthesia in the general operating room area with anesthesia support and then transport the patent to the radiology suite. Newer institutions have begun to address this issue by placing interventional suites closer to the operating rooms.

Visceral Procedures

BILIARY PROCEDURES

Biliary Angiography and Drainage

Percutaneous biliary procedures can determine the presence of biliary obstruction, infection, or malignancy. Patients undergoing biliary drainage because of obstruction may be critically ill from sepsis and too unstable to tolerate operative cholecystectomy. Patients are placed in the supine position with the right arm placed above the head and a needle inserted at or below the 10th rib via the liver into the biliary system. Although moderate sedation is usually administered for this procedure, stimulation from dilation of transhepatic tracts can be significant, and neuraxial analgesia has been successfully used for these procedures.[14] Contraindications for the procedure include uncorrected coagulopathy, contrast reaction, hydatid disease, a vascular hepatic lesion, and undrained ascites.

TRANSVENOUS BILIARY PROCEDURES

Transvenous biliary procedures include hepatic venography, hepatic hemodynamic pressure measurements, liver biopsy, and TIPS. Indications for hepatic hemodynamic pressure measurements include assessing the presence of hepatic venous pathology and the severity of portal venous hypertension.

Indications for TIPS are recurrent esophageal variceal bleeding, bridge to liver transplantation to prevent variceal bleeding, and large ascites or hydrothorax that is not amenable to medical therapy.[18] Absolute contraindications to TIPS are primary prevention of variceal bleeding, congestive heart failure, multiple hepatic cysts, uncontrolled infection or sepsis, unrelieved biliary obstruction, and severe pulmonary hypertension. Creation of the portal shunt may lead to significantly greater venous return and may strain a failing right heart.

The procedure involves cannulating the right or left jugular vein using ultrasound guidance and placing a sheath. The hepatic vein is then canalized, a catheter is wedged, and carbon dioxide is injected as contrast for a hepatic venogram. The venogram outlines the portal venous system and guides the interventionalist for the liver puncture. The portal system is then accessed, a tract is dilated, and a covered metal stent is left in place to maintain patency of the shunt. After the stent is deployed, pressure measurements and portal venography are repeated. A decrease in the portosystemic gradient to less than 12 mm Hg is considered a successful procedure, because this leads to a decreased incidence of variceal bleeding and decreased recurrence of ascites (Figure 17-3).[19]

Patients with refractory ascites are likely to have poor pulmonary compliance, compressive atelectasis, pleural effusions, and hepatopulmonary syndrome, with hypoxemia secondary to pulmonary arteriovenous malformations.[20] Some centers require an echocardiogram before TIPS to investigate for portopulmonary hypertension; this is an absolute contraindication to TIPS, and the incidence may be up to 16% in the cirrhotic population.[21]

TIPS has been performed under sedation, monitored anesthesia care, and general anesthesia.[22-24] The risk for aspiration, difficult access to the airway, hepatic encephalopathy, and other significant comorbidities make a general anesthetic the prudent choice.[25] An emergency TIPS procedure for acute variceal bleeding should be performed under general anesthesia because of the increased risk for aspiration and hemorrhage. Fluid administration should be kept to a minimum because of worsening ascites and edema formation. Complications from transvenous biliary procedures include hepatic bleeding into the portal tract, biliary leak, sepsis, capsular bleeding, hemothorax, pneumothorax, and contrast reaction.

Chalasani et al[26] retrospectively reviewed morbidity after TIPS procedures and found that an emergency procedure for variceal hemorrhage, alanine aminotransferase greater than 100 international units/L, bilirubin >3.0 mg/dL, and the presence of pre-TIPs encephalopathy were independent predictors for 30-day mortality.[26] Of the four risk factors, emergency procedure for variceal hemorrhage was the strongest predictor of mortality.

GENITOURINARY PROCEDURES

Percutaneous nephrostomy is performed for direct access to the renal pelvis to provide urinary drainage in the setting of obstruction and allow for direct extraction or destruction of large renal calculi. The patient is placed in the prone position, and a subcostal or supracostal approach is taken to access the kidney. A significantly higher incidence of pulmonary injuries, such as pneumothorax and hydrothorax, occur in patients undergoing the supracostal approach, so breath-holding or apnea should be initiated during cannulation to decrease the incidence of pulmonary complications.[27] A chest radiograph is recommended after every percutaneous nephrolithotomy, regardless of access site.[27] The anesthesiologist should be diligent in monitoring for increased peak airway pressures, hypoxemia, and increasing arterial carbon dioxide tension ($PaCO_2$). Anemia from blood loss and hemodilution may be profound as a result of absorption of the irrigation fluids, with an average decrease in hemoglobin of 2.8 g/dL.[28] Although general anesthesia is typically employed, neuraxial anesthesia and sedation have been shown to be appropriate for this type of procedure (Figure 17-4).[15]

Vascular Procedures

Diagnostic peripheral angiography and angioplasty are most commonly performed on the lower extremities for claudication secondary to peripheral vascular disease. A vascular sheath is usually introduced into the femoral artery, but the brachial artery also can be accessed. Light sedation and generous local anesthetic administration at the site of cannulation are usually all that is required for these procedures, and an anesthesiologist typically is not

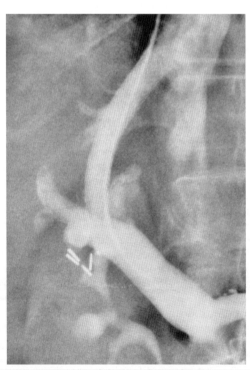

Figure 17-3 Portal venogram immediately after transjugular intrahepatic portosystemic shunt placement showing excellent shunt patency with minimal portal flow to the liver. (From Rosch J, Keller FS. Transjugular intrahepatic portosystemic shunt: present status, comparison with endoscopic therapy and shunt surgery, and future prospectives. *World J Surg.* 2001;25[3]:339.)

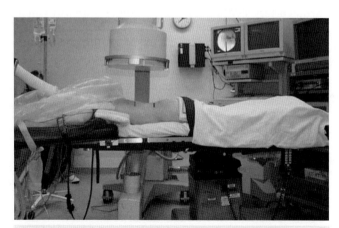

Figure 17-4 Patient and fluoroscope positioning for a prone percutaneous nephrostomy tube placement. (From Ray AA, Chung DG, Honey RJ. Percutaneous nephrolithotomy in the prone and prone-flexed positions: anatomic considerations. *J Endourol* 2009;23[10]:1609.)

involved.[12,13] If an obstruction is noted, balloon angioplasty with a subsequent stent may be performed to improve blood flow for symptomatic claudication. General anesthesia is rarely needed for these procedures, unless the patient cannot tolerate the supine position for even short periods.

CATHETER-DIRECTED THROMBOLYSIS

Arterial thrombolysis is accomplished by mechanical disruption of the clot and infusion of a thrombolytic agent such as recombinant tissue plasminogen. A catheter is advanced through the clot to increase exposure to the thrombolytic, or it may stop just proximal to the clot. The catheter is then left in place and the medication allowed to infuse until perfusion is restored or the clot is determined not to be resolving. Similar to angiography, this procedure is typically performed with generous local anesthesia and mild sedation. Anesthesia is seldom required, but if it is, the anesthetic depends on patient comorbidities and avoiding trauma during airway maneuvers.[12,13] Neuraxial regional anesthesia is contraindicated because of the use of thrombolytic medication.[29]

VENOUS ACCESS

Vascular access constitutes a large part of interventional radiology practice in some settings. Catheters range in size and purpose and are typically placed for intermittent hemodialysis or long-term infusion of medications. Patients are supine during the procedure to decrease the risk for venous air embolism during cannulation.[30] Sedation should be light enough to allow patients to comply with holding their breath. Judicious use of local anesthesia significantly decreases the amount of sedation required for the procedure. Adverse reactions that can occur during the procedure are bleeding, vessel injury, pneumothorax, venous air embolism, and contrast reaction.

Neurological Procedures

CAROTID ARTERY STENTING

Carotid artery stenting (CAS) is a minimally invasive alternative to an open carotid endarterectomy (CEA) for severe carotid artery stenosis. This endovascular approach is preferred in patients with difficult cervical anatomy, stenosis that is above the mandible or below the clavicle, radiation to the neck area, and significant comorbidities that may increase the risk for surgery.[31] In high-risk patients, no significant difference was found between long-term incidence of stroke, myocardial infarction, and risk for death in patients randomized to receive CAS or CEA.[32] The periprocedural stroke rate is higher in patients undergoing CAS, but they have a lower incidence of periprocedural myocardial infarction than those undergoing CEA. These outcome differences disappear over 4 years.[33]

CAS is performed through an arterial sheath that is placed in the femoral artery with the patient supine. Heparin is given after femoral artery cannulation, and activated clotting time is titrated to between 200 and 300 seconds. In the event of significant hemorrhage, protamine should be immediately available. A catheter is advanced to the site of the lesion, and an emboli-protection device (e.g., Spider FX Embolic Protection Device, Covidien, Mansfield, Mass.) may be deployed to decrease the incidence of periprocedural stroke. A balloon angioplasty is performed, leaving a stent in place to maintain patency of the carotid artery. CAS is almost always performed under light sedation, because this allows monitoring for any neurological changes during the procedure.[34,35] If the patient cannot tolerate light sedation, employing a cerebral monitoring device such as an electroencephalograph is prudent.[36] Distention of the carotid artery and activation of the baroreceptor reflex may cause significant bradycardia and hypotension that can be treated with anticholinergic medications but may require external pacing if it is severe.[37] Postprocedure hypertension should be avoided to prevent cerebral hyperemia and neurological complications. Patients are usually continued on aspirin and clopidogrel to prevent stent thrombosis.

ACUTE STROKE REVASCULARIZATION

"Time is brain" is the critical factor in the setting of an acute stroke. Revascularization is always an emergency procedure, and the faster the procedure is performed from the onset of symptoms the greater is the chance for neurological recovery.[38] The two most common methods of revascularization are intraarterial thrombolysis and endovascular thrombectomy. Intraarterial thrombolysis is performed when intravenous recombinant tissue plasminogen activator (rt-PA)—a protein that breaks down blood clots and is used in medicines to treat clots—has failed to improve the neurological deficit, no intracranial hemorrhage is present, and imaging confirms a lesion in the M1 or M2 segment, internal carotid artery, or posterior circulation.[39] Current guidelines restrict the use of intraarterial thrombolysis to 6 hours from the onset of symptoms and up to 24 hours in the posterior circulation.[39] Intraarterial thrombolysis allows for higher local concentrations of rt-PA, direct administration over the thrombus, and mechanical disruption of the clot to improve exposure to the thrombolytic agent.[40]

Endovascular thrombectomy is employed as a first-line treatment in patients with a contraindication to administration of thrombolytics or as an adjunct if intraarterial thrombolysis is unsuccessful. The devices work by grasping the clot proximally, distally sweeping the clot into a basket, or aspiration of the clot with balloon occlusion of the proximal vessel. Endovascular thrombectomy allows for a longer therapeutic window in the setting of acute stroke of up to 8 hours, because it does not use thrombolytics.[39] Complications with mechanical approaches include excessive trauma to the vasculature that may include vasospasm, vessel dissection, perforation, or rupture and thrombus fragmentation causing distal embolization (Figure 17-5).

Because the procedure is time-sensitive, little may be known about the patient's medical or surgical history other than the presenting condition. Patients are usually unable to answer questions, and family or caregivers may not be available. A preoperative evaluation focusing on whatever history is available, airway examination, physical examination, and preprocedural mental status should be performed in a timely manner and must not significantly delay the procedure. Assessment of mental status should include

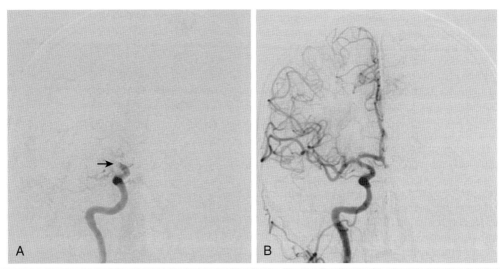

Figure 17-5 The Mechanical Embolus Retrieval in Cerebral Ischemia (Merci) retriever. **A,** Baseline angiogram demonstrates complete occlusion of the right internal carotid artery (ICA) terminus *(black arrow)*. **B,** Posttreatment angiogram demonstrates complete reperfusion of the right ICA territory after 1 pass of the Merci L6 device. (From Nogueira RG, Schwamm LH, Hirsch JA. Endovascular approaches to acute stroke. I. Drugs, devices, and data. *AJNR Am J Neuroradiol.* 2009;30[4]:654.)

risk for aspiration, ability to protect the airway, and ability to follow commands and remain motionless during imaging. Common comorbidities found in patients with acute stroke are hypertension, diabetes, atrial fibrillation, coronary artery disease, peripheral vascular disease, chronic obstructive pulmonary disorder, and smoking.[41] Hyperglycemia is found in one third of all patients with stroke and is associated with worse neurological outcomes. Glucose levels should be decreased to below 140 mg/dL, and some patients may require an insulin infusion.[39] The physical examination may be the most helpful part of the preoperative evaluation in identifying other medical conditions.

Sedation or general anesthsia can be safely performed in patients with acute stroke, but patient selection for each technique is critical.[42-44] The two most important variables for determining the level of anesthesia are whether patients can remain motionless and apneic during imaging and whether they can protect their airway. Because the procedure is time-sensitive, in the presence of any doubt a general anesthetic with endotracheal intubation is indicated. Additionally, any worsening of preprocedural neurological status may require that the airway be secured and a general anesthetic administered. Recent literature suggests that relative hypotension (systolic blood pressure <140 mm Hg) and general anesthesia may worsen outcomes after endovascular therapy for acute stroke.[44,45] This study should be viewed as inconclusive because of the numerous limitations in the study, including small sample size, a sicker patient population undergoing general anesthesia, and no standardized general anesthesia technique.[44] Also, the retrospective analysis precludes definitive conclusions about the relationship between general anesthesia and worse neurological outcomes in the setting of revascularization in acute stroke.

Evidence to guide treatment for pharmacologically induced hypotension in the setting of an acute stroke is lacking. Current understanding of altered cerebral autoregulation in the setting of acute stroke suggests that hypotension during a general anesthetic should be avoided, but the level of hypotension that decreases cerebral blood flow is unknown. Preprocedural blood pressure may be used as a guide to help the anesthesiologist determine the appropriate target blood pressure during the procedure. Overt hypertension, defined as a systolic blood pressure greater than 185 mm Hg or diastolic greater than 110 mm Hg, should be avoided because it has been shown to worsen outcomes in stroke and is a contraindication for intravenous rt-PA.[39] Discussion should be ongoing throughout the procedure between the neurointerventionalist and anesthesiologist regarding the optimal blood pressure. Blood pressure monitoring with an arterial line may be benefical because of the likelihood of significant lability in blood pressure and the need to avoid pressure extremes, but placement of the catheter should not be at the expense of delaying the procedure. Ideally, the neurointerventional team and the anesthesia team should work in parallel as they prepare the patient for the procedure.

CEREBRAL ARTERIOVENOUS MALFORMATION THERAPY

Cerebral arteriovenous malformations are congenital collections of arteries that lead into a venous system with a large collection of noncapillary vessels, termed a nidus, interspersed between them. Endovascular therapy is performed as either primary therapy to embolize the nidus of vessels or in combination with a surgical resection. Preoperative embolization is performed to decrease arteriovenous malformation bleeding and to size and target vessels that are not amenable to surgical resection.[46] During embolization, solid occlusive devices (coils, balloons), particulates (polyvinyl alcohol particles), or liquid embolic agents (onyx glue) via flow-directed catheters are fluoroscopically positioned in the arterial feeders or the nidus.

Anesthetic considerations for arteriovenous malformation embolization focus around lowering arterial blood pressure to aid embolization.[47,48] Decreasing arterial pressure causes a decrease in blood flow across the arteriovenous malformation, allowing for a more controlled deployment of embolization devices. General anesthesia is typically employed, and volatile agents can be used to help decrease blood pressure. Controlled ventilation also allows for mild hypoventilation (Paco$_2$ 50-60 mm Hg) and cerebral vasodilatation, which helps to further decrease flow across an arteriovenous malformation. Complications of the procedure include embolization of particulate matter in the pulmonary circulation, hemorrhage, thrombosis, and cerebral infarction. Hypertension after embolization should be avoided, because this may precipitate hemorrhage and edema in adjacent cerebral parenchyma as a result of normal perfusion pressure breakthrough. Normal vasculature surrounding the arteriovenous malformation is chronically vasodilated to divert cerebral blood flow to healthy tissue. Cerebral autoregulation may be impaired, and the resulting hyperemia may result in hyperperfusion injury.[49]

ANEURYSM EMBOLIZATION

Over the past decade, endovascular aneurysm embolization has become the primary treatment for many cerebral aneurysms. Regardless of the approach—surgical or endovascular—the goal of aneurysm embolization is to remove the communication between the cerebral vasculature and the aneurysm sac. Initial endovascular embolizations in the 1970s were performed using detachable balloons to occlude either the aneurysm sac or the parent vessel supplying the aneurysm.[50] Guido Guglielmi et al[51] revolutionized the treatment of endovascular embolization in 1991 with the use of detachable thrombogenic platinum coils for the treatment of a carotid-cavernous fistula. Using a metallic guidewire, a coil can be positioned in the aneurysm sac, where a small electrical current is used to detach it and leave it in place. Multiple Guglielmi detachable coils (GDC, Boston Scientific, Natick, Mass.) are used for each aneurysm, with the goal of producing a thrombus to exclude it from the circulation. Endovascular embolization became the primary treatment for both ruptured and unruptured aneurysms after the International Subarachnoid Aneurysm Trial proved short-term efficacy for endovascular treatment by showing a decreased mortality and dependence in the endovascular treatment group after 1 year.[52] Middle cerebral artery aneurysms may be the exception to the "coil first" approach because of the unfavorable endovascular anatomy, and these aneurysms may be primarily treated using surgical clipping.

Anesthetic considerations for elective endovascular coiling include blood pressure control, imaging requirements, discomfort during coiling, and expected length of the procedure. Hypertension and acute changes in systolic pressure should be avoided during endotracheal intubation if a general anesthetic is used, because this can increase the risk for rupture.[53] DSA and road-mapping techniques are used to help guide the catheters to the aneurysm sac, and patients must remain motionless with periods of apnea for image acquisition and catheter advancement. During injection of contrast material, awake patients may experience a warm sensation accompanied by a headache, and the electrical current that is generated when detaching the GDC can be painful.[54] Endovascular procedures may be quite long, especially if the aneurysm sac is difficult to

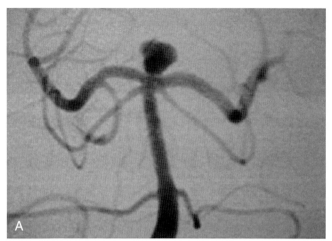

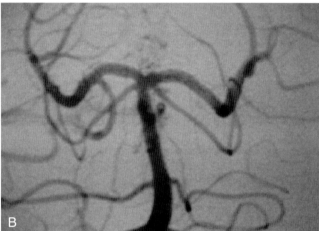

Figure 17-6 Angiographic view of basilar artery aneurysm before and after coiling with detachable platinum coils. (From Johnston SC, Higashida RT, Barrow DL, et al. Recommendations for the endovascular treatment of intracranial aneurysms: a statement for healthcare professionals from the Committee on Cerebrovascular Imaging of the American Heart Association Council on Cardiovascular Radiology. *Stroke.* 2002;33(10):2537.

access or the coils are not conforming appropriately. Given the needs of imaging requirements, discomfort of the procedure, and expected length, general endotracheal anesthesia is often chosen for this procedure, but it can be successfully performed under local anesthesia with or without sedation.[55] A general anesthetic with endotracheal intubation should be used for all ruptured aneurysms. Patients who are to undergo emergency aneurysm coiling typically have altered mental status, increased intracranial pressure, and hemodynamic instability. Arterial pressure monitoring typically is not necessary for elective procedures because of the low risk for hemorrhage, unless patient comorbidities warrant more aggressive monitoring, but it may be beneficial in emergencies (Figure 17-6).

Complications include thrombosis, aneurysmal rupture, vasospasm, perforation of normal vessels, and contrast reaction. Rupture can be detected by extravasation of contrast or hemodynamic changes (i.e., hypertension or bradycardia) secondary to raised intracranial pressure. If rupture occurs during a procedure performed under sedation, immediate conversion to general anesthesia is advised, being mindful not to cause hypertension, which may exacerbate the hemorrhage. Heparin should be immediately reversed with protamine, and blood pressure should be controlled to prevent worsening hemorrhage while still maintaining adequate cerebral perfusion pressure.[54,56] Communication between the anesthesiologist and interventionalist should include the extent of the hemorrhage and the plan for further management. Further coiling can be performed to attempt to obliterate the aneurysm and prevent further hemorrhage. If this fails, the patient may require an operative intervention, including surgical clipping, craniectomy, or placement of a ventricular drain.[56] Measures to decrease intracranial pressure, such as administration of mannitol and mild hyperventilation, should be considered in the event of a large rupture.

Certain aneurysms are not amenable to embolization without sacrificing the parent artery. In these situations a parent vessel occlusion test is performed before embolization to determine if adequate collateral circulation exists to avoid cerebral infarction. The procedure is always performed on an awake patient to provide the sensitivity required in the neurological examination to detect changes caused by ischemia. The patient is given heparin for anticoagulation, and an intravascular balloon is placed at the base of the parent artery. A baseline neurological examination is done, the balloon is inflated, and continuous neurological examinations are performed to search for any new deficits. A new deficit shows that collateral flow is inadequate and a cranial bypass needs to be placed before embolization. Some centers will induce hypotension to detect the ischemic threshold in patients and further quantify the adequacy of collateral flow.

VASOSPASM

Cerebral vasospasm is a clinically significant vasoconstriction of the cerebral vessels in the circle of Willis that causes worsening neurological status precipitated by extravasated blood in the subarachnoid space. Vasospasm is a neurological emergency and is primarily treated by augmenting cerebral blood flow, decreasing intracranial pressure and decreasing cerebral metabolic rate.[57] The mainstay of improving cerebral blood flow is triple H therapy (i.e., hypertension, hemodilution, and hypervolemia) by increasing cerebral perfusion pressure, decreasing blood viscosity, and improving cardiac output. Patients presenting to the interventional suite with vasospasm will have failed conventional therapy and are critically ill, with neurological deficits. A general anesthetic should be administered for this procedure because of the urgency of the procedure and ongoing neurological deficits. Endovascular therapy involves the infusion of vasodilators and angioplasty of the affected vessels.[58] Infusion of calcium channel blockers can cause significant bradycardia and hypotension, which should be aggressively treated in the patient with vasospasm because this can exacerbate cerebral ischemia.[59] Angioplasty is a last resort for the treatment of vasospasm because of the risk for vessel rupture and hemorrhage.

References

1. Bush WH, Swanson DP. Acute reactions to intravascular contrast media: types, risk factors, recognition, and specific treatment. *AJR Am J Roentgenol*. 1991;157(6):1153–1161.

2. Beaty AD, Lieberman PL, Slavin RG. Seafood allergy and radio-contrast media: are physicians propagating a myth? *Am J Med*. 2008;121(2):e1–e4.

3. American College of Radiology Committee on Drugs and Contrast Media. *ACR manual on contrast media*. 8th ed; 2012. http://www.acr.org/~/media/ACR/Documents/PDF/QualitySafety/Resources/Contrast%20Manual/2013_Contrast_Media.pdf.

4. Pannu N, Wiebe N, Tonelli M. Prophylaxis strategies for contrast-induced nephropathy. *JAMA*. 2006;295(23):2765–2779.

5. Tepel M, van der Giet M, Schwarzfeld C, Laufer U, Liermann D, Zidek W. Prevention of radiographic-contrast-agent-induced reductions in renal function by acetylcysteine. *N Engl J Med*. 2000;343(3):180–184.

6. Merten GJ, Burgess WP, Gray LV, Holleman JH, et al. Prevention of contrast-induced nephropathy with sodium bicarbonate: a randomized controlled trial. *JAMA*. 2004;291(19):2328–2334.

7. McCartney MM, Gilbert FJ, Murchison LE, Pearson D, McHardy K, Murray AD. Metformin and contrast media: a dangerous combination? *Clin Radiol*. 1999;54(1):29–33.

8. Anastasian ZH, Strozyk D, Meyers PM, Wang S, Berman MF. Radiation exposure of the anesthesiologist in the neurointerventional suite. *Anesthesiology*. 2011;114(3):512–520.

9. Kemerink GJ, Frantzen MJ, Oei K, et al. Patient and occupational dose in neurointerventional procedures. *Neuroradiology*. 2002;44(6):522–528.

10. Standards for basic anesthetic monitoring. Approved by the American Society of Anesthesiologists House of Delegates October 21, 1986, and last amended on October 20, 2010, with an effective date of July 1, 2011. In: *ASA standards, guidelines and statements*. October 2010. http://www.asahq.org/For-Members/Standards-Guidelines-and-Statements.aspx.

11. Arepally A, Oechsle D, Kirkwood S, Savader SJ. Safety of conscious sedation in interventional radiology. *Cardiovasc Intervent Radiol*. 2001;24(3):185–190.

12. Haslam PJ, Yap B, Mueller PR, Lee MJ. Anesthesia practice and clinical trends in interventional radiology: a European survey. *Cardiovasc Interv Radiol*. 2000;23(4):256–261.

13. Mueller PR, Wittenberg KH, Kaufman JA, Lee MJ. Patterns of anesthesia and nursing care for interventional radiology procedures: a national survey of physician practices and preferences. *Radiology*. 1997;202(2):339–343.

14. Harshfield DL, Teplick SK, Brandon JC. Pain control during interventional biliary procedures: epidural anesthesia vs I.V. sedation. *AJR Am J Roentgenol*. 1993;161(5):1057–1059.

15. Kuzgunbay B, Turunc T, Akin S, Ergenoglu P, Aribogan A, Ozkardes H. Percutaneous nephrolithotomy under general versus combined spinal-epidural anesthesia. *J Endourol*. 2009;23(11):1835–1838.

16. Schenker MP, Martin R, Shyn PB, Baum RA. Interventional radiology and anesthesia. *Anesthesiol Clin*. 2009;27(1):87–94.

17. Statement on nonoperating room anesthetizing locations. Approved by the American Society of Anesthesiologists House of Delegates October 15, 2003, and amended on October 22, 2008. In: *ASA standards, guidelines and statements*. October 2008. http://www.asahq.org/For-Members/Standards-Guidelines-and-Statements.aspx.

18. Boyer TD, Haskal ZJ. American Association for the Study of Liver Diseases practice guidelines: the role of transjugular intrahepatic portosystemic shunt creation in the management of portal hypertension. *J Vasc Interv Radiol*. 2005;16(5):615–629.

19. Haskal ZJ, Martin L, Cardella JF, et al. Quality improvement guidelines for transjugular intrahepatic portosystemic shunts. *J Vasc Interv Radiol*. 2003;14(9 Pt 2):S265–S270.

20. Rodríguez-Roisin R, Krowka MJ. Hepatopulmonary syndrome: a liver-induced lung vascular disorder. *N Engl J Med*. 2008;358(22):2378–2387.

21. Hoeper MM, Krowka MJ, Strassburg CP. Portopulmonary hypertension and hepatopulmonary syndrome. *Lancet*. 2004;363(9419):1461–1468.

22. DeGasperi A, Corti A, Corso R, et al. Transjugular intrahepatic portosystemic shunt (tips): the anesthesiological point of view after 150 procedures managed under total intravenous anesthesia. *J Clin Monit Comput*. 2009;23(6):341–346.

23. Yonker-Sell AE, Connolly LA. Mortality during transjugular intrahepatic portosystemic shunt placement. *Anesthesiology*. 1996;84(1):231–233.

24. Scher C. Anesthesia for transjugular intrahepatic portosystemic shunt. *Int Anesthesiol Clin*. 2009;47(2):21–28.

25. Pivalizza EG, Gottschalk LI, Cohen A, Middelbrook M, Soltes G. Anesthesia for transjugular intrahepatic portosystemic shunt placement. *Anesthesiology*. 1996;85(4):946–947.

26. Chalasani N, Clark WS, Martin LG, et al. Determinants of mortality in patients with advanced cirrhosis after transjugular intrahepatic portosystemic shunting. *Gastroenterology*. 2000;118(1):138–144.

27. Rozentsveig V, Neulander EZ, Roussabrov E, et al. Anesthetic considerations during percutaneous nephrolithotomy. *J Clin Anesth*. 2007;19(5):351–355.

28. Stoller ML, Wolf Jr JS, St. Lezin MA. Estimated blood loss and transfusion rates associated with percutaneous nephrolithotomy. *J Urol*. 1994;152(6 Pt 1):1977–1981.

29. Horlocker TT, Wedel DJ, Rowlingson JC, et al. Regional anesthesia in the patient receiving antithrombotic or thrombolytic therapy: American Society of Regional Anesthesia and Pain Medicine evidence-based guidelines (third edition). *Reg Anesth Pain Med*. 2010;35(1):64–101.

30. Vesely TM. Air embolism during insertion of central venous catheters. *J Vasc Interv Radiol*. 2001;12(11):1291–1295.

31. Erickson KM, Cole DJ. Carotid artery disease: stenting vs endarterectomy. *Br J Anaesth*. 2010;105(suppl 1):i34–i49.

32. Gurm HS, Yadav JS, Fayad P, et al. Long-term results of carotid stenting versus endarterectomy in high-risk patients. *N Engl J Med*. 2008;358(15):1572–1579.

33. Brott TG, Hobson 2nd RD, Howard G, et al. Stenting versus endarterectomy for treatment of carotid-artery stenosis. *N Engl J Med*. 363(1):11–23.

34. Reddy U, Smith M. Anesthetic management of endovascular procedures for cerebrovascular atherosclerosis. *Curr Opin Anaesthesiol*. 2012;25(4):486–492.

35. Lewis SC, Warlow CP, Bodenham AP, et al. General anaesthesia versus local anaesthesia for carotid surgery (gala): a multicentre, randomised controlled trial. *Lancet*. 2008;372(9656):2132–2142.

36. McFarland HR, Pinkerton Jr JA, Frye D. Continuous electroencephalographic monitoring during carotid endarterectomy. *J Cardiovasc Surg (Torino)*. 1988;29(1):12–18.

37. Lin PH, Zhou W, Kougias P, et al. Factors associated with hypotension and bradycardia after carotid angioplasty and stenting. *J Vasc Surg*. 2007;46(5):846–853. discussion 853–854.

38. Baron JC, von Kummer R, del Zoppo GJ. Treatment of acute ischemic stroke: challenging the concept of a rigid and universal time window. *Stroke*. 1995;26(12):2219–2221.

39. Adams Jr HP, del Zoppo G, Alberts MJ, et al. Guidelines for the early management of adults with ischemic stroke: a guideline from the American Heart Association/American Stroke Association Stroke Council, Clinical Cardiology Council, Cardiovascular Radiology and Intervention Council, and the Atherosclerotic Peripheral Vascular Disease and Quality of Care Outcomes in Research Interdisciplinary Working Groups: the American Academy of Neurology affirms the value of this guideline as an educational tool for neurologists. *Circulation*. 2007;115(20):e478–e534.

40. Nogueira RG, Schwamm LH, Hirsch JA. Endovascular approaches to acute stroke. I. Drugs, devices, and data. *AJNR Am J Neuroradiol*. 2009;30(4):649–661.

41. Grau AJ, Weimar C, Buggle F, et al. Risk factors, outcome, and treatment in subtypes of ischemic stroke: the German Stroke Data Bank. *Stroke*. 2001;32(11):2559–2566.

42. Brekenfeld C, Mattle HP, Schroth G. General is better than local anesthesia during endovascular procedures. *Stroke*. 2010;41(11):2716–2717.

43. Gupta R. Local is better than general anesthesia during endovascular acute stroke interventions. *Stroke*. 2010;41(11):2718–2719.

44. Davis MJ, Menon BK, Baghirzada LB, et al. Anesthetic management and outcome in patients during endovascular therapy for acute stroke. *Anesthesiology*. 2012;116(2):396–405.

45. Jumaa MA, Zhang F, Ruiz-Ares G, et al. Comparison of safety and clinical and radiographic outcomes in endovascular acute stroke therapy for proximal middle cerebral artery occlusion with intubation and general anesthesia versus the nonintubated state. *Stroke*. 2010;41(6):1180–1184.

46. Gobin YP, Laurent A, Merienne L, et al. Treatment of brain arteriovenous malformations by embolization and radiosurgery. *J Neurosurg*. 1996;85(1):19–28.

47. Osborn IP. Anesthetic considerations for interventional neuroradiology. *Int Anesthesiol Clin*. 2003;41(2):69–77.

48. Jaeger K, Ruschulte H, Herzog T, Heine J, Leuwer M, Piepenbrock S. Anaesthesiological and criterial care aspects regarding the treatment of patients with arteriovenous malformations in interventional neuroradiology. *Minim Invasive Neurosurg*. 2000;43(2):102–105.

49. Heidenreich JO, Hartlieb S, Stendel R, et al. Bleeding complications after endovascular therapy of cerebral arteriovenous malformations. *AJNR Am J Neuroradiol*. 2006;27(2):313–316.

50. Serbinenko FA. Balloon catheterization and occlusion of major cerebral vessels. *J Neurosurg*. 2007;107(3):684–705.

51. Guglielmi G, Vinuela F, Briganti F, Duckwiler G. Carotid-cavernous fistula caused by a ruptured intracavernous aneurysm: endovascular treatment by electrothrombosis with detachable coils. *Neurosurgery*. 1992;31(3):591–596. discussion 596–597.

52. Molyneux A, Kerr R, Stratton I, et al. International Subarachnoid Aneurysm Trial (ISAT) of Neurosurgical Clipping Versus Endovascular Coiling in 2143 Patients with Ruptured Intracranial Aneurysms: a randomized trial. *J Stroke Cerebrovasc Dis*. 2002;11(6):304–314.

53. Juvela S. Prehemorrhage risk factors for fatal intracranial aneurysm rupture. *Stroke*. 2003;34(8):1852–1857.

54. Jones M, Leslie K, Mitchell P. Anaesthesia for endovascular treatment of cerebral aneurysms. *J Clin Neurosci*. 2004;11(5):468–470.

55. Ogilvy CS, Yang X, Jamil OA, et al. Neurointerventional procedures for unruptured intracranial aneurysms under procedural sedation and local anesthesia: a large-volume, single-center experience. *J Neurosurg*. 2011;114(1):120–128.

56. Tummala RP, Chu RM, Madison MT, Myers M, Tubman D, Nussbaum ES. Outcomes after aneurysm rupture during endovascular coil embolization. *Neurosurgery*. 2001;49(5):1059–1066.

57. Macdonald RL. Management of cerebral vasospasm. *Neurosurg Rev*. 2006;29(3):179–193.

58. Eddleman CS, Hurley MC, Naidech AM, Batjer HH, Bendok BR. Endovascular options in the treatment of delayed ischemic neurological deficits due to cerebral vasospasm. *Neurosurg Focus*. 2009;26(3):E6.

59. Rosenberg N, Lazzaro MA, Lopes DK, Prabhakaran S. High-dose intra-arterial nicardipine results in hypotension following vasospasm treatment in subarachnoid hemorrhage. *Neurocrit Care*. 2011;15(3):400–404.

18 Pediatric Anesthesia in the Radiology Suite

CHRISTINA D. DIAZ and ROSE CAMPISE-LUTHER

The pediatric patient population presents unique challenges to its anesthesia providers. These challenges are multiplied when administering an anesthetic in a non-—operating room anesthesia (NORA) location. Evidence indicates that NORA procedures have an increased risk for patients, especially with regard to respiratory events. "Inadequate oxygenation/ventilation was the most common respiratory related remote location claim in the ASA closed claims database, occurring seven times more frequently than in [the] operating room."[1] Other respiratory events include difficult intubation, esophageal intubation, and aspiration of gastric contents.[1] "One out of 200 sedations required some form of airway rescue ranging from bag masking to emergency intubation."[2] In part, the increased risk to the patient is due to inadequate monitoring,[1] the limited availability of specialized equipment, and decreased access to skilled assistance. Other concerns include oversedation and failure to adequately assess the patient's comorbidities and risks. Children with coexisting diseases as reflected by a higher American Society of Anesthesiologists (ASA) physical status, children under the age of 1 year, and patients presenting for emergent procedures are also at higher risk for adverse events.[3]

The NORA arena is often unpredictable because of urgent or emergent add-on cases with changing procedural requirements, varying locations, and inadequate preprocedural preparation time. The remote location personnel often lack experience with critical situations and may not be able to appropriately assist with or anticipate the anesthesiologist's needs. In summary, these challenges require the anesthesiologist to be self-reliant, flexible, familiar with the procedures, and prepared for the unexpected.

Pediatric Anesthesia in Remote Locations

When working with children, the anesthesiologist needs to take into consideration the age-dependent physiology, psychological state, and pediatric comorbidities.

Preoperative Considerations

Children have distinctively different anesthetic requirements than adults. The preoperative considerations will be largely influenced by the child's physiology and preexisting medical conditions.[4] Neonates aged 0 to 28 days have a transitional physiology while adapting to extrauterine life. This period may be prolonged depending on the gestational age at delivery. The respiratory, circulatory, and metabolic systems are affected during this transitional phase. Because of an immature central nervous system, young infants are at risk for central apnea, as well as apnea in response to hypoxia and hypothermia.[5] This risk is increased by anemia, younger gestational age at birth, and a history of apneic periods. In addition, administration of sedatives, opioids, or volatile anesthetics significantly increases the risk for postprocedural apneic episodes.[6] Rather than an increase in respiration and sympathetic tone, hypoxia can lead to bradycardia and hemodynamic depression. Cardiac output in young infants is largely heart rate–dependent; thus a heart rate under 60 beats/min necessitates chest compression to maintain end-organ perfusion.[7] Other differences to consider in the neonatal cardiovascular physiology include the presence of a patent foramen ovale and patent ductus arteriosus (PDA). Anesthesia induction generally decreases systemic vascular resistance. Because neonates have a higher pulmonary vascular resistance than older children and adults, which can further increase during a stressful induction, potential exists for reversal of the typically left-to-right to a right-to-left shunt.[8] A shunt reversal should be considered in all cases of unexpected arterial oxygen desaturation. This is of particular interest in children who receive large amounts of intravenous fluids, because this can lead to a reopening of a functionally closed PDA within the first 2 weeks of life and lead to shunt reversal. Desaturations because of shunt reversal or inadequate oxygen supply are particularly pronounced in small children because of their high metabolic rate. Oxygen consumption is up to three times higher than in adults.[9]

Another important factor in the anesthetic management of neonates is temperature control. Because of its large ratio of body surface area to volume, lack of subcutaneous fat, and poor temperature regulation, the neonate is prone to heat loss.[10] Hypothermia again predisposes the neonate to apnea and bradycardia. Other side effects of hypothermia include shivering with increased oxygenation consumption, potential coagulation abnormalities, and increased discomfort during emergence. For these reasons, monitoring and maintenance of normal temperature remains important for all age groups.

As children's physiology transitions from neonatal to adult state, their respiratory, cardiac, and central nervous systems mature. Some of the characteristics of the neonate may persist. For example, 50% of children 1 year of age have a probe patent foramen ovale and 30% of the adult population still has a probe patent foramen ovale.[11] This necessitates meticulous avoidance of air bubbles in all intravenous lines to prevent a potentially dangerous paradoxical air embolus.

The normal vital signs in children will approach adult values over time, but vary significantly across age groups (Table 18-1).

The most common medical conditions that one will encounter while taking care of children include respiratory infections, asthma, obstructive sleep apnea, and more common congenital diseases such as Down syndrome (trisomy 21) and sickle cell disease.

A child in daycare or school may have up to 14 upper respiratory tract infections (URIs) per year.[12] A respiratory tract infection increases the perioperative risk for respiratory complications, such as laryngospasm, bronchospasm, thick airway secretions, mucous plugs, and croup.[3] The risk may be increased by the choice of anesthetic (i.e., airway manipulation) and the age of the patient. Younger children are at higher risk, mainly because of the smaller airway diameter.[13] All children with a URI develop an increased airway reactivity that can persist for 6 weeks after the initial symptoms. In cases of severe symptoms, an elective procedure probably should be postponed for 4 weeks.[14]

Another risk group is the increasing number of children with preexisting reactive airway disease. Among patients with asthma, great variability exists in disease severity and compliance with medications. A thorough history concerning triggering agents and the frequency and severity of attacks should be obtained, and an elective procedure should potentially be postponed until optimal pulmonary status is achieved.[15]

A third group at risk for airway complications is children with obstructive sleep apnea and/or upper airway obstruction secondary to airway hypotonia or adenotonsillar hypertrophy. These children are exquisitely sensitive to the respiratory depressant effects of sedatives, anesthetics, and opioids and are at risk for complete upper airway obstruction and respiratory arrest. They require a high level of vigilance, meticulous drug titration, and a low threshold for advanced airway management to ensure adequate ventilation and oxygenation.[3,16,17] Children with developmental delays such as cerebral palsy may be at higher risk for airway obstruction because they are known to have up to a 40% decrease in their palatal width.[18]

Among the commonly encountered congenital problems is Down syndrome. These children are prone to upper airway obstruction secondary to a small midface structure, a large tongue, and in some cases low baseline muscle tone. They also have a smaller-than-normal trachea, which requires downsizing the expected endotracheal tube size for age by 0.5 to 1.[19] Another feature of the syndrome is a connective tissue abnormality that can make intravenous catheter placement a challenge and lead to atlantooccipital instability. The latter can place the child at risk for cord compression during intubation and should be evaluated after 1 year of age. In addition, children with Down syndrome may present with hypothyroidism and congenital heart defects. Even without a documented congenital heart defect, these patients have a high incidence of bradycardia with higher doses of anesthetics.[20]

Another frequently encountered genetic problem is sickle cell disease. The tendency to develop vasoocclusive crisis with stress, hypothermia, anemia, hypercarbia, and hypoxia makes these patients a high-risk group. A thorough history concerning the severity and frequency of vasoocclusive crises should be obtained, and the transfusion thresholds should be discussed with the patient's hematologist before the procedure. Preoperative determination of a hemoglobin level may be helpful. The anesthetic management needs to focus on keeping these children warm, well hydrated, comfortable, and well oxygenated.[21]

An understanding of a child's psyche and developmental age is imperative in planning an anesthetic. Reasoning with a child may not be possible, depending on the child's age and general fear of the unknown.[22] Parental influence will have a great impact on the overall experience as well as the anesthesiologist's ability to interact with the child. Parental separation from the child can be a significant stressor to a young child.[3] Children are able to feel the parent's fear and anxiety, even if neither child nor parent is verbalizing it. The parent's honest and appropriate preparation of the child for the procedure will allow the anesthesiologist more flexibility in choosing the anesthetic. Parental dishonesty about the procedure can cause unnecessary trauma and undermine the ability to form a trusting relationship with the treating physician. Patients who require multiple anesthetics, such as those undergoing radiation therapy, may develop a distrust that can complicate further treatments and patient care.[23]

The stress of a traumatic anesthesia induction can lead to maladaptive behavior in more than half of the children who experience it.[24] The anesthesiologist should employ comfort measures in light of the child's potential anxiety. Measures may include parental presence, the use of a premedication, or walking the child through the procedure before the actual event. The appropriate comfort measure must be chosen to match the setting. For example, a parent who may become incapacitated or obstructive may not be suited to be present at induction. Premedication with oral midazolam has been shown superior to parental presence during induction[24] but may lead to prolonged sedation after a short procedure. Even with a preoperative plan in place, the anesthesiologist must exhibit situational flexibility.[18]

In planning the anesthetic, the anesthesiologist needs to know the procedure to be performed, the location of the procedure, and the age, physiology, and medical history of the

Table 18-1   Normal Range of Vital Signs in the Pediatric Patient

Age Group	Heart Rate (beats/min)	Systolic Blood Pressure* (mm Hg)	Respiratory Rate (breaths/min)
Neonate (<30 days)	120-160	60-75	40-60
1-6 mo	110-140	65-85	25-40
6-12 mo	100-140	70-90	20-35
1-2 yr	90-130	75-95	20-30
3-5 yr	80-120	80-100	18-28
6-8 yr	75-115	85-105	18-25
9-12 yr	70-110	90-115	15-25
13-16 yr	60-110	95-120	9-15
>16 yr	60-100	100-125	9-15

*As measured using an oscillometric blood pressure device.
Modified from Gottlieb EA, Andropoulos DB. Pediatrics. In: Miller R, ed. *Basics of anesthesia*. 6th ed. Philadelphia: Saunders; 2011:548, 550.

patient.[4] The anesthesia equipment necessary will largely depend on the location and type of procedure. There will be compatibility problems with the equipment in some locations. In other locations, problems of space availability due to the presence of other equipment may be an issue. Access to the patient may also be limited.

When preparing for the anesthetic, the age and weight of the patient will dictate the sizes of the equipment. Variability is greater in children than in adults in the sizes of airway equipment, intravenous setups, vascular access, fluid requirements, and drug dosages.[25] The preparation of the endotracheal tube should include the availability of the calculated tube size and one size larger and smaller than calculated (Table 18-2). When using a cuffed endotracheal tube, the calculated tube size should be decreased by 0.5. In cases of procedures with an unsecured airway, the appropriate-size airway equipment must still be present.

The availability and quality of the ventilators can significantly vary, depending on the institution and location. The anesthesiologist may be faced with older and less sophisticated equipment in contrast to the operating room. These ventilators may not be able to adequately accommodate the needs of the neonates or patients requiring special ventilation settings. For example, the requirement for a longer circuit may lead to rebreathing without using higher gas flows, inadequate tidal volume delivery, and erroneous end-tidal gas readings. High-frequency /oscillator ventilation may not be possible in many remote locations. Even if a ventilator is present, the appropriate size bag-valve-mask and oxygen source must always be available.

The intravenous catheter placement may be significantly more challenging in the pediatric patient secondary to lack of cooperation and smaller vasculature. Additional personnel will be necessary to hold the child, place, and secure the intravenous line. The parents may or may not be helpful. If the intravenous line is going to be placed awake, comfort measures in the form of local analgesics and distraction techniques should be used if possible. The available local anesthetics may include a eutectic cream, lidocaine applied via a needleless system, or an intradermal injection of lidocaine. Another option may be the use of a vapocoolant spray.[22] One should have a variety of catheter sizes and the appropriate fluid setup ready before starting. At our institution, a large tertiary care children's hospital, we use a buretrol intravenous line setup for children 5 years of age and under or weighing under 20 kg to prevent accidental overhydration. For children under 5 kg, the buretrol is initially filled with only 50 mL of crystalloid and in children over 5 kg it is filled with 100 mL.

The requirements of different age groups must be considered when choosing IV fluids. Most children will do well with a balanced salt solution such as 0.9 percent normal saline, lactated Ringer's solution, or Plasmalyte.[26] A good guideline for the calculation of the maintenance fluid is the 4-2-1 rule: 4 mL/kg for the first 10 kg, an additional 2 mL/kg for the second 10 kg, and an additional 1 mL/kg for each kilogram over 20 kg. The amount of fluid to be administered depends on the time of the last oral intake. The nil per os (NPO) guidelines for radiology procedures are the same as for operating room procedures (Table 18-3), but parents may not adhere to these guidelines.[4,27] Reasons for the noncompliance include a fear of the child suffering while NPO

Table 18-2 Endotracheal Tube Sizes

Age Group	Uncuffed ETT Size (ID mm)	Cuffed ETT Size (ID mm)
Preterm	2.5-3.0	NA
Term	3.0-3.5	3.0-3.5
1-6 mo	3.5	3.5
7-12 mo	4.0	3.5-4.0
1-2 yr	4.5	4.0-4.5
3-4 yr	4.5-5.0	4.5
5-6 yr	5.0-5.5	4.5-5.0
7-8 yr	5.5-6.0	5.0-5.5
9-10 yr	6.0-6.5	5.5-6.0
11-12 yr	6.5-7.0	6.0-6.5
13-14 yr	7.0-7.5	6.5-7.0
14+ yr	NA	7.0-7.5

Calculation of appropriate tube size for uncuffed endotracheal tubes
Divide the age by 4 and add 4 (for ages >1 yr). *Example for a 8 year old:*
$8 \div 4 + 4 = 6$

Depth of insertion
Multiplying the ID of the ETT by 3 yields the proper depth of insertion to the lips in cm. *Example:*
4 mm ETT × 3 = 12 cm for depth of insertion.

ETT, Endotracheal tube; *ID,* internal diameter.
Modified from Gottlieb EA, Andropoulos DB. Pediatrics. In: Miller R, ed. *Basics of anesthesia.* 6th ed. Philadelphia: Saunders; 2011:554.

Table 18-3 American Society of Anesthesiologists Nil Per Os Guidelines

Ingested Material	Minimum Fasting Period (hr)
Clear liquids Examples include water, juice without pulp (apple or white grape juice), clear tea, black coffee	2
Breast milk	4
Infant formula	6
Nonhuman milk Nonhuman milk is similar to solids in gastric emptying time; the amount ingested must be considered when determining the appropriate fasting time	6
Light meal Typically toast and clear liquids. Meals including fatty foods or meat may prolong gastric emptying time. Both the amount and type of foods ingested must be considered when determining the appropriate fasting time	6

These recommendations apply to healthy patients of all age groups scheduled to undergo elective procedures. They are not intended for women in labor. Following these guidelines does not guarantee complete gastric emptying.
Modified from Practice guidelines for preoperative fasting and the use of pharmacologic agents to reduce the risk of pulmonary aspiration: application to healthy patients undergoing elective procedures. *Anesthesiology.* 1999;90(3):896-905.

and the perception that radiology procedures are not equal to surgical procedures. A careful history of the patient's last oral intake should be obtained. In cases of an NPO violation, the procedure should be postponed or the airway secured with an endotracheal tube. Some evidence in the literature indicates that hyperhydration with 20 mL/kg perioperatively may be beneficial in the prevention of postoperative nausea and vomiting.[28]

Neonates are at risk for hypoglycemia because of their immature liver function and lack of glucose storage capability. Unless frequent glucose monitoring can be provided, neonates in the first week of life should receive $D_{10}W$ at the maintenance rate (4 mL/kg/hr). After the first week, full-term babies who have been fed will tolerate a fast of several hours and will not require dextrose in their fluids.[29] It is essential to avoid administering bolus doses of dextrose-containing fluids because of the risk of hyperglycemia. Children with metabolic disorders that lack gluconeogenesis, such as with acyl coenzyme A (CoA) dehydrogenase deficiency disorders and glycogen storage diseases, also may require supplemental glucose.

Drug dosages must be adjusted for the pediatric population. Factors that affect the dosage include weight, volume of distribution, and liver and kidney function. "Although children need higher doses by body weight than adults, they also react with respiratory depression and airway obstruction more quickly than adults do."[18] The medications and their indication may differ from those in adult practice.

Because of the higher incidence of laryngospasm and bradycardia in the pediatric patient, succinylcholine (2 mg/kg/dose intramuscularly or 0.5 to 2 mg/kg intravenously) and atropine (0.02 mg/kg intramuscularly or intravenously) must always be available. The first drug of choice during resuscitation is epinephrine. The resuscitation dose for pediatric patients is 10 mcg/kg. Most other vasoactive drugs are not commonly used in this population.[30] The most frequently used medications for procedural sedation in radiology include chloral hydrate, midazolam, methohexital, pentobarbital, dexmedetomidine, fentanyl, and ketamine. A newer agent that is gaining popularity for imaging studies is dexmedetomidine.[31] For a general anesthetic, inhalational agents or intravenous medications can be used. In certain locations outside the operating room, a total intravenous anesthetic (TIVA) with a hypnotic agent may be the only option. Common choices for TIVA include propofol, midazolam, and methohexital (Table 18-4).

The intraoperative management and the choice of anesthetic depend on the procedure and the child. Factors that influence the choice between a general anesthetic and procedural sedation include the invasiveness, length, and level of stimulation of the procedure. Even though some procedures can be done with the patient awake or with sedation, a general anesthetic may still be required if a child cannot cooperate.[22]

When inducing for a general anesthetic, we often choose an inhalational induction for pediatric patients to spare them the stress of an awake intravenous catheter placement. The exception is children who are at risk for aspiration or have preexisting conditions that preclude an inhalational induction. A mask induction has a higher risk for laryngospasm and other adverse respiratory events because of its slower transition through the stages of anesthesia.[13]

Intraoperative monitoring should follow the ASA standard guidelines whenever possible. At a minimum, heart rate, oxygen saturation, end-tidal carbon dioxide, and blood pressure should be monitored routinely.[32,33] During procedures with limited patient access, such as radiation therapy and magnetoencephalography (MEG) scans, it is necessary to ensure that the monitors are visible from outside the procedure room at all times. Efforts need to be made to protect the child and the anesthesiologist in locations with radiation exposure.

The patient recovering from a NORA procedure presents unique challenges. A dedicated area or personnel may not be available for the patient's recovery. The nurses assisting the anesthesiologist during sedation or administration of an anesthetic often cannot stay with the recovering patient because they have to participate in the next scheduled procedure. Using the operating room postanesthesia care unit for recovery after a NORA procedure involves transporting the patient to that area during a vulnerable phase. Younger children are also at risk for emergence delirium. Although not always present, emergence delirium occurs most commonly between the ages of 2 and 5 years and is a state of significant agitation, inconsolability, and, frequently, unawareness of their surroundings. While not completely understood, emergence delirium has been linked to painful procedures, inhalational anesthetics, and shorter anesthesia times.[3]

Adequate monitoring of the patient has to be ensured. The disposition of the patient after recovery needs to be discussed with the proceduralist and family of the patient before the procedure. Patients are discharged home after the majority of NORA procedures. The discharge criteria depend again on the procedure, the anesthetic, and the child. The risk for postoperative apnea and bradycardia will determine if the ex-premature infant can be discharged or has to be observed for 23 hours. In general, the younger the patient's gestational and postconceptual ages, the greater the risk for postoperative apnea.[6] Other patients who may require postoperative observation are those with obstructive sleep apnea or sickle cell disease and children who have undergone a procedure with increased risk for postoperative bleeding, such as liver biopsy or arterial angiography. (See Box 18-1 for a Preoperative Checklist.)

Specific Areas of Radiology Procedures

MAGNETIC RESONANCE IMAGING

Magnetic resonance imaging (MRI) is a medical imaging technique using a strong magnetic field and radio waves to create two- or three-dimensional images of the soft tissue and bony structures of the body. To generate the images, coils sometimes need to be placed over the body area of interest. This may interfere with airway devices and patient positioning.

The magnetic field warrants special precautions to avoid injuries to patients and personnel. Ferromagnetic objects will be pulled into the magnetic field of the scanner. If the object, such as surgical implants or shrapnel, is embedded in the patient, the scanner may move it or generate heat

Table 18-4 Common Hypnotic Drugs, Dosages, Duration, and Properties

Drug	Dosage and Route	Onset and Duration	Of Note
Chloral hydrate	50-100 mg/kg PO	Onset: 10-20 min Maximal effect: 30-60 min Duration: 4-8 hr	Oral medication. Commonly used on children under 10 kg Prolonged sedation
Midazolam	0.5-0.75 mg/kg PO 0.025-0.5 mg/kg IV 0.2-0.3 mg/kg intranasal 0.1-0.15 mg/kg IM	PO: onset 10-20 min, duration 1-2 hr IV: Onset 1-3 min, duration 20-30 min Intranasal: Onset 5 min, duration 30-60 min IM: Onset 5min, duration 2-6 hr	Versatile administrative routes Caution when combined with other sedatives Intranasal route is very irritating May have paradoxical reaction
Pentobarbital	2-6 mg/kg PO 1-3 mg/kg IV	IV: Onset 3-5 min, duration 15-45 min Oral: Onset 15-60 min, duration 1-4 hr	Long history of use for radiological imaging Prolonged wake-up time Children often irritable on emergence
Methohexital	0.75-2 mg/kg IV 20-35 mg/kg rectal	IV: Onset 1 minute, duration 7-10 min Rectal: Onset <10 min	Shorter duration of action, good for CT scans Rectal route associated with apneas
Fentanyl	1-3 mcg/kg IV	IV: Onset 1 min, duration 30-60 min	Used primarily as an adjunct to sedation when performing painful procedures Risk for hypoventilation and apnea when used in conjunction with other sedatives
Etomidate	0.1-0.4 mg/kg IV	IV: Onset 30-60 seconds, duration 2-10 min	Minimal effect on hemodynamics Can suppress adrenal axis Generally used for induction of an anesthetic
Ketamine	6-10 mg/kg PO 3-7 mg/kg IM 1-2 mg/kg IV	PO: Onset 30 min IV: Onset 30 seconds, duration 5-10 min IM: Onset 3-4 min, duration 15-30 min	Maintains respiration unless combined with other sedatives Possible hallucination and delirium Associated with drooling Analgesic properties
Nitrous oxide	Up to 50% in 50% oxygen for sedation Up to 70% in 30% oxygen for induction of anesthesia	Rapid onset Requires continuous flow for maintenance	The patient desaturates quickly when apneic Analgesic properties Odorless May cause nausea and vomiting
Dexmedetomidine	Load 0.5-1 mcg/kg over 10 min Infusion 0.2-1 mcg/kg/hr	Slow onset, usually requires load	Maintains respiration Risk for bradycardia Minimal analgesic properties.
Propofol	1-3 mg/kg boluses 100-200 mcg/kg/min	Onset 30 seconds Duration 3-10 min depending on single dose	Should be used only by practitioners skilled at airway management/intubation Can easily achieve general anesthetic levels and loss of airway reflexes Painful on injection
Sevoflurane	2%-3% in oxygen MAC 2.5-3.3	Rapid onset Requires continuous flow	Exclusively used by anesthesiologists Always a general anesthetic Loss of airway reflexes, increased risk for laryngospasm at lighter levels of anesthesia

CT, Computed tomography; MAC, monitored anesthesia care.
Modified from Cravero JP, Blike GT. Review of pediatric sedation. *Anesth Analg.* 2004;99:1355-1364; Lexicomp Pharmacopeia. http://www.lexi.com.

and cause thermal injury. Ferromagnetic objects outside the scanner such as oxygen tanks and laryngoscopes may turn into projectiles. The Joint Commission published a Sentinel Event Alert in 2008 listing eight types of potential injuries (Box 18-2).

Another area of concern in the MRI suite is the potential interference by the electromagnetic field with the monitoring equipment. All medical equipment must be MRI compatible or used only outside the scanner area. The monitoring equipment may not be optimal for the pediatric patient because only limited sizes are available. Because of the smaller size of the pediatric patient, a child placed in the scanner will be physically farther away from the anesthesiologist than an adult patient and therefore less accessible should an issue arise.[34]

Younger children may require sedation and/or anesthesia for an MRI scan because of the associated loud noises and lack of understanding of the foreign environment. The procedure is not painful, so neonates are frequently able to sleep through the scan after being fed. This action is known in our institution as "feed and bundle." Infants weighing 10 kg or less may require only oral chloral hydrate for sedation. Children weighing more than 10 kg commonly receive intravenous anesthetics such as pentobarbital, midazolam, or dexmedetomidine.[3] The anesthetic sometimes needs to be escalated to a general anesthetic with propofol

Box 18-1   Pediatric Anesthesia Preoperative Checklist for Outside the Operating Room

Preoperative

- Thorough review of medical history and physical assessment of patient
- Consider upper respiratory tract infection, obstructive sleep apnea, syndromes, comorbidities, age-related concerns
- Understand the anticipated procedure
- Discuss the needs of the proceduralist and anesthesiologist with staff
- Obtain anesthesia consent
- Verify procedure consent
- Premedication and/ or parental presence

Setup

ASA monitoring: capnography, pulse oximeter, electrocardiography, blood pressure, temperature
- Need appropriate sizes
- Able to view monitors at all times
- May need to be MRI compatible
- May need to be viewed by video camera or remote viewer
- Machine check and scavenging system
- Bag-valve-mask (either self-inflating or flow-regulated)
- Suction
- Oxygen source (central gas supply or tank with sufficient residual gas)
- Infusion pumps
- Appropriate fluids and intravenous access supplies
- Appropriate-sized airway equipment
  - Calculated endotracheal tube size (±1 size)
  - Difficult airway cart (if needed)
- Drugs (know the appropriate doses)
  - Hypnotics
  - Opioids
  - Paralytics

- Infusions (depending on case: vasopressors, inotropes, vasodilators)
- Emergency drugs

Location

- Examine resources and available personnel
- Consider lighting (flashlight backup)
- Check positioning of anesthesia equipment
- Prepare for accessibility of the patient during the procedure
- Examine the ability to see procedure and monitors during anesthesia
- General anesthesia versus monitored anesthesia care and sedation
- Induction
- Placement of ASA monitors
- Mask or intravenous induction
- Place or confirm intravenous access
- Airway management

Maintenance

- Positioning
- Inhalationals, infusions, intermittent boluses
- Blankets or warming devices (e.g., Bair Hugger, 3M, St. Paul, Minn.)

Recovery

- Possible parental presence
- Timing and location of emergence
- Location of recovery (recovery room, day surgery, or procedure location)
- Transport with oxygen and monitors
- Discharge criteria: special considerations
  - Former premature infant
  - Apneas, croup, laryngospasm, upper or lower respiratory tract infection
  - Increased bleeding risk
  - Other comorbidities

ASA, American Society of Anesthesiologists.

or inhalational agents. Because of the lack of stimulation during the procedure, the general anesthetic bears the risk for significant hypotension, necessitating careful titration of medications used. Parental presence, watching a movie, and rewards such as stickers and toys may help older children undergo the scan without sedation. (See Box 18-3 for a Magnetic Resonance Imaging Checklist.)[35]

COMPUTER TOMOGRAPHY

Computer tomography (CT) uses computer-processed x-ray images to generate two- and three-dimensional pictures. The scan is painless but involves a significant exposure to radiation. It is of short duration, allowing even younger patients with some parental coaching to complete the scan without sedation. Additionally, the placement of sandbags on children's extremities can limit movement. In the neonate, the feed and bundle technique may be an option. However, if sedation is required, the anesthetic should be chosen carefully and with consideration of the short duration of the procedure. Because many CTs are scheduled as an outpatient procedure, parents frequently expect to leave shortly after completion of the scan.[36]

When a CT scan requires intravenous contrast, placement of a large antecubital intravenous line is preferred to allow for administration by a power injector and the quick

distribution to the central vascular system. When performing a cardiac CT, the anesthesiologist may be asked to slow or briefly arrest the heart to produce optimal imaging. This can be achieved with esmolol or adenosine but will require a general anesthetic. For three-dimensional reconstruction images, the child needs to be completely immobile and may require a general anesthetic as well.[35]

Because of radiation, the patient and anyone staying in the room during the scan should have appropriate shielding. If the anesthesiologist chooses to leave the room, the monitors must always be clearly visible. (See Box 18-4 for a Computed Tomography Checklist.)

RADIATION THERAPY

Radiation therapy uses focused beams of ionized photons to target tumor cells in specific areas of the body. Because the ionized energy destroys all tissue in its path, the patient must remain immobile to avoid excess damage of healthy tissue and limit the side effects. The radiation therapist will calculate the allowable total dose of radiation per patient. When the patient moves, the radiation therapy lost to the healthy tissue may not be repeated. A simulation session usually precedes the initiation of therapy. Molds and masks are created during that time to limit movement by the patient and determine the coordinates of the treatment

Box 18-2   Joint Commission Sentinel Event Alert: Preventing Accidents and Injuries in the Magnetic Resonance Imaging Suite

The following types of injury can and have occurred during the MRI scanning process:

1. "Missile effect" or "projectile" injury, in which ferromagnetic objects (those having magnetic properties) such as ink pens, wheelchairs, and oxygen canisters are pulled into the MRI scanner at rapid velocity.
2. Injury related to dislodged ferromagnetic implants, such as aneurysm clips, pins in joints, and drug infusion devices.
3. Burns from objects that may heat during the MRI process, such as wires (including lead wires for both implants and external devices) and surgical staples, or from the patient's body touching the inside walls (the bore) of the MRI scanner during the scan.
4. Injury or complication related to equipment or device malfunction or failure caused by the magnetic field. For example, battery-powered devices (laryngoscopes, microinfusion pumps, monitors, etc.) can suddenly fail to operate; some programmable infusion pumps may perform erratically; and pacemakers and implantable defibrillators may not behave as programmed.
5. Injury or complication due to failure to attend to patient support systems during the MRI. This is especially true for patient sedation or anesthesia in MRI arenas. For example, oxygen canisters or infusion pumps run out and staff must either leave the MRI area to retrieve a replacement or move the patient to an area where a replacement can be found.
6. Acoustic injury from the loud knocking noise that the MRI scanner makes.
7. Adverse events related to the administration of MRI contrast agents.
8. Adverse events related to cryogen handling, storage, or inadvertent release in superconducting MRI system sites.

From The Joint Commission Sentinel Event Alert, *issue 38, February 14, 2008.*

Box 18-3   Magnetic Resonance Imaging Checklist

Remove all metal objects and cards with magnetic strips (credit cards, badges) from patient, parent, and self
Use magnetic resonance imaging–compatible equipment only
Use appropriate-size monitoring equipment
Provide ear plugs or headphones for patients and parents staying in the magnetic resonance imaging suite
Determine anesthetic technique: Sedation or general (with or without secured airway)
Discuss with team any special requirements (e.g., breath holds, contrast [oral or intravenous], positioning, coil placement)

Box 18-4   Computed Tomography Checklist

Shield patient and parents
Use appropriate-size monitoring equipment
Ensure monitor is visible to anesthesiologist
Determine anesthetic technique: Sedation or general
  ▪ May be short

Box 18-5   Radiation Therapy Checklist

Ensure that patient remains immobile
Prepare for anesthesiologist being unable to stay in room
Ensure visibility of patient and monitor via camera
Use appropriate-size monitoring equipment
Consider positioning devices (e.g., face mask)
Determine anesthetic technique: Sedation or general

patient, a video camera needs to be focused on the patient, and an additional camera needs to be focused on the monitor. The ASA recommended standard monitors should be used, including end-tidal carbon dioxide monitoring.[36]

Radiation therapy is painless, but the positioning of the patient, especially while in a face mask, may cause some discomfort. Some patients have reported an unusual odor when undergoing radiation therapy of the brain. Older patients are generally able to participate in the therapy, but younger patients commonly need an anesthetic. The need for immobility should be a consideration when choosing the anesthetic. A general anesthetic can be instituted using TIVA, with or without a secured airway, or an inhalational anesthetic, which would require placement of an airway device. Children undergoing radiation therapy may be inpatients or outpatients and usually have a permanent central venous access, which minimizes the trauma associated with repeated intravenous line placements and the trauma of the anesthetics. Because nausea is frequently associated with radiation therapy, antinausea medication should be available.

As mentioned previously, recovering these patients can be challenging. There may be no additional personnel available to watch the recovering patient in the radiation therapy area. It may be necessary to transport these patients to the postanesthesia care unit of the operating room on a monitor with available oxygen. (See Box 18-5 for a Radiation Therapy Checklist.)

INTERVENTIONAL RADIOLOGY

A variety of procedures are performed in the interventional radiology suite. They can range from a gastrostomy tube exchange to the coiling of intracranial arteriovenous malformations. Some procedures are done under ultrasound guidance, and others require the use of fluoroscopic imaging. Depending on the procedure, varying degrees of pain may be associated with it. The parents often expect their children to be asleep or at least unaware of the procedure and without any distress or pain.[18]

Most interventional radiology suites are not designed to accommodate anesthesiologists and their equipment,

area. Radiation therapy also may be used to eradicate bone marrow stem cells before a bone marrow transplant. Radiation therapy usually involves daily treatments, 5 days per week, for a variable number of successive weeks.[37] For bone marrow eradication, the patient may have to undergo multiple treatments per day.

Because of the large amounts of radiation used during a treatment, the patient is the only person who may remain in the room. The room is sealed with a large leaded door, and access to the patient is limited. To appropriately monitor the resulting in limited space and access to the patient. The procedures are usually performed with dimmed lights to optimize visualization for the radiologist. It can be very difficult to follow the procedure because the monitor displaying the procedural images may not be visible where the anesthesiologist is located.

Unless located in a children's hospital, the staff in the radiology suite may not be familiar with the needs of a pediatric patient. Cases are often posted on short notice and at any time of day, limiting the preoperative preparation time.

Within the interventional radiology suite, the procedures may be grossly divided into two categories: endovascular and lymphatic procedures and nonvascular procedures. Examples of endovascular procedures include vascular access, coiling of vascular malformations, and sclerotherapy. During these procedures, intravenous contrast is used to visualize the structures. When using these contrast dyes in children, it is important to calculate the allowable dye load before the start of the procedure. Reactions to the intravascular contrast include nausea, vomiting, bronchospasm, hypertension, hypotension, flushing, renal failure, seizures, anaphylaxis, and cardiac arrest. Some reactions may occur immediately upon administration, while others may appear later.[38]

Sclerotherapy is used to treat vascular and lymphatic malformations. The procedure involves accessing the malformation, potentially draining its contents, and injecting various agents aimed at causing an inflammatory process and the eventual scaring and shrinkage of the lesion. Accessing the pediatric vessels can be more challenging because of their overall smaller size in contrast to those of adults. Ethanol can be used as a sclerosing agent. Problems encountered with high doses of ethanol can include intoxication, coagulopathy, increased pulmonary artery pressures, and possible cardiovascular collapse. Another common sclerotherapy agent is sodium tetradecyl sulfate (STS). It is a detergent-based chemical that disrupts the lining of the vessel and may result in urticaria, necrosis, and allergic reactions. Additional sclerosing agents include hypertonic saline and other osmotic agents, other detergents, and chemical irritants such as erythromycin, polyiodinated iodine, and chromated glycerin. All sclerosants produce hemolysis when injected into the vascular bed, leading to hematuria. The child should be adequately hydrated and the urine alkalinized to prevent precipitation of hemoglobin in the renal tubules and to prevent renal failure. Because of the risk for extravasation and possible reactions to the sclerosing agents, the patient needs to remain motionless. Therefore a general anesthetic is recommended for sclerotherapy procedures.[39]

For intracranial vascular malformations, the common treatment modality is endovascular coiling and glue. Before the treatment of the malformation, examination of the lesion usually involves a cerebral angiogram or other imaging modality (MRI angiogram). The diagnostic imaging may be accomplished with sedation or a general anesthetic. Because of the risk for intravascular injury and hemorrhage with movement, a general anesthetic is usually required during the treatment. In light of the potential hemodynamic instability involved with the procedure, an arterial line may be a useful tool, and vasoactive agents should be immediately available. As with sclerotherapy, the anesthesiologist

should be cognizant of the maximum amount of dye allowable for the child. Because of the large variability in patient sizes, the fluid boluses accompanying the administration of dye need to be carefully accounted for to diminish the risk for fluid overload, especially in infants.[40]

The nonvascular procedures in the interventional radiology suite may range from gastric or duodenal tube exchanges to biopsies of the liver, kidneys, bones, or tumors and drainage of abscesses and pleural effusions. The anesthetic strategy has to be adapted to the needs of the proceduralist, the invasiveness of the procedure, and the ability of the child to cooperate.[18] (See Box 18-6 for an Interventional Radiology Checklist.)

NUCLEAR MEDICINE

Nuclear medicine or nuclear imaging produces images by detecting radiation emitted from radioactive tracer material injected into the bloodstream. The materials, depending on the compound, can evaluate the function of different organ systems and diagnose disease processes. Nuclear imaging is used in the surveillance and diagnosis of cancer (bone scan), detection of seizure foci and evaluation of cerebrovascular disease (single-photon emission computer tomography [SPECT] and positron emission tomography[PET]),[41] and evaluation and follow-up of urinary reflux disease (renal scans). Nuclear imaging is one of the oldest imaging modalities and is painless except for the placement of an intravascular catheter. The radionuclides are physiologically harmless and nonallergenic, but all bodily fluids should be handled with radiation safety precaution.[42]

Children have to remain motionless during the scan, which in younger children usually requires sedation or a general anesthetic. It is necessary to be aware of the timing of the imaging when planning the anesthetic. Children are injected with the radioactive tracer and then imaged at exact predetermined intervals to optimize the diagnostic value of the scan. (See Box 18-7 for a Nuclear Medicine Checklist.)

Box 18-6   Interventional Radiology Checklist

Shield patient and self
Calculate allowable dye load
Determine anesthetic technique: Sedation or general
Consider need for pain management
Use appropriate-size monitoring equipment
Discuss need for complete immobility
Discuss positioning of the patient and equipment

Box 18-7   Nuclear Medicine Checklist

Place peripheral intravenous access and administer tracer before scan
Time the scan appropriately after tracer administration
Determine anesthetic technique: Sedation or general
Discuss need for patient to remain motionless for the scan
Use appropriate-size monitoring equipment

Box 18-8 Magnetoencephalography Scan Checklist

Understand implications of shielded room
- No access to patient
- Monitors outside the room, with cables and circuit threaded through wall

Use appropriate-size monitoring equipment

Avoid magnetic dust being introduced into room (i.e., no shoes)

Remove all metal objects

Allow parental presence if room is large enough

MAGNETOENCEPHALOGRAPHY

The magnetoencephalography (MEG) scan is the measurement of magnetic fields produced by naturally occurring electrical currents of the brain to map brain activity. The fields are measured by using magnetometers that are formed by superconducting quantum interference devices.[43] MEG scans are used to localize diseased areas of the brain, such as localizing epileptic foci before surgery. Because the magnetic fields produced by the electrical currents of the brain are minuscule, extensive shielding from interfering magnetic fields of the earth and electrical equipment is required. Therefore equipment used to monitor the patient must be located outside the MEG scanner.[44]

During the scan, the patient is placed into the shielded and sealed room, which allows minimal access to the patient. When the room is opened, magnetic interference enters the room and requires recalibration of the scanner before proceeding with the examination. No metallic material can be taken into the room. The examination is painless and quiet, and the bed and scanner do not move. The exam may require electrodes to be glued to the patient's scalp, which in younger patients may have to be done under anesthesia.

The choice of anesthetic agents should be influenced by the drug's effect on brain activity. Midazolam should be avoided when using the MEG scan to localize epileptic foci because of the high failure rate associated with its use. Chloral hydrate used as premedication seems to have only a small effect on the scan. The scan can be performed using sedation or a general anesthetic, but the anesthetic must ensure that the child remains motionless for at least 1 hour. Lighter levels of anesthesia should be used to reduce the potential for interference with electrical brain activity. Dexmedetomidine has been shown not to suppress brain activity but to ensure patient immobility.[45,46] Older children may be able to tolerate the scan without sedation. As with any procedural sedation or anesthetic, appropriate monitoring needs be ensured.

Monitoring the patient in the MEG scanner involves cables threaded through shielded channels in the wall. The oxygen supply, breathing circuit, and end-tidal gas sampling line are also fed through this channel to the equipment located outside the scanner. (See Box 18-8 for a Magnetoencephalography Scan Checklist.)

Conclusion

The remote location of the NORA area is a special challenge to the pediatric anesthesiologist. Sick children, poor access, and locations distant from the operating room with unfamiliar personnel can add to the stress of the procedure. Although stated earlier in the chapter, it bears repeating that the challenges presented in the NORA suite require the pediatric anesthesiologist to be self-reliant, flexible, and familiar with the procedures to provide the best possible patient care. When rendering a pediatric anesthetic in the NORA suite, the practitioner must expect, and be prepared, for the unexpected.

References

1. Metzger J, Posner KL, Domino KB. The risk and safety of anesthesia at remote locations: the U.S. closed claim analysis. *Curr Opin Anesthesiol.* 2009;22(4):502–508.
2. Cravero JP. Risk and safety/anesthesia for procedures outside the operating room. *Curr Opin Anesthesiol.* 2009;22(4):509–513.
3. Collins CE, Everett LL. Challenges in pediatric ambulatory anesthesia: kids are different. *Anesthesiol Clin.* 2010;28(2):315–328.
4. Gozal D, Gozal Y. Pediatric sedation/anesthesia outside the operating room. *Curr Opin Anesthesiol.* 2008;21(4):494–498.
5. Rigatto H, Brady JP, de la Torre Verduzco R. Chemoreceptor reflexes in the preterm infant: the effect of gestational age and postnatal age on ventilatory response to inhalation of 100% and 15% oxygen. *Pediatrics.* 1975;55(5):604–613.
6. Coté CJ, Zaslatsky A, Downes JJ, et al. Postoperative apnea in former preterm infants after inguinal herniorrhaphy: a combined analysis. *Anesthesiology.* 1995;82(4):809–822.
7. Kattwinkel J, Perlman JM, Aziz K, et al. Neonatal resuscitation: 2010 American Heart Association guidelines for cardiopulmonary resuscitation and emergency cardiovascular care. *Pediatrics.* 2010;126(5):1400–1413.
8. De Souza D, McDaniel G, Baum V. Cardiovascular physiology. In: Davis P, ed. *Smith's anesthesia for infants and children.* 8th ed. St. Louis: Mosby; 2008:87.
9. Sands SA, Edwards BA, Kelly VJ, et al. A model analysis of arterial oxygen desaturation during apnea in preterm infants. *PLoS Comput Biol.* 2009;5(12):e1000588.
10. Sinclair JC. Thermal control in premature infants. *Annu Rev Med.* 1972;23:129–148.
11. Hasan A, Parvez A, Ajmal MR. Patent foramen ovale: clinical significance. *J Ind Acad Clin Med.* 2004;5(4):339–344.
12. Revai K, Dobbs LA, Nair S, et al. Incidence of acute otitis media and sinusitis complicating upper respiratory tract infection: the effect of age. *Pediatrics.* 2007;119(6):e1408–e1412.
13. Lerman J. Perioperative respiratory complications in children. *Lancet.* 2010;376(9743):745–746.
14. Tait AR, Malviya S. Anesthesia for the child with an upper respiratory infection: still a dilemma? *Anesth Analg.* 2005;100(1):59–65.
15. Woods BD, Sladen RN. Perioperative considerations for the patient with asthma and bronchospasm. *Br J Anaesth.* 2009;103(suppl 1):i57–i65.
16. Brown KA, Laferrière A, Lakheeram I, Moss IR. Recurrent hypoxemia in children is associated with increased analgesic sensitivity to opiates. *Anesthesiology.* 2006;105(4):665–669.
17. Sander JC, King MA, Mitchell RB, et al. Perioperative complications of adeno-tonsillectomy in children with obstructive sleep apnea syndrome. *Anesth Analg.* 2006;103(5):1115–1121.
18. Kannikeswaran N, Mahajan PV, Sethuraman U, et al. Sedation medication received and adverse events related to sedation for brain MRI in children with and without developmental disabilities. *Pediatr Anesth.* 2009;19(3):250–256.
19. Shott SR. Down syndrome: analysis of airway size and a guide for appropriate intubation. *Laryngoscope.* 2000;110(4):585–592.
20. Kraemer FW. Bradycardia during induction of anesthesia with sevoflurane in children with Down syndrome. *Anesth Analg.* 2012;111(5):1259–1263.
21. Firth PG. Anesthesia and hemoglobinopathies. *Anesth Clin.* 2000;27:321–336.
22. Neuhäuser C, Wagner B, Heckmann M, Weigand MA, Zimmer KP. Analgesia and sedation for painful interventions in children and adolescents. *Dtsch Aerztebl Int.* 2010;107(14):241–247.
23. Chorney JM, Kain ZN. Family-centered pediatric perioperative care. *Anesthesiology.* 2010;112(3):751–755.

24. Kane ZN, Caldwell-Andrews A, Blount R, et al. Parental presence during induction during anesthesia versus sedative premedication: which intervention is more effective? *Anesthesiology.* 1998;89:1147–1156. discussion 9-10A.

25. Committee on Drugs. Section on Anesthesiology, American Academy of Pediatrics. Guidelines for the elective use of conscious sedation, deep sedation and general anesthesia in pediatric patients. *Pediatrics.* 1985;76(2):317–321.

26. Paut O, Lecroix F. Recent developments in the perioperative fluid management of the pediatric patient. *Curr Opin Anesth.* 2006;19(3):268–277.

27. American Society of Anesthesiologists Committee. Practice guidelines for preoperative fasting and the use of pharmacologic agents to reduce the risk of pulmonary aspiration: application to healthy patients undergoing elective procedures: an updated report by the American Society of Anesthesiologists Committee on Standards and Practice Parameters. *Anesthesiology.* 2011;114(3):495–511.

28. Yogedran S, Asokumar B, Cheng DC, Chung F. A prospective randomized double blind study of the effect of intravenous fluid therapy on adverse outcomes on outpatient surgery. *Anesth Analg.* 1995;80(4):682–686.

29. Bennett EJ, Daughety MJ, Jenkins MT. Fluid requirements for neonatal anesthesia and operation. *Anesthesiology.* 1970;32(4):343–350.

30. Kleinman ME, Chameides L, Schexnayder SM, et al. Pediatric advanced life support: 2010 American Heart Association guidelines for cardiopulmonary resuscitation and emergency cardiovascular care. *Pediatrics.* 2010;126(5):1361–1399.

31. Metzner J, Domino KB. Risks of anesthesia or sedation outside the operating room: the role of the anesthesia care provider. *Curr Opin Anesthesiol.* 2010;23:523–531.

32. Standards for basic anesthetic monitoring (last amended by the House of Delegates October 20, 2010). http://www.asahq.org/for-members/standards-guidelines-and-statements.aspx.

33. American Academy of Pediatrics, American Academy of Pediatric Dentistry, Coté CJ, Wilson S, Work Group on Sedation. Guidelines for monitoring and management of pediatric patients during and after sedation for diagnostic and therapeutic procedures: an update. *Pediatrics.* 2006;118(6):2587–2602.

34. Laurence AS. Sedation, safety and MRI. *Br J Radiol.* 2000;73:575–577.

35. Macias C, Chumpitazi C. Sedation and anesthesia for CT: emerging issues for providing high-quality care. *Pediatr Radiol.* 2011;41(suppl 2):S517–S522.

36. Eichhorn V, Henzler D, Murphy M. Standardizing care and monitoring for anesthesia or procedural sedation delivered outside the operating room. *Curr Opin Anesthesiol.* 2010;23:494–499.

37. McFayden G, Pelly N, Orr RJ. Sedation and anesthesia for the patient undergoing radiation therapy. *Curr Opin Anesthesiol.* 2011;24(4):433–438.

38. Singh J, Daftary A. Iodinated contrast media and their adverse reactions. *J Nucl Med Technol.* 2008;36:69–74.

39. Berenguer B, Burrows PE, Zurakowski D, Mulliken JB. Sclerotherapy of craniofacial venous malformations: complications and results. *Plast Reconstr Surg.* 1999;104(1):1–11.

40. Dorairaj IL, Hancock SM. Anesthesia for interventional neuroradiology. *Contin Educ Anaesth Crit Care Pain.* 2008;8(3):86–89.

41. Chiron C, Raynaud C, Dulac O, et al. Study of the cerebral blood flow in partial epilepsy of childhood using the SPEC. *J Neuroradiol.* 1989;16(4):317–324.

42. Mason KJ, Koka BV. Anesthesia outside the operating room. In: Coté CJ, ed. *A practice of anesthesia for infants and children.* 4th ed. Philadelphia: Saunders; 2009:998.

43. Cohen D. Magnetoencephalography: detection of the brain's electrical activity with a superconducting magnetometer. *Science.* 1972;175:664–666.

44. Szmuk P, Kee S, Pivalizza EG, et al. Anesthesia for magnetoencephalography in children with intractable seizures. *Pediatr Anesth.* 2003;13(9):811–817.

45. Talke P, Stapelfeldt C, Garcia P. Dexmedetomidine does not reduce epileptiform discharges in adults with epilepsy. *Neurosurg Anesthesiol.* 2007;9:195–199.

46. Koenig M, Mahmoud MA, Fujiwara H, et al. Influence of anesthetic management on quality of magnetoencephalography scan data in pediatric patients. *Anesthesiol Clin.* 2009;27(2):321–336.

19 Anesthesia Concerns in the Magnetic Resonance Imaging Environment

RAMON MARTIN

Providing anesthesia in the magnetic resonance imaging (MRI) environment differs from that in the operating room. The static magnetic field necessitates that all monitors, devices, and machines be nonferrous. The gradient magnetic field can interfere with electrocardiographic (ECG) tracing and is the main source of acoustic noise. Radiofrequency field energy is transferred into heat, so the patient usually becomes warm when more energy is absorbed. If too much heat is transferred to the patient, burns may occur.

Because of the desire to minimize ionizing radiation and the ability of MRI to provide better imaging of some tissues and tissue planes, a gradual increase has occurred in the use of MRI not only for diagnosis but also as a part of treatment procedures.[1] In a tertiary care hospital in which a sick patient population often has multiple comorbidities, patients are frequently unable to lie flat, still, or comfortably. Thus a corollary increase is seen in the request for anesthetic support.

This chapter presents some of the issues faced when anesthetizing a patient in the MRI suite. Training and preparation are needed before caring for a patient in the MRI environment. The MRI room should be inspected to make sure it is suitably prepared for the emergency and contingency situations, such as airway difficulty and cardiorespiratory collapse requiring resuscitation. Primarily because of acoustic noise during MRI, staff must be prepared to monitor the patient remotely after the onset of the anesthetic. Constant vigilance is required before bringing anything into the MRI room, because several commonly used anesthetic devices have not been tested to determine if they are even conditionally MRI safe.

With the increase in the number and type of interventional procedures done in the MRI suite, a corresponding rise has occurred in the amount of anesthetic support needed. The MRI suite should be viewed as a non–operating room anesthesia location that requires not only an anesthetic machine, monitors, cart, and drugs but also constant vigilance for the safety of both patients and staff.

Training and Personnel

As a requirement to practice anesthesia in MRI in our institution, individuals must attend an orientation lecture and video about MRI safety. This orientation includes a tour of the facility to highlight areas of concern, such as the magnetic zone and corresponding safety zones. The operating room safety checklist[2] has been expanded for MRI to include not only the patient's MRI checklist but also a personal patdown before entering zone 4 with the patient. Table 19-1 lists the zones in the MRI area.

In addition to the MRI technologist, our institution requires that a nurse be present whenever an anesthetic is administered. This policy applies to both diagnostic scans and procedures. Having a nurse assist during the anesthetic administration acknowledges the fact that the patient who requires an anesthetic for a diagnostic scan often has comorbidities. This practice began after a situation in which a patient needed a preoperative MRI for surgical planning. Administration of a general anesthetic began with the anesthesiologist and an MRI technologist present in the room. The patient developed cardiopulmonary arrest after the induction of general anesthesia. The ensuing resuscitation was unsuccessful. A review of the events led to the requirement to treat such cases as they would be handled in the main operating room. Whenever a therapeutic procedure is performed, the interventionalist must also be present in the MRI suite.

The Magnetic Resonance Imaging Suite

Although the operating room table is the center of the operating room, the magnet is the central, space-occupying mass in the MRI suite. The two issues that must be addressed are whether the patient bed is fixed or can be docked and undocked and whether access to the patient exists for emergent exit.

If the bed is fixed to the MRI scanner, a general anesthetic will require induction of the patient on an MRI-compatible stretcher before being transferred to the bed. The stretcher is left in MRI zone 4 in case the patent must be quickly evacuated. A bed that docks and undocks allows for mobility to position the patient as needed for induction of an anesthetic and quick transfer from the bore of the magnet.

Emergency access always should be assessed when a patient enters zone 4. An area in zone 3 should be available with adequate space, oxygen, suction, and outlets for resuscitation of a patient if needed. An MRI bay must meet basic criteria that allow for an anesthetic to be provided safely. For example, if an MRI bay does not allow adequate space for entry and exit of zone 4 or fails to provide an adequate number of electrical outlets for standard

Table 19-1   Magnetic Resonance Imaging Zones

Zone	Description
Zone 1	Zone 1 consists of all areas freely accessible to the general public. This zone includes the entrance to the MRI facility, and the magnet poses no hazards in these areas.
Zone 2	Zone 2 acts as a buffer between zone 1 and the more restrictive zone 3. Here, patients are under the general supervision of MRI personnel. Normally, these areas are also safe from the magnet. Zone 2 may include the reception area, dressing room, and interview room.
Zone 3	Access to zone 3 should be restricted by a physical barrier. Only approved MRI personnel and patients who have answered a medical questionnaire and interview are allowed inside zone 3. The MRI control room and/or computer room are located within zone 3.
Zone 4	Zone 4 is strictly the area within the walls of the MRI scanner room, sometimes called the magnet room. Access into the MRI scanner room should be available only by passing through zone 3. Zone 4 is sometimes considered to be inside zone 3 because it does not have a direct entrance to unrestricted areas. Zones 3 and 4 are sometimes collectively referred to as the MRI suite.

anesthesia equipment necessary in zone 3 for a resuscitation, that bay should considered unsafe and not used as an anesthetic site. In some institutions, older MRI bays do not fit these criteria. For all new construction, a member of the anesthesia staff should be involved in the planning stages to ensure there is no compromise for providing a safe anesthetic.

MRI zone 3 is the buffer zone where resuscitation should be done. Most of the emergency scenarios such as cardiopulmonary collapse, difficult airway, and allergic or anaphylactic reactions require instruments that might not be MRI safe, as well as a variety of support personnel, not all of whom may be cognizant of MRI safety, and the patient should be moved as quickly as possible to zone 3. Although zone 2 is preferred for resuscitation, the urgency of the situation might dictate a short transit to begin emergent resuscitative maneuvers.

Patient Selection

A poor quality of continuous ECG tracing is one the most serious limitations in monitoring an anesthetized patient in the MRI suite. If a patient is at risk for cardiac ischemia or further injury in the setting of recent ischemic stress, the benefit of anesthetizing the patient for MRI should be weighed against that risk. Technological advances will eventually overcome this limitation.[3] Cardiac MRI does allow for visualization of global cardiac function. This type of MRI requires frequent breath-holding, but techniques that allow for free breathing have been reported.[4,5]

Known difficult intubation or prior history of allergic reaction to medication or contrast dye must be considered before entering zone 4. However, unanticipated difficult intubation or an anaphylactic reaction to contrast dye requires quick action and exit from zone 4. Plans to deal with contingency situations should be in place before a patient is brought into the MRI suite.

Remote Monitoring

The biological effects of magnetic and radiofrequency currents are subtle and continue to be studied.[6-8] The acoustic noise, mainly from gradient magnetic fields, leads to the need to remotely monitor the patient. The Occupational Noise Exposure Standard states that a permissible exposure limit over 8 hours is 90 dBA.[9] More than 85 dBA requires a hearing protection program. In our institution, the 8-hour equivalent sound levels in the three MRI bays that regularly provide anesthesia are between 87 and 93 dBA. Although comfortable hearing protection is available for patients, anesthesia providers often have difficulties hearing the pulse oximeter tone when more than 1 or 2 feet from the monitor. Although developing technologies will allow for sound deadening with transmission of monitor tones through headphones, this technology is not widely available. Remote monitoring is routinely done in these cases.

Remote monitoring is accomplished by a slave monitor that displays vital signs and end-tidal gases, a view of the anesthesia ventilator and settings by either direct line of sight or a remote camera, and a view of the patient in the bore of the magnet by a camera linked to a display next to the vital signs monitor. This is generally done when the patient is stable after the induction of the anesthetic. If an intervention is needed during the course of the scan, the scan is halted until the issue is resolved.

Devices in Magnetic Resonance Imaging

In addition to standard monitoring devices, patients with multiple comorbidities or who are in the recent postoperative period may require or have already attached to them monitors or devices that have not been screened for MRI safety.[10] In response to emergent situations, devices may be used that have not been assessed for MRI safety. The following case report illustrates such an instance.

A 62-year-old man was scheduled for MRI of the brain and total spine after a fall. He became restless and occasionally combative, and anesthesia support was requested to ensure that the patient held still and remained comfortable for the duration of the examination. Because of the uncertainty of his nil per os (NPO) status and the length of the examination, the patient received a general anesthetic with a rapid sequence induction. The airway examination did not raise any preoperative concerns before intubation. After taking the patient into the MRI room, standard monitors were attached. The patient was preoxygenated before a rapid sequence induction was performed. The vocal cords were not visualized on the first and second attempts at intubation. A Fastrach laryngeal mask airway (LMA, San Diego, Calif.) was placed. After breath sounds were auscultated, an endotracheal tube (ETT) was uneventfully placed. The patient was placed on the ventilator and, with stable vital signs, the scan was initiated. Figure 19-1 shows the

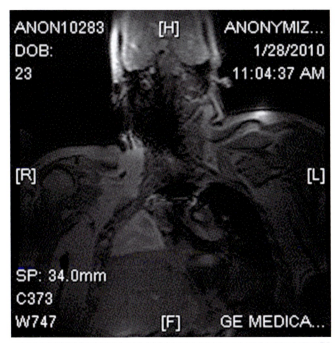

Figure 19-1 Magnetic resonance imaging of the brain and cervical and thoracic spine with a Fastrach endotracheal tube (LMA, San Diego, Calif.) in place.

Table 19-2 Degrees of Deflection and Force for Commonly Used Devices

Device	α(°)	Force [=mg tan(α)]
Sheridan ETT	5	1.9458
LMA	2	1.7475
Fastrach ETT	90	3.1769
Reinforced ETT	90	4.9923
Laser Shield ETT	0	0
Laser Flex ETT	30	2.0866
Arrow Central Line	0	0
Edwards Swan Gantz	15	5.2146
Edwards Swan Gantz CCO	12	7.0912
B. Braun Epidural Catheter	0	0
Arrow Epidural Catheter	2.5	1.2138
Epimed Epidural Catheter	90	4.5385
Medtronic Atrial Wire	90	4.5385
Medtronic Ventricular Wire	90	4.5385

scan obtained. After discussion with the MRI technologist, it was decided that the ETT was probably the reason for the signal drop out. The scan was halted, and with a tube changer the Fastrach ETT was replaced with a Sheridan ETT (Teleflex, Research Triangle Park, NC). An examination of the packaging for the Fastrach gave no indication of MRI safety. An examination of the actual Fastrach ETT, however, showed a reinforced coil running the length of the tube. A hand-held magnet placed close to the ETT revealed magnetic attraction.

This event led to an appraisal of other devices and monitors used or encountered in the operating room. Devices that contained no markings about MRI safety were given particular scrutiny. Table 19-2 lists the gradient magnetic attraction of commonly used devices, none of which are listed in the 2009 Edition of the *Reference Manual for Magnetic Resonance Safety Implants and Devices.*[11] Only the Epimed epidural catheter (Johnstown, NY) is actually labeled as not being safe for use in the MRI environment. Many devices that are used frequently and ubiquitously were found to have some magnetic attraction. The Sheridan ETT has a valve for the pilot balloon that, when left lying against the face (Figure 19-2), may account for artifact in a scan of the brain. Testing is being done to measure heat generated by each of these devices. Methods are being developed to standardize a testing system to quickly evaluate any monitor or device for which there is no readily identifiable information about MRI safety.[12]

Drug delivery to patients, either as a part of the anesthetic or for delivery of ongoing medications and fluids, requires planning as well. Commonly used infusion pumps are not MRI safe. These pumps are left outside of zone 4 and continue to function with extra lengths of tubing to reach the patient. These pumps should never be brought into the room because magnetic attraction causes imaging distortion and

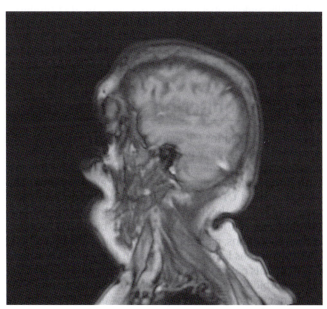

Figure 19-2 Magnetic resonance imaging of the brain in a patient intubated with a Sheridan endotracheal tube (Teleflex, Research Triangle Park, NC). The pilot balloon is lying against the right cheek.

possible pump malfunction. MRI-compatible pumps are under development. Current models on the market are the B. Braun SpaceStation MRI pump (Melsungen, Germany), the Covidien MRidium IV pump (Mansfield, Mass.), and the Harvard Apparatus MRI Syringe Pump (Holliston, Mass.). These pumps can be used for the delivery of intravenous anesthetic agents because they have adequate drug libraries or flexible dosing parameters. The cartridges and tubing for these pumps are not compatible with conventional MRI-unsafe pumps. If a patient is receiving a continuous infusion of medication through a conventional pump, the pump must be left outside the MRI room in zone 3, using extra tubing, or the infusion must be switched to an MRI-compatible pump.

Table 20-1   Daily Schedule of Coverage for Outside the Operating Room

Time	Monday	Tuesday	Wednesday	Thursday	Friday
AM	Endo (2 rms)	Endo (2 rms)	Endo (2 rms)	Endo (2 rms)	Endo (2 rms)
PM	Endo (2 rms)	Endo (2 rms)	Endo (2 rms)	Endo (2 rms)	Endo (2 rms)
AM		FPC		FPC	
PM			FPC		
AM	Rad Onc		Rad Onc	Rad Onc	
PM	Rad Onc		Rad Onc	Rad Onc	
AM		MRI		MRI	
PM					
AM	CT	CT	CT	CT	
PM				CT	
AM	Angio	Angio	Angio		Angio
PM	Angio			Angio	Angio
AM	INR				INR
PM			INR		
AM	Cath	Cath	Cath	Cath	Cath
PM	Cath	Cath	Cath	Cath	Cath
AM	EP	EP	EP	EP	EP
PM	EP	EP	EP	EP	EP
AM	CVRR	CVRR	CVRR	CVRR	CVRR
PM	CVRR	CVRR	CVRR	CVRR	CVRR
AM	AMIGO	AMIGO		AMIGO	AMIGO
PM	AMIGO	AMIGO		AMIGO	AMIGO

Radiation Oncology (L2): Rad Onc
Angiography/Interventional Radiology (L2): Angio
Cardiac Cath Laboratory (L2): Cath
Electrophysiology Laboratory (L2): EP
Interventional Neuroradiology (L1): INR
CT Scan for Ablations, etc. (L1): CT
Magnetic Resonance Imaging (L1): MRI
Endoscopy Suite (ASB2): Endo
Family Planning Clinic (A Main): FPC
Cardiovascular Recovery Room (Shapiro L2): CVRR
Advanced Multi-Image Guided Operating Suite (L2): AMIGO

with and signed off by the corresponding financial section of each department where services are provided. As mentioned earlier, even though the contract is negotiated and signed yearly, it is amended if substantive changes are needed in clinical coverage.

The impact of this fixed or block schedule for NORA has been widely felt. As mentioned earlier, the increased visits to the PES are being mitigated by an evolving non–operating room preoperative assessment service. This is being developed in conjunction with the main operating room to take care of both elective and last-minute in-house patients for both the non–operating room location and the main operating room. Just as has been demonstrated for the PES, it is hoped that the service will prove its worth by decreasing the incidence of last-minute case cancellations so that more cases can be handled efficiently.

The expansion of anesthesia to non–operating room locations has resulted in the establishment of area-specific postanesthesia care units in high-volume areas. These operate not only during the day, Monday through Friday, but also nights and weekends. The cardiovascular recovery

room (CVRR) takes patients from the catherization and electrophysiology laboratories, angiography suite, and the interventional neuroradiology (INR) suite. The anesthesia attending physician who provides support for transesophageal echocardiography and cardioversions also covers the CVRR. The endoscopy suite has its own recovery area. Anesthetic coverage is provided by attending physicians assigned to endoscopy procedures for the day. After hours, requests for assistance are covered by the main operating room call team.

Along with the scheduled non–operating room cases, a steady increase has occurred in the number of procedures performed during nights and weekends. These are covered by the main operating room call team. Some procedures such as endoscopic retrograde cholangiopancreatography and some angiography procedures can be done in the main operating room, in a hybrid operating room that has built-in fluoroscopic equipment. The number of procedures in the remaining areas is relatively small and is still handled by the main operating room call team. This is being followed closely to determine if and when either a separate non–operating room call team or an extra attending specifically for those cases is needed. Requests to provide anesthetic support for diagnostic tests (MRI and positron emission tomography [PET]) during nights and weekends are receiving increased scrutiny, with attending-level discussions taking place before each case.

The expansion of anesthesia care in the non–operating room setting has sparked the realization that a lot of interaction occurs between the main operating room and non–operating room settings, which thus provides an opportunity for anesthesiologists to be the brokers for these transfers. Examples are as follows:

1. Preoperative angiogram and embolization of large vascular tumors before surgical excision.
2. Perforated viscus in the endoscopy suite that needs to be transferred emergently to the main operating room for exploration.
3. A patient with a pelvic crush injury secondary to a motor vehicle accident who goes to the angiography/invasive radiology suite first for angiographic embolization of pelvic bleeding vessels before going to the main operating room for stabilization of long-bone fractures.
4. Cerebral angiogram and possible coiling of a ruptured aneurysm. If the aneurysm cannot be coiled, the patient is transferred to the main operating room for a craniotomy and aneurysm clipping.
5. Tract preparation in the angiography suite before going to the main operating room for lithotripsy of a renal calculus.

Operating rooms have only recently begun to incorporate imaging techniques into their design and function, and a steady, consistent advance has been seen in techniques outside the main operating room. These advances include the activities of interventional pulmonologists, as well as advances in cervical and prostate brachytherapy, chemoembolization, and various ablation techniques for solid tumors. Advances in imaging technology, such as 7-tesla MRI and functional imaging with PET and CT, still require a patient to be very still, occasionally with

MEMORANDUM

TO: Executive Director, Surgical Services and Imaging

FROM: Executive Director, Anesthesiology

DATE:

RE: Anesthesia Services Agreement

The purpose of this memorandum is to specify the terms of agreement between Brigham and Women's Hospital (BWH) and the Brigham and Women's Physicians Organization – Anesthesia (BWPOA) relative to providing anesthesia care for _____ patients provided at the Brigham and Women's Hospital.

Coverage/Financial Arrangement:

1. BWPOA will provide anesthesia services for BWPOA in a room exclusively for _____ from 7:00 a.m. to 4:00 p.m. Monday through Thursday (9:00 a.m. to 5:00 p.m. on Wednesday).

2. BWH will reimburse BWPOA a total of $_____ for each physician, each day (estimated at $_____ per month) less related professional receipts billed by BWPOA (estimated at $_____ per month). In the event a session exceeds the scheduled timeframe, BWH will compensate BWPOA at the rate of $_____ per hour.

3. Each month BWH will initiate a transfer of $_____ from _____ to _____ to fund the current month per the rates outlined in item #2 above.

4. Patient receipts associated with this activity have been considered in the monthly transfer. Any surplus or deficit resulting from actual patient receipts vs. estimates outlined above will be settled on a quarterly basis in arrears.

Operations/Reporting:

1. BWHE will schedule patients through the operating room scheduling office (2-7448) at least 48 hours in advance. If within 48 hours the slots for patient bookings for BWHE have not been utilized, the anesthesia staff will be deployed elsewhere. BWHE will be charged the agreed upon day rate unless the BWPOA Scheduling Office and BWPOA Finance Manager have been notified in writing at least 48 hours in advance that the Anesthesia services are not required.

2. Bookings that occur after the 48-hour deadline must be handled via discussion with the Anesthesia Clinical Director or his/her designee. Although every effort will be made to provide anesthesia services as requested, no guarantees are made for bookings less than 48 hours in advance.

3. Anesthesia staff will be available for the _____ Suite during the agreed upon blocks. Block time utilization will be reviewed quarterly to optimize scheduling for BWH and BWPOA.

4. BWPOA will send a quarterly report to you summarizing case volume, billing and collections for anesthesia related services provided in the _____ suite.

Term: One-year agreement beginning October 1, 20__ automatically renewed on May 1st for the following fiscal year. Notice of termination given by BWH required before May 1st for termination effective the following September 30th.

Agreed: _____   Agreed: _____

Date: _____   Date: _____

Figure 20-1 Anesthesia services agreement for outside the operating room.

breath-holding; this frequently requires anesthetic support because these techniques are increasingly aligned with procedures. This also provides opportunities for anesthesiologists to be involved in discussions with interventionalists about what they are doing and about planning for new procedure areas.

As non–operating room activities continue to increase, there might be a question as to whether the non–operating room should be separate from the main operating room. The integration of main operating room and non–operating room activities does not support this suggestion. The schedule should be integrated and accessible by all parties involved. However, the following differences still exist between the two:

1. Separate preanesthetic and postanesthetic care areas are used in high-volume locales. With the regular presence of anesthesiologists, this separation also provides support for nurses who provide moderate sedation.
2. A mobile preanesthetic assessment service is used to ensure that both inpatients and outpatients receive a thorough evaluation before their procedure to address any medical issues and minimize the chances of last minute cancellations.
3. If current trends continue, it may be necessary to add another call position for nights and weekends to do non–operating room procedures. The physical distance to some locations, combined with the potential acuity of patients with multiple comorbidities, makes it impractical and unsafe for a staff to cover both the main operating room and remote locations with residents.

4. Effects of bundled payments on the flow of care must be assessed. This might shift some treatments from the main operating room to the non–operating room location, where the overall cost of some procedures is less.

These points require regular reflection as to their efficacy and cost-effectiveness when all costs are included and should evolve in parallel with changes in health care.

Summary

The "schedule" for the non–operating room is more than a daily and weekly list of procedures to be anesthetized. It is the codification of a shift in diagnostic and treatment areas where care was initially provided by nurses using moderate sedation. More complex procedures and sicker patients have led to the increasing need for anesthetic support. The driving engine behind this is the development of proceduralists using imaging techniques. Although some techniques are being incorporated into operating rooms, the interventionalists are varied and well into a movement that will continue to increase. The schedule reflects the breadth of this movement, and anesthesiologists have a significant role in this shift.

References

1. Macario A. Proper scheduling of anesthesiology services outside of the operating room suite. *Medscape Anesthesiology*. December 29, 2009.
2. Anastasian ZH, Strozyk D, Meyers PM, Wang S, Berman MF. Radiation exposure of the anesthesiologist in the neurointerventional suite. *Anesthesiology*. 2011;114(3):512–520.
3. Dexter F, Epstein RH. Scheduling of cases in an ambulatory center. *Anesthesiol Clin North Am*. 2003;21:387–402.

21 Financial and Operational Analysis for Non–Operating Room Anesthesia

CAITLIN J. GUO and ALEX MACARIO

Approximately 20,000 medical students take the Hippocratic Oath each year.[1] They vow to spend the next 10 years learning the art and science of medicine, but little do they know that reality also involves economics and administrative problem-solving. In today's world of bulging hospital networks and multitiered reimbursements, the days of doctors making house calls are long gone. Consolidation in health care is transforming medicine as hospitals, private firms, and even health insurance companies acquire physician practices at a rapidly growing rate. The shift away from independent physician solo practices to systems that employ doctors is intended to make health care less fragmented and less expensive by building infrastructures that foster better care coordination and take advantage of economies of scale. Health care is a $2.8 trillion business, according to the 2012 Centers for Medicare & Medicaid Services, and it operates on the same set of principles that run Fortune 500 companies.[4]

Similar to the growth of ambulatory surgeries in the 1990s, an explosive growth of non–operating room procedures has occurred over the past decade. Today, medical proceduralists perform a wide variety of procedures, ranging from simple needle biopsies to complicated vascular stents. From 1996 to 2006, the volume of surgical and nonsurgical procedures performed at freestanding ambulatory centers tripled, largely as a result of procedures performed outside the operating room, whereas those performed at hospitals remained the same.[2] The most common procedures performed include endoscopy of large intestine (5.7 million), endoscopy of small intestine (3.5 million), extraction of a lens (3.1 million), injections of agent into spinal canal (2.0 million), and insertion of a prosthetic lens (2.6 million).[2]

The current challenge and concurrent opportunity for anesthesiologists is to decide how to expand our services in a changing health care environment that is safe, efficient, and financially sound. The goal of this chapter is to examine the financial and operational implications of non–operating room anesthesia. It is presented in the format of a business plan, starting with market analysis and opportunity, competitive landscape, comparative advantage, and a logistics section with a focus on financial analysis and operational infrastructural analysis. Other issues such as scheduling and staffing are discussed in other chapters.

Market Analysis

MARKET TRENDS

Some argue that fee-for-service fuels much of U.S. health care spending and results in excessive usage, but it is also important to recognize that the same financial incentive also propels medical advances. In the 1990s, minimally invasive surgical techniques led to a growth in ambulatory surgeries. Fast-forward 20 years to 2013, the next set of innovations prompting changes is minimally invasive procedures performed outside the operating room.

These nonsurgical procedures are appealing. From the patient's perspective, it means a less invasive approach and faster recovery. It also appeals to the patient who is too sick to undergo a traditional surgical treatment. From the hospital's perspective, minimally invasive procedures mean shorter length of stays, higher volume, less overhead cost, and of course the satisfaction of making medical advancements. While market forces are at work, as long as there is a demand, there will be a supply to meet. As a result, the demand for anesthesia outside the operating room also has grown. And yet, many practices may be in a difficult situation if they are unable to staff these procedures efficiently. The failure to properly manage these procedures creates erratic coverage and unhappy proceduralists.

NEW CUSTOMERS

The operating room has traditionally served as the anesthesiologist's home. Anesthesiologists are increasingly perceived as natural masters of operating room management as they make strides in leadership, efficiency, scheduling, and cost effectiveness. Customers traditionally have included patients, surgeons, and hospital management. With the rise of non–operating room anesthesia (NORA) cases, the specialty now has an additional set of nonsurgical customers that demand and value anesthesiologists' services.

Unlike surgeons, proceduralists such as medical interventionists and radiologists have different needs. For example, they do not perform painful procedures that require multimodal postoperative pain management. In addition, they and the nurses around them are often unused to working with anesthesiologists and thus unfamiliar with their particular needs. Given that NORA cases are often short procedures, they demand faster room turnover and rapid recovery.

AN OPPORTUNITY

As the aging population grows older and sicker, it is inevitable that the number of procedures performed outside the operating room will continue to increase in the next decade. The chart in Figure 21-1 shows the large increases in the population aged 65 and older from 3.1 million people in 1900 to 35 million in 2000 and projected to 72 million in 2030.

Table 21-1 illustrates the dramatic increase in anesthesia professional participation in the two most common NORA procedures, esophagogastroduodenoscopy and colonoscopy. By 2015, anesthesia services will be involved in over half of these procedures.

The anesthesiology community is adjusting its practice to meet the NORA demand. Without appropriate preprocedural and postprocedural care, cancellation and rescheduling from unanticipated medical complexity will certainly rise. Thus early risk stratification of patients and planned anesthesia service can greatly improve efficiency and reduce cost. Most surgical patients currently undergo a preoperative assessment by a member of the anesthesia team. In contrast, the evaluation of patients for NORA procedures may be lacking despite the fact that some of these patients are ill enough to be hospitalized. The anesthesia group needs to work with the hospital and proceduralists to ensure that proper infrastructure is in place to optimize scheduling and provide safe care of these patients. The question "Is it safe for proceduralists with minimal training in airway and pharmacology to perform the procedure, manage comorbidities, and supervise administered sedation?" is often raised. Everyone wants to avoid the use of unplanned anesthesia on an emergency basis.

When tallied together, the costs of procedural cancellation, emergent anesthesia usage, and unforeseen hospitalizations are expensive and should be minimized. Thus it is important that anesthesiologists take a leadership role by creating appropriate policies and systems of care to preemptively avoid complications and delays and improve efficiency.

Competitive Landscape

COMPETITORS

Many providers such as registered nurses, dentists, and oral surgeons deliver sedation that might be considered competition to anesthesiologists. However, many NORA cases require deep sedation or general anesthesia, in particular patients with complex comorbidities or those who previously failed routine sedation. Because of difficulty in coordination of services or resources, some hospitals may elect to outsource contracts with an outside anesthesia group to provide consistent and reliable services. This represents a loss of business for the existing group. Thus when faced with the question "Can you provide coverage to our new location outside the operating room?" the answer should be yes, "Let's get together and discuss how we can optimally do this for everyone involved."

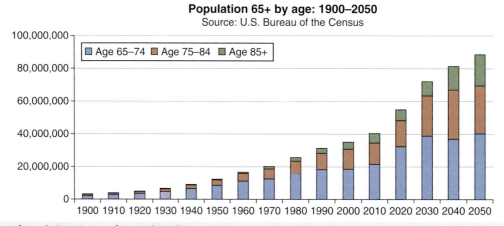

Population 65+ by age: 1900–2050
Source: U.S. Bureau of the Census

Figure 21-1 Chart of population 65 years of age and over by age: 1900 to 2050. (Compiled by the U.S. Administration on Aging. Projected future growth of the older population: chart of population 65 and over by age: 1900 to 2050. Compiled by the U.S. Administration on Aging using the Census data. Department of Health & Human Services, Administration on Aging. http://www.aoa.gov/aoaroot/aging_statistics/future_growth/future_growth.aspx.)

Table 21-1 Predicted Anesthesia Professional Participation Rates (%) for Colonoscopy and Esophagogastroduodenoscopy by Year

Condition	2007	2008	2009	2010	2011	2012	2013	2014	2015
Colonoscopy (%)	23.9	27.6	31.3	34.9	38.6	42.3	46.0	49.7	53.4
EGD (%)	24.4	28.0	31.5	35.1	38.7	42.2	45.8	49.3	52.9

EGD, Esophagogastroduodenoscopy.
From Inadomi JM, Gunnarsson CL, Rizzo JA, Fang H. Projected increased growth rate of anesthesia professional–delivered sedation for colonoscopy and EGD in the United States: 2009 to 2015. *Gastrointest Endosc.* 2010;72(3):580-586.

BARRIERS TO ENTRY

The addition of anesthesia service is perceived to add time and cost. As a result, many proceduralists have historically been reluctant to ask for coverage. In addition, unfamiliarity with anesthesia care also causes reluctance.

From an anesthesia perspective, cultural and operational barriers exist to practicing outside the comfort zone of the surgical suite. Traditionally, anesthesiologists reside in the operating room. Most find experiences outside the operating room to be unpleasant because of ergonomically unfavorable physical space, poor ancillary support, lack of backup equipment, distance from the recovery room, and dealing with a new set of providers who may not understand anesthesiologists' approach to safe care. In regard to staffing, too few anesthesiologists are available to provide guaranteed coverage to all of the subspecialists. This lack creates delays and frustration, especially when dealing with add-on cases. Financially speaking, proceduralists may find it more economically favorable to rely on sedation nurses for most of their cases and use emergent anesthesia on demand. This situation may worsen when procedure reimbursements are bundled into one case payment.

Comparative Advantages

As anesthesiologists, our knowledge and technical skills in providing anesthesia are without peer. Patient safety is undoubtedly the most important service we offer. Although it may be unrealistic to always have anesthesia coverage for every proceduralist because the cost would be too high, it is possible to take an active role in designing the appropriate infrastructure to maximize efficiency and reduce cost.

As the line between surgery and procedure blurs, it is more important than ever to engage the proceduralists to obtain anesthesia evaluations. The goal is to identify the medically complex patients early and match them with appropriately trained providers to better risk-stratify their comorbidities.

It is important that we apply the same concepts of management to settings outside the operating room with the goal being to improve coordination and efficiency. The current system is chaotic. Most proceduralists and anesthesiologists share common frustrations of difficult scheduling and frequent delays. We must integrate ourselves in the procedural suites permanently, the same way we did in the operating room many decades ago.

Financial Considerations

BILLING AND MONITORED ANESTHESIA CARE REIMBURSEMENT

Unlike routine anesthesia billing, procedures performed outside the operating room are confronted with a different set of rules. Most surgical anesthetics are provided in a form of general or regional technique. In contrast, the majority of procedures performed outside the operating room are carried out with sedation. For simple procedures such as gastrointestinal endoscopies, sedations provided by anesthesiologists may not be easily reimbursed. Instead, the fees are bundled with the professional fees and paid to the proceduralists. Because of the lack of financial incentives, anesthesia coverage has been slow to grow.

Monitored anesthesia care services are payable only if medically reasonable and necessary. Indications for monitored anesthesia care include the nature of the procedure, patient's clinical condition, and potential need to convert to a general or regional anesthetic. It is a billable service when provided by a qualified member of the anesthesia team.

BASIC ECONOMICS

The three simple variables in managerial economics are cost, revenue, and volume. The three are intimately related; careful planning and optimizing of these variables are greatly beneficial.

Cost

Traditional cost accounting includes variable and fixed costs (Figure 21-2).

$$\text{Total cost} = \text{Fixed cost} + \text{Variable cost} \times \text{Volume}$$

The fixed cost remains constant, whereas the variable cost is directly related to volume.

Fixed costs, also known as overhead costs, do not vary with patient encounters and are shared among the group. They remain constant even if anesthetics are not provided. These costs include administrative overhead, facilities cost, utilities, and upkeep of shared equipment such as anesthesia machines, monitors, bronchoscopes, and echo machines. Although fixed costs are generally viewed as constant in the short run or within a given surgical volume, it is important to remember that they are long-term variable costs. As an organization grows, it is inevitable that overhead and capital costs will grow.

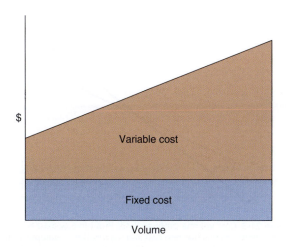

Figure 21-2 Total cost as a function of volume, including fixed and variable costs.

Variable costs, on the other hand, are those associated with each patient encounter and are thus volume dependent. Typical variable costs of providing an anesthetic are the wages of the anesthesiology team, wages of the preoperative and postoperative recovery staff, drugs administered, laboratory or diagnostic studies, and equipment used in the preoperative, intraoperative, and postoperative care settings. Unlike a manufacturing plant, in which end products are identical, the variable cost per patient can differ significantly from one patient to another.

Revenue

Revenue is a function of price and volume. The more volume a practice sees, the more revenue it generates. A key variable in this equation is the payer mix, which affects the price; a favorable ratio benefits a practice.

$$\text{Total revenue} = \text{Price} \times \text{Volume}$$

This is a relative simplification of the revenue equation. In reality, many variables are involved in anesthesia billing, including relative value units (RVUs), time, case mix, patient mix, and payer mix.

Cost Volume Profit Analysis

Putting the previously mentioned three variables together is the cost volume profit analysis. The cost volume profit model is often used in managerial economics for short-run decision-making. It is used to calculate the break-even point and help a firm project a target volume. By changing the variables in the model, break-even points can be obtained (Figure 21-3).

Although the model demonstrates a simple economic theory clearly, it does carry the following several linearizing assumptions:

- Constant sales price
- Constant total fixed cost
- Constant variable cost per unit
- Units sold equals units produced
- Constant sales mix

Because the end products in health care are not identical, the unit variable cost and sales price are not constant. In addition, the payer mixes can differ significantly and are constantly in flux. The model can be adapted to use the average cost and price for a given institution. In addition, the cost volume profit model assumes a clear division between fixed and variable costs, which may be true in the short run. However, in the long run, all costs are variable as the group brings in additional staff and invests in new capital.

An Example Analysis

Let's take the cost volume profit model and apply it to an anesthesia group that is considering off-site expansion to determine the optimal committed coverage.

When faced with an expansion, most anesthesia groups will start with on-demand services, which minimize fixed cost and accrue only variable cost. At the early stages, this is a sensible approach. The demand for our services is largely unknown because the proceduralists are also at their initial stages of expansion. Committing scheduled blocks may be unnecessary.

Although cost efficient, on-demand services are often associated with significant delays and frustration and are not long-term solutions. In addition, the costs associated with overuse of staff are expensive. It is therefore important for the practice to constantly reevaluate its position on committed versus on-demand coverage (Figure 21-4).

A Toward B. Moving from point A toward B represents a practice that was previously at its break-even point and is now providing on-demand coverage for the new procedural suite. In the short term, moving from point A to B reflects a profit as the practice is using its staff from 80% to 90%, but in reality, this is a short-lived effect because of burdensome cost associated with overuse.

POINT B. Let's assume growth of volume has occurred from the proceduralist side, the practice is now providing 1 day per week of committed coverage, and it hired a new anesthesiologist and bought a new anesthesia machine,

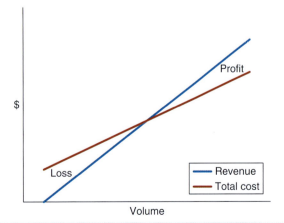

Figure 21-3 Cost volume profit analysis. Profit in $ (y-axis) is the difference between revenue and cost and is a function of volume in units (x-axis). At low volume, there is a loss as total cost exceeds revenue. At the break-even point, cost is equal to revenue. Volume beyond the break-even point generates a profit.

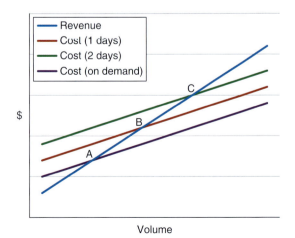

Figure 21-4 Cost volume analysis for variable coverage. In this model, revenue curve remains constant, Total revenue = price × volume, and the cost curve varies depending on how much coverage is provided.

thus establishing cost curve 1 and point B as the new break-even point.

From a management perspective, the practice should consider committed coverage when volume approaches the break-even point of the new cost curve to allow more growth.

B Toward C. Similar break-even analysis can be carried out for 2, 3, 4, or 5 days of committed coverage. The previously described analysis provides a dynamic view of the relationships among cost, revenue, and volume. It can be used to guide a practice in defining the optimal committed coverage when negotiating with the hospital and the proceduralist group.

Operational Infrastructure

UTILIZATION RATE

Anesthesia administered outside the operating room covers a variety of specialties, each with its own scheduling needs, so early planning is crucial. Specialty-specific anesthesia usage rates can be very useful in distributing staff efficiently and committing to blocked coverage. Both underusage and overusage are costly and unproductive. Most operating room management sources quote an optimal utilization rate of 0.8.[3] Rates lower than 0.8 are associated with wasted resources in which staff are paid until 5 PM and often leave at 3 PM, while rates higher than 0.9 leave very little room for add-on cases and are associated with overusage when procedures run overtime.

Tools such as surgical score cards promote transparency and adequate reporting, and they can be easily implemented to use outside the operating room. They can track core measures such as usage, on-time starts, and delays. Specialties that underuse their block time should have less committed coverage, whereas specialties that overuse their block time should have more committed coverage. Of course, this is a dynamic process and should be constantly reassessed.

STAFFING

Optimal distribution of staffing to match workload is important. Underusage represents a scenario in which a team is scheduled to work 10 hours but works only 8 hours. Overusage represents a team that is scheduled to work 10 hours but in reality works 12 hours and incurs costs of overtime pay. It is thus important to match the staff availability to workload.

To illustrate, we will schedule two interventional radiology cases into room 1, each lasting 2.5 hours. We will schedule three cases into room 2, with the first two lasting 2.5 hours and the last one 4 hours (Figure 21-5).

In both scenarios, the anesthesia team is scheduled to work a 9-hour day. Matching of workload to staffing has not been optimized. In scenario 1, there are 3 hours of underusage. In scenario 2, there are 2 hours of overusage. Awakening patients more quickly or reducing the turnover time will not improve the overall efficiency.

The key to maximizing resources is to allocate appropriate time to each service. Optimizing staffing costs is finding the best balance between overtime and finishing early. In examining historic data, if one service is consistently

running late, the allocated anesthesia block should be extended. For example, if a radiologist performs 12 hours' worth of cases once every other week, it is more optimal to assign a 12-hour anesthesia block on those days. That way, the team is expected to stay for 12 hours when they arrive and will not be frustrated by having to stay late. From a financial perspective, the cost of overusage will be reduced as well.

The next step when considering whether to expand current staff involves examination of existing usage by comparing scheduled anesthesia time with actual used time. A group with high overusage cost will have a difficult time expanding without new staff and capital cost. Such expansion will involve the addition of both fixed and variable costs and may involve negotiating a subsidy from the hospital. In a fee-for-service environment facility, fees to the hospital may be large enough to subsidize anesthesia staffing care in locations outside the operating room, especially if this staffing leads to increased service throughout NORA cases. Because of the large overhead of hospitals, hospital managers aim to have a high census and high turnover of cases in the NORA suite.

A group with lower staff usage can expand easily with only variable cost. In this scenario, initial coverage is provided by using existing resources. However, as the volume for off-site services grows over time, the cost of overusage will inevitably burden the existing staff and should prompt the group to add new shifts or members if needed.

EQUIPMENT AND ANCILLARY SUPPORT

Although the bulk of anesthesia cost involves staffing, equipment and ancillary support also add costs, especially

Scenario #1: Under-utilization (each case is 2.5 hrs plus 1 hr turnover)

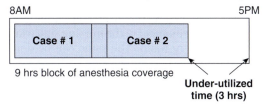

Scenario #2: Over-utilization

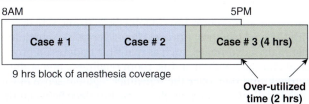

Figure 21-5 Underused hours reflect how early the room finishes. In scenario 1 in the figure, if an anesthesiologist and a radiology nurse were scheduled to work from 8 AM to 5 PM and instead the room finished at 2 PM (including 1 hour turnover time), this would result in 3 hours of underused time. The excess staffing cost would be 33% (3 hours/9 hours). In contrast, for scenario 2, 11 hours of cases handled outside the operating room are performed with staff scheduled to work 9 hours. This means that the excess staffing cost is 44% (2 hours/9 hours = 22%, which is then multiplied by a "fudge" factor of 2 to include the additional monetary and morale cost of staff staying late). (From Macario A. Staffing and case scheduling for elective out-of-operating room cases. *ASA Refresher Course.* 2009;37:129-140.)

in off-site care. With the expansion of NORA procedures, a need is developing for more easily mobile anesthesia machines and monitoring and equipment setups. If a location is sufficiently busy, having an anesthesia machine permanently there may be optimal. Such a setup must take into account the smaller geographical spaces and multiple off-site locations. In addition, support staff such as anesthesia technicians and pharmacy staff allocated to the surgical suite may not be available to support the team providing anesthesia care outside the operating room in a timely fashion. Thus development of infrastructures, such as mobile anesthesia machines, onsite automated drug dispensers, and stocked supply carts that allow the anesthesiologist to efficiently turn over rooms, is crucial.

POSTOPERATIVE CARE AND RECOVERY

Along with the challenge of being in a remote location with poor ancillary support, perhaps the greatest difficulties most anesthesiologists face in locations outside the operating room are preprocedure evaluation and postoperative care. Although most procedural suites have recovery units that care for patients after receiving sedation provided by the proceduralist, the units are not equipped to deal with patients with high American Society of Anesthesiologists (ASA) classifications or those who have undergone deep sedation or received a general anesthetic. Thus anesthesiologists may find themselves having to transport their patients from the procedural suite to a distant recovery room. This process causes significant delay and negatively affects the overall work flow.

Flexible nursing staff handling patients in recovery in both the main and procedural recovery units can help alleviate this issue. Many operating rooms that handle cases in two locations already employ flexible nursing staff to work in both the ambulatory and the main recovery rooms. The ambulatory surgery center closes down after all the patients have recovered, and the remainder of the nursing staff transition to the main recovery room. The same can be done with procedures outside the operating room, with recovery nurses assigned to work in both the procedure suite and the main recovery room.

ELECTRONIC SCHEDULER

Many operating rooms have adopted electronic schedulers with the goal to improve process flow. Electronic schedulers offer many advantages, such as real-time updates on procedural changes, patient status, room readiness, and staffing changes, and they offer the scheduler a global sense of the workday. Features such as electronic interface between the procedural and anesthesia scheduler can further improve real-time communication.

However, scheduling for off-site locations at many facilities is still completed on paper, even in institutions that have adopted an electronic scheduler. The process often involves multiple pieces of paper being faxed back and forth and finally taped to the operating room schedule on the day of the procedure. Taking this one step further, in institutions that have already implemented the electronic medical record (EMR), incorporating the scheduler into the EMR can be advantageous. Linking the scheduler

with the medical record allows providers direct access to patient charts and can help identify patients with particular preoperative and postoperative needs, such as a history of malignant hyperthermia or postoperative nausea and vomiting. Because remote locations are often distant from the operating room, tools that facilitate communication can reduce delays and foster a better working relationship.

OPTIMAL UTILIZATION OF RESOURCES

In an ideal world, staffing and cash flow are unlimited and constant anesthesia coverage can be provided anywhere and at any time. In reality, resources are scarce and must be prioritized.

For an anesthesia group that is looking at expansion for off-site procedures for the first time, taking into consideration all of the financial and operational implications, the goal should be to maximize the existing infrastructures and accrue only variable cost. At the early stages of expansion, it is unclear how much coverage will be needed. Because most proceduralists are also in their early stages of expansion, on-demand coverage may be the simplest form of meeting the need. From a staffing and ancillary support perspective, on-demand coverage involves increasing current usage rates and possibly overuse of manpower. From a financial perspective, savings from fixed cost can offset the cost of overuse. Although wage is technically a variable cost, in reality the cost of an anesthesia provider falls somewhere between a variable and a fixed cost. Thus the addition of staff may not be the first step in providing coverage for groups that do not have preexisting high usage rates.

Assume that same anesthesia group is approaching the second stage of expansion where there is a continued demand for its services from the proceduralists. Using the cost volume profit analysis, we see that volume is approaching the breakeven point. The group is now looking into investing in more capital and adding new staff, thus shifting the cost curve upward to allow growth. From a staffing and scheduling perspective, the group is now considering committed coverage. Such analysis should be further used for multiple days of blocked time as volume continues to grow.

In reality, expansion is multifaceted; the same anesthesia groups are concurrently asked to provide coverage for radiology, gastroenterology, and cardiology. The cost volume profit analysis can be carried out across the various specialties to determine the best strategy for providing simultaneous coverage. Using tools such as surgical scorecards, the group can analyze the true anesthesia usage rates across the different specialties and determine what the optimal committed coverage should be and negotiate appropriately.

Take the example of MRI and electroconvulsive therapy (ECT). Both are typically elective procedures that do not have high demand for anesthesia; thus daily 9 o'clock to 5 o'clock committed coverage may not be necessary. Instead, staff can be shared; the same staff can provide ECT care in the morning and transition to MRI in the afternoon. The key is to match staff with predicted demand. Because both procedures are elective and can be scheduled ahead of time, having an electronic scheduler that enables all involved parties to see the allotted appointments can be valuable (Table 21-2).

Table 21-2   Sample Weekly Schedule for Procedures Outside the Operating Room*

Day	GI	Cardiology/EP	IR	Neurological IR	Vascular IR	Bronchoscopy	MRI/CT	ECT
Mon	8-5	8-5	1-5	8-5			1-5	8-12
Tues	8-5	8-5	1-5		8-5	8-12		
Wed	8-5	8-5	1-5	8-5				
Thurs	8-5	8-5	1-5		8-5	8-12		
Fri	8-5	8-5	1-5	8-5			1-5	8-12

CT, Computed tomography; *ECT*, electroconvulsive therapy; *EP*, electrophysiology; *GI*, gastroenterology; *IR*, interventional radiology; *MRI*, magnetic resonance imaging.
*This is an example of a defined schedule for procedures outside the operating room that allows committed coverage across multiple specialties. The schedule can be adjusted over time to account for any changes in volume or new specialties that may get added.

Conclusion

Going forward, NORA procedures will be an integral part of every anesthesia practice. As medical proceduralists continue to advance their skills, the line between surgery and procedure narrows. Although anesthesia coverage is often fragmented today, NORA can be provided in a safe, efficient, and financially sound way with the appropriate setup and financial incentives. As proceduralists continue to build NORA suites, it is important for anesthesiologists to take initiatives to shape the infrastructure and integrate other anesthesiologists to assume leadership roles so that our services become indispensable, like those in an operating room.

References

1. Association of American Medical Colleges. Table 1: U.S. medical school applications and matriculants by school, state of legal residence, and sex. 2013. https://www.aamc.org/download/321442/data/2013factstable1.pdf.
2. Cullen K, Hall M, Golosinskly A. Ambulatory surgery in the United States, 2006. National Health Statistics Reports. http://www.cdc.gov/nchs/data/nhsr/nhsr011.pdf.
3. Tyler DC, Pasquariello CA, Chen C. Determining optimum operating room utilization. *Anesth Analg*. 2003;96:1114–1121.
4. Centers for Medicare & Medicaid Services. National health expenditures 2012 highlights. 2012. http://www.cms.gov/Research-Statistics-Data-and-Systems/Statistics-Trends-and-Reports/NationalHealthExpend-Data/Downloads/highlights.pdf.

22 Anesthesia and Competitive Strategies

JOHN M. TRUMMEL and SOPHIA VAN HOFF

Sedation for medical procedures performed outside the operating room has been traditionally provided by proceduralists and their proxies. However, as these procedures have steadily increased in both number and complexity, anesthesiologists have been increasingly asked to provide care in non–operating room settings. Given the technical demands of many of these procedures and the comorbidities of the patient population, this increase makes sense. Unfortunately, the cost of anesthesiologist-directed care and the availability of anesthesia providers have limited the use of anesthesia-provided sedation in many non–operating room settings. This chapter reviews the various options for procedural sedation by non–anesthesia providers, the data on effectiveness and safety of these practices, available policies and guidelines, and the cost considerations involved.

Traditionally, sedation for off-site procedures is typically achieved with a benzodiazepine (midazolam) and opioid (fentanyl or meperidine) combination,[1] targeted to moderate sedation[2] and overseen by the proceduralist. These agents often provide effective and safe sedation.[3] However, because of the increasing number and sophistication of many non–operating room procedures, deficiencies related to this approach have emerged. The onset of sedation can be delayed, and some patients cannot be sedated adequately and/or have a poor experience with the procedure. In addition, significant postsedation side effects occur, including nausea, vomiting, and prolonged sedation.

Another problem encountered during non–operating room procedures involves controlling the depth of sedation. The American Society of Anesthesiologists (ASA) endorses a continuum of depth of sedation, ranging from minimal sedation to general anesthesia (Table 22-1).[2] Patients may be inadvertently sedated to a depth greater than planned; therefore the American Society of Anesthesiologists (ASA) states that providers must be able to rescue patients from at least one depth greater than the intended level. In most care settings, proceduralists are credentialed to provide moderate sedation without further assistance. Unfortunately, the fact remains that many procedures require deep sedation to achieve adequate procedural conditions and patient comfort.

A study from the Cleveland Clinic evaluated the occurrence of deep sedation in patients having several standard endoscopic procedures. Eighty healthy outpatients were evaluated for the frequency of inadvertent deep sedation when patients were sedated with midazolam and meperidine targeted to achieve moderate sedation.[4] Deep sedation occurred at some time during the procedure in 68% of all patients, but varied by procedure type—45% for colonoscopy, 60% for esophagogastroduodenoscopy (EGD), 80% for endoscopic ultrasound (EUS), and 85% for endoscopic

retrograde cholangiopancreatography (ERCP). ERCP and EUS were independent predictors of deep sedation. This study confirms what many providers involved in endoscopy already know—many patients receive deep sedation for their procedures despite the goal of moderate sedation.

As a result of these deficiencies, alternatives to "traditional" moderate sedation have developed and include a variety of sedative agents and techniques. Approaches to improving sedation by nonanesthesiologists focus on three generic categories: using different agents to improve moderate sedation, using other techniques for reducing pain and anxiolysis, or using propofol (2,6-diisopropylphenol). Propofol is a sedative that is nearly ideal for many non–operating room procedures because it has rapid onset and offset of deep sedation with minimal side effects. Because it routinely leads to deep or greater depths of anesthesia, its use for non–operating room procedures is a potential problem for those not trained in the provision of anesthesia. However, given the advantages of propofol, extensive investigation into its use has been done by nonanesthesiologists. The remainder of this chapter explores in more detail the approaches to procedural sedation used by nonanesthesia providers, with an emphasis on the use of propofol. Although a majority of the information can be applied to generic non–operating room procedures, most of the available data are specific to gastrointestinal (GI) endoscopy.

Practice Patterns in Non–Operating Room Sedation

Sedation practice in the non–operating room setting varies widely throughout the world. This is exemplified by routine diagnostic GI endoscopy. In the United States, it is frequently assumed most patients want sedation for endoscopy. A study of U.S. gastroenterologists found that more than 98% of routine endoscopies are performed with sedation and approximately 25% of these providers now use propofol sedation.[5] In addition, 68% of gastroenterologists using conventional sedation would consider using propofol if it were easily available. When propofol was used, it was provided by anesthesia-trained personnel in almost 90% of cases, with the remainder being directed by the endoscopist. Large regional variations are seen in the use of propofol from a low of 7% in the Northeast to a high of 37% in the Mid-Atlantic region. This variation appears to be driven by local reimbursement policies for sedation. In addition, an increasing number of more complex non–operating room procedures are performed in the United States.[6] These factors have led to a dramatic increase in the need for high-quality sedation.

Table 22-1   Continuum of Depth of Sedation: Definition of General Anesthesia and Levels of Sedation and Analgesia

	Minimal Sedation (Anxiolysis)	Moderate Sedation/Analgesia ("Conscious Sedation")	Deep Sedation/Analgesia	General Anesthesia
Responsiveness	Normal response to verbal stimulation	Purposeful* response to verbal or tactile stimulation	Purposeful* response following repeated or painful stimulation	Unarousable even with painful stimulus
Airway	Unaffected	No intervention required	Intervention may be required	Intervention often required
Spontaneous ventilation	Unaffected	Adequate	May be inadequate	Frequently inadequate
Cardiovascular function	Unaffected	Usually maintained	Usually maintained	May be impaired

Committee of Origin: Quality Management and Departmental Administration.
*Reflex withdrawal from a painful stimulus is *not* considered a purposeful response.
Approved by the American Society of Anesthesiologists House of Delegates on October 27, 2004, and amended on October 21, 2009. Table from ASA statement on continuum of depth of sedation. http://www.asahq.org.

A review of sedation practice in 1998[7] revealed that in much of the world outside the United States and United Kingdom, the norm was for unsedated routine endoscopy. However, by 2006 this standard had begun to change in Europe; an observational study of 6004 patients undergoing colonoscopy[8] found that 17% of patients had no sedation, 53% had moderate sedation, and 30% had deep sedation. More recently, Ladas et al[9] collected data regarding the sedation rate for EGD and colonoscopy in Europe, North America, Asia, Africa, and Australia. No data were available from the last three continents, so questionnaire surveys were mailed to gastroenterologists in those locations. For upper GI endoscopy, rates of sedation varied in European countries from less than 20% to more than 75%; in the United States and Australia, over 98% of upper GI endoscopies were performed with sedation; in Asian countries many areas performed upper GI endoscopies without sedation, although some centers reported a 100% sedation rate. Finally, the surveys showed that 25% to 50% of patients received sedation in African countries. The authors note that the survey respondents reported that in as many as 46% of the countries, monitoring was not available in the majority of endoscopy suites; this lack of monitoring could be a factor in the low sedation rate. The rates of sedation for colonoscopy were shown to be quite variable among countries and among centers within each country. Sedation medication varied as well, although it was noted that propofol has been used in each country that responded to the survey. These data support an increasing expectation and use of sedation for endoscopy worldwide.

Propofol Use by Nonanesthesiologists

Propofol is used extensively in non–operating room sedation practice by both anesthesia-trained and nonanesthesiologist providers. Non–operating room settings where propofol frequently is given by nonanesthesiologists include the GI endoscopy suite, the electrophysiology laboratory, and, to a lesser degree, both diagnostic and interventional radiology areas. Propofol is a unique intravenous medication available as an oil-in-water emulsion for induction or maintenance of moderate-to-deep sedation and general anesthesia through facilitation of inhibitory neurotransmission mediated by gamma–aminobutyric acid (GABA). It is highly lipid-soluble,

which results in an onset of action that is rapid; awakening from a single bolus dose is very rapid as well, because of a short initial redistribution half-life of 2 to 8 minutes. Propofol is cleared partly via hepatic conjugation and renal elimination of those inactive metabolites, but it also likely has a component of extrahepatic metabolism as the clearance of propofol exceeds hepatic blood flow. Propofol has many effects on the organ systems. It decreases arterial blood pressure as a result of a drop in systemic vascular resistance, cardiac contractility, and preload. It is a profound respiratory depressant and causes dose-dependent apnea while it inhibits hypoxic ventilatory drive and depresses the normal response to hypercarbia at sub–general anesthetic doses. It has antipruritic properties as well as antiemetic effects.[10]

Propofol is preferred by many endoscopists and patients and has been shown in multiple studies to be associated with a faster induction of sedation and faster full recovery time, higher postprocedure patient satisfaction, and quicker anticipated return to baseline function. Dewitt et al[11] demonstrated these findings in a prospective randomized, single-blinded trial of 80 consecutive patients who were randomized to receive either sedation with nurse-administered propofol sedation or midazolam and meperidine for EUS procedures. Nayar et al[12] performed a retrospective analysis comparing outcomes of 1000 EUS procedures performed with anesthesia-assisted propofol sedation (propofol deep sedation) and 1000 EUS procedures performed under conventional sedation using midazolam and meperidine titrated to moderate sedation and found that sedation time, induction time, and intraprocedural time were significantly shorter in the propofol group. Randomized trials by Cohen,[13] Sipe et al,[14] and Ulmer et al[15] that compared endoscopist-directed propofol (EDP) with traditional sedation with opioids and benzodiazepines in patients undergoing endoscopy or colonoscopy found that EDP resulted in faster onset of sedation, faster recovery, and similar or better patient satisfaction.

Not surprisingly, the use of propofol by non–anesthesia trained providers has led to some controversy. Anesthesiologists are concerned that propofol can induce general anesthesia and apnea very rapidly and that nonanesthesiologists lack sufficient airway expertise to rescue patients who receive propofol. The package insert for propofol states that propofol should be administered only by persons trained in rescue from unintended general anesthesia. At least 12 states in the United States have laws or regulations regarding nursing practice that prevent the administration

maintained stable heart rate, invasive arterial blood pressure, and oxygenation. They concluded that deep sedation by nonanesthesiologists was safe and that consultation of an anesthesiologist was not necessary for this procedure.

Very limited data exist on comparison of NAAP to anesthesiologist-directed care. A recent randomized controlled trial evaluated whether there was a difference in endoscopist-administered versus anesthetist-administered propofol in terms of safety and patient satisfaction.[30] Although the study included only 90 ASA class 1 or 2 patients, the authors found that patient satisfaction scores were slightly higher in the endoscopist group, despite actually having higher pain scores in that group. They also found that the occurrence of minor sedation-related complications (hypotension requiring increased crystalloid and desaturation of below 95% for 30 seconds) was higher in the anesthetist group. The study was quite limited by the small number of patients, and using this study to conclude that it is safer to undergo propofol sedation with an endoscopist may not be advisable because the overall rate of serious complications in patients with ASA class 1 and 2 undergoing routine endoscopy is so low. Furthermore, their definition of "complications" was not consistent with events that many anesthetists would consider complications.

A small observational study published in 2009 attempted to evaluate and compare the quality of sedation provided for upper EUS using anesthesiologist-directed propofol versus standard moderate sedation provided by the endoscopy team.[31] Quality was determined using expert video analysis of the procedural sedation using a validated scoring system. The study included 50 patients with 25 in each group and found that 52% of patients receiving moderate sedation exhibited an uncontrolled patient state (significant undersedation or oversedation) at some time during the procedure versus 28% of the propofol group. Of more significance, patients receiving midazolam and an opioid spent 7.1% of the procedure in an uncontrolled patient state, whereas patients in the propofol group experienced an uncontrolled state approximately 1% of the procedure time. Overall efficiency was also considerably better in the propofol group; these patients experienced significantly less in-hospital and at-home nausea and vomiting and fell back to baseline status more quickly. Finally, patient satisfaction was improved in the propofol group: 60% thought the procedure was better than anticipated versus 21% in the standard group. It would be interesting to have similar data on NAAP versus anesthesiologist-directed care, but this type of information is currently unavailable.

Many studies have been done to date supporting the safety of nonanesthesiologist administered propofol. The available data suggest that rates of complications are no greater for NAAP compared to moderate sedation using a benzodiazepine/opioid combination and that NAAP seems to be safe for specific procedures, such as routine GI endoscopy, with appropriately trained personnel and appropriate patient selection. However, certain patients (e.g. those with ASA class 3 status or greater, chronic opioid use, elevated BMI) and advanced procedures (e.g., EUS, ERCP, biventricular pacemakers) may be at higher risk and warrant anesthesiologist-directed care. In addition, it is difficult to come to clear conclusions regarding the use of NAAP in other settings such as electrophysiology or radiology because

the data are limited. Despite the apparent safety of NAAP, questions remain: Is it beneficial from an efficiency or quality standpoint to use anesthesiologists or anesthetists in the non–operating room setting? Should anesthesia professionals be involved in overseeing or training nonanesthesiologists providing sedation? What type of presence should anesthesia providers have in a stand-alone endoscopy setting where sedation is provided but immediate access to a "code" or "STAT airway" team may not be available? These questions become more important as NAAP appears to be safe and pressure to provide this type of care may become more common. If this practice is to be continued, careful patient and procedure selection is necessary and must be clearly defined.

Economic Considerations

Demand for anesthesia services for non–operating room procedures is increasing.[32] From 2003 to 2009 the proportion of gastroenterology procedures using anesthesia services increased from approximately 14% to more than 30% and more than two thirds of anesthesia services were delivered to low-risk patients (ASA class 1 or 2), as determined from both Medicare and commercially insured patients.[33] The use of anesthesia service had significant cost; payments for anesthesia over this time doubled for Medicare patients and quadrupled for commercially insured patients. Every procedure that uses an anesthesia provider generates an additional fee. The Centers for Medicare & Medicaid Services (CMS) pays an average of $155 to an anesthesia specialist for monitored anesthesia care for endoscopy, and private insurers pay an average of $437.[34] Cohen[16] notes that the average cost of anesthesia-assisted sedation during an endoscopic procedure is approximately $400 per case.[16] Many gastroenterologists argue that the best method of sedation for most endoscopy patients is NAAP, because they believe this modality retains the advantages of propofol-based sedation while maintaining patient safety and lowering the cost. EDP results in no additional charge for sedation because it is covered under the professional fee for performance of the sedation.

Several studies have attempted to estimate the costs associated with NAAP sedation in contrast to that administered by an anesthesia provider. Rex et al[21] estimated the cost of using anesthesia specialists instead of EDP in their study looking at 646,080 cases of EDP that had four deaths possibly related to sedation. Their estimate is based on many assumptions; the added cost to use an anesthesia specialist for all 646,080 procedures would be $286 per procedure and thus $184,778,880 total. If each four decedents lived to be 85 years of age, resulting in 72 life-years saved, had anesthesia specialists prevented these deaths, the cost per life year saved is $2.6 million. If however, anesthesia specialists were used only for patients with ASA class 3 or higher (estimated 10% of all patients), the added cost per life-year would be $257,000. Most experts agree that an acceptable cost-effectiveness range is from $50,000 to $100,000 per life-year saved.

More recently Hassan et al[35] studied the cost-effectiveness of EDP versus anesthesiologist assistance for colonoscopy. They estimated the cost of anesthesiologist assistance for

Medicare beneficiaries at $95 and the non-Medicare cost of $450, the proportion of colonoscopies with anesthetist assistance (34.8%), and the cost of training the nurses in EDP. Their model outputs were projected onto the U.S. population and showed a 10-year saving of $3.2 billion. Assuming a 0.0008% mortality rate (the rate found by Rex et al[21]), the incremental cost-effectiveness of anesthetist-assisted colonoscopy versus an EDP policy was $1.5 million per life-year gained. A 31-fold increase of EDP-related mortality would be required for EDP to become not cost-effective (incremental cost-effectiveness ratio <$50,000 per life-year saved). The authors do note that for EDP implementation to be permitted in the United States, further political steps may be needed because the revised CMS Hospital Conditions of Participation and Interpretive Guidelines have rules addressing nonanesthesiologist and nonphysician practitioners' administration of anesthesia.

Several deficiencies exist with these cost analyses. First, only the present care models are evaluated and the cost impact is based on billing and a fee-for-service anesthesia care model. Going forward, most care will be compensated by bundled payments, so there will be no additional charge for sedation service. These bundled payments will drive care models that prioritize overall cost efficiency while maintaining quality. For example, the addition of an anesthesia provider may allow the elimination of the sedation nurse, which would reduce overall cost. In addition, many important contributions of the anesthesia provider in the GI endoscopy suite are not accounted for, including assistance with the preprocedural assessment; preparation of the patient, including intravenous equipment and monitor placement; intraprocedural monitoring and administration of drugs; and recovery room care. The presence of an anesthesia provider also reduces some of the patient care burden from the proceduralist. These factors may help improve overall efficiency in the endoscopic suite. If anesthesia-provided care can eliminate some cost and improve efficiency, it may not be as expensive as portrayed by these studies.

Policy Considerations and Guidelines for the Use of Propofol

The ASA endorses the concept of a continuum of sedation (reviewed previously) and in its 2009 Statement on Safe Use of Propofol[36] recommends that patients given propofol should receive care consistent with that required for deep sedation, which would be care by an anesthesia professional.[37] The ASA argues that propofol requires special attention because of the potential for rapid, profound changes in sedative or anesthetic depth and the lack of antagonist medication. Furthermore, the ASA recommends that the practitioner monitoring the patient should be present throughout the procedure and be completely dedicated to that task. This has led to opposition by the ASA to the use of propofol by nonanesthesiologists in non–operating room settings.

This position is opposed by many gastroenterologists. Also in 2009, four major gastroenterology groups, the American Association for the Study of Liver Disease, the American College of Gastroenterology, the American Gastroenterological Association, and the American Society

for Gastrointestinal Endoscopy, published a position statement on the use of propofol by the nonanesthesiologist.[38] The statement made several significant claims about NAAP based on the group's understanding of the literature. In terms of safety, NAAP is equivalent to standard sedation for upper endoscopy and colonoscopy. It appears to be equivalent for ERCP and EUS as well, but data are insufficient to draw definitive conclusions at this time. NAAP is more effective than standard sedation and more cost effective than both standard sedation and, for healthy, low-risk patients undergoing routine endoscopy, anesthesiologist-administered sedation. Although the paper concluded with the findings that with appropriate training and patient selection, NAAP was safe practice, the statement fell short of openly advocating this practice.

In December of 2009 the CMS issued a publication with a key provision that only a trained medical doctor or doctor of osteopathy not involved in the performance of a procedure could administer deep sedation or general anesthesia for procedural sedation.[39] The American Association of Nurse Anesthetists took credit for the policy shortly after it was issued, indicating that it was the result of years of advocacy. In January 2011 the CMS issued a revised appendix that removed mention of propofol; however, it continues to endorse that deep sedation can be administered only by a medical doctor or doctor of osteopathy not involved in the performance of the procedure. The ASA considers that propofol implies deep sedation; thus it becomes problematic for hospitals to allow nonanesthesiologists to use propofol. The CMS publication also states that it is not possible to predict how an individual patient will respond to medications administered to provide sedation and that hospitals must ensure that procedures are in place to rescue patients from a deeper level of sedation than was originally intended. This "rescue" requires an intervention from a practitioner with "expertise in airway management and advanced life support." The CMS states that this is also consistent with the requirements under the Patients' Rights standard, guaranteeing patients care in a safe setting. At this point, it is unclear where this finding leaves the future of NAAP in the United States.

European guidelines are also in a state of flux. In 2010 a guideline for the nonanesthesiologist administration of propofol for GI endoscopy was developed through a collaborative effort by representatives of the European Society of Gastrointestinal Endoscopy, the European Society of Gastroenterology and Endoscopy Nurses and Associates, and the European Society of Anesthesiology (ESA).[40] The guideline provides nonanesthesiologists with a comprehensive framework for propofol sedation during digestive endoscopy. The authors concluded, after evaluating the available literature, that propofol-based sedation presents rates of adverse events similar to those with traditional sedation. However, for specific high-risk patients (ASA class 3 or greater, Mallampati class 3 or greater, other conditions that put the patient at risk for airway obstruction, patients on significant chronic pain medication, or anticipated lengthy procedures), care should be provided by an anesthesiologist. Further recommendations include patient monitoring by a person dedicated to NAAP and that this monitoring should include pulse oximetry and noninvasive blood pressure measurement in all patients and electrocardiography in selected patients; capnography is not recommended as standard. Confusing the picture, the ESA general assembly voted to retract its endorsement of the guideline on June 15, 2011.[41] The initial support by the ESA was voted on by the board of directors and was unanimous, based on scientific evidence; however, a majority of national societies of the ESA were unable to support the guideline and voted to retract the statement. It is unclear at this time where this leaves the use of propofol in many European countries.

Moderate Sedation

Although many providers would prefer to use propofol for off-site procedures, they are often credentialed to provide moderate sedation only and do not have access to propofol or anesthesia services for various reasons. As previously mentioned, the use of a benzodiazepine and opioid combination remains the mainstay for the provision of moderate sedation in non–operating room anesthesia care. However, several studies have attempted to improve on traditional moderate sedation by using other sedative agents instead of or as an adjunct to a benzodiazepine and/or narcotic in the hopes of producing better sedation and reducing adverse effects. One major complication of combining opioids and benzodiazepines is respiratory depression. Dexmedetomidine is a highly selective alpha-2–adrenoreceptor agonist that typically maintains respiration while achieving a responsive sedative state. Jalowiecki compared dexmedetomidine to either a combination of meperidine and midazolam or fentanyl only for sedation for outpatient colonoscopy.[42] Although dexmedetomidine has been successfully used for certain types of intraoperative sedation, this study found it was inferior to both comparison groups. Dexmedetomidine produced significant hemodynamic instability, frequently required the addition of fentanyl to complete the procedure, produced prolonged recovery, and was complicated to administer. It appears unsuitable for use in endoscopy.

Ketamine is an N-methyl-D-aspartate antagonist used for sedation and analgesia. For adults, data are limited on the use of ketamine or combination therapy involving ketamine for non–operating room procedures. This limitation is likely due to the dysphoria often associated with ketamine, which may make it unsuitable for this use. In pediatric patients, some of the literature suggests ketamine is useful as a sedative outside the operating room.[43] The following three studies evaluated ketamine for sedation in pediatric GI endoscopy. Gilger et al[44] compared it to a midazolam and meperidine combination and found statistically significantly fewer complications and better sedation, although that improvement was found to be not statistically significant. Brecelj[45] evaluated ketamine versus ketamine/midazolam given by nonanesthesiologists for upper and lower endoscopy and found that the combination provided excellent sedation without significant dysphoria, in contrast to ketamine alone. Finally, a study by Tosun et al[46] found that both propofol with midazolam and propofol with ketamine were effective in pediatric upper endoscopy but that the ketamine group had more side effects. Perhaps ketamine may be useful in contrast to moderate sedation with an opioid and benzodiazepine combination but not for cases in which propofol is used. One side effect frequently noted with ketamine is laryngospasm.

Two studies evaluated the potential for the potent but short-acting opioid remifentanil for endoscopic sedation. Moerman et al[47] found that remifentanil was effective in colonoscopy but was associated with a higher incidence of patient recall and significant respiratory depression in contrast to propofol. A more recent study by Akcaboy et al[48] was designed to avoid these problems. Patients were randomly assigned to either low-dose remifentanil to avoid respiratory depression or a continuous propofol infusion with supplemental bolus as needed. To decrease procedural awareness, all patients also received 2 mg of midazolam. Low-dose remifentanil infusion was found to be effective, with excellent patient satisfaction, faster recovery, and no significant difference in respiratory depression. The discharge times were similar, but a higher incidence of nausea and vomiting occurred in the remifentanil group. This study was relatively small, and it is not clear that remifentanil offers any significant advantage over standard agents.

Two additional studies evaluated modifications to traditional sedation. The first study replaced fentanyl with oral tramadol; both were paired with midazolam. Fentanyl provided significantly better analgesia with fewer postprocedural side effects.[49] No patients in either group had hemodynamic or respiratory complications, and the authors concluded that fentanyl was superior to tramadol. The second study evaluated the effect of adding diphenhydramine to midazolam and meperidine for colonoscopy and found an improvement in the quality of sedation while allowing a reduction in the use of midazolam and meperidine[50]; no change was seen in the length of recovery. However, closed claims data suggest that sedative combinations increase the risk for sedation-related complications,[51] so caution when using more than two agents at a time is warranted.

Other Modalities

Alternatives and additions to intravenous sedation are available for GI endoscopy. Outside the United States a substantial number of patients undergo EGD without sedation.[52] Hypnosis has been used to facilitate endoscopy, although its use was unsurprisingly associated with greater patient discomfort and less amnesia in contrast to midazolam.[53] The use of pharyngeal local anesthetic sprays is relatively common, and a meta-analysis of five randomized controlled trials showed that the use of spray led to less procedure-related discomfort and less technical difficulty.[54] A small risk for methemoglobinemia and aspiration may be more likely after pharyngeal anesthesia. Another adjunct that has been used and evaluated is music in the endoscopy suite. It has been shown that listening to music before the procedure was associated with lower doses of analgesia and shorter procedure times, as well as lower patient anxiety levels.[55] Another modality that may become available in the future is patient-controlled sedation in which the patient controls the level of sedation, typically with propofol. This is discussed in more detail in another chapter. Although these modalities may be useful in certain cases, they will not supplant traditional sedation methods in the near future.

Conclusion

To date, no studies offer a clear alternative to propofol for sedation in non–operating room procedures in safety, efficiency, or effectiveness. In addition, with the possible exception of ketamine and midazolam for pediatric patients and outside of propofol-based strategies, there appears to be limited ability to improve on moderate sedation with a benzodiazepine and opioid combination. Thus, unless other medications become available, propofol is by far the best procedural sedative agent for routine use in most non–operating room cases. The unresolved and controversial question at this time is who should be using this agent, in which settings, and for which patients.

Considerable data are available on the use of propofol by nonanesthesiologists that appear to support NAAP for routine GI endoscopy in healthy patients (ASA class 1 or 2) by appropriately trained personnel. However, for patients with ASA class 3 and greater or those having prolonged and advanced procedures, caution may be warranted. In addition, policy considerations and regulations may affect who can provide sedation in the non–operating room setting. This may lead to medicolegal concerns with nonanesthesiologist use of propofol for sedation. As this practice increases, so does the potential for an adverse outcome or injury. Malpractice lawyers will undoubtedly scrutinize these cases to determine whether the duty of care between patient and clinician has been breached.[56] Because the U.S. Food and Drug Administration product labeling for propofol states that propofol "should be administered only by persons trained in the administration of general anesthesia and not involved in the conduct of surgical/diagnostic procedure," the decision to proceed without an anesthesiologist for GI endoscopy may be challenged.

Although it is difficult to predict the future in the field of medicine, several trends in non–operating room sedation are likely to continue. First, the trend toward increasingly complex non–operating room procedures on increasingly sick patients will continue. This will lead to an increasing demand for high-quality and cost-effective sedation for these procedures. In addition, significant pressure will continue to be placed on cost containment in medical care. Finally, the debate concerning who should provide sedation for which patients having what procedures will continue. As sedation experts, anesthesiologists need to maintain a clear voice on this issue. Until now, anesthesiologists have generally allowed nonanesthesiologists to control the debate. In the future, it is incumbent on the anesthesia community to be proactive in the sedation debate and to define ways in which anesthesia care adds value in the non–operating room setting. This includes exploring ways to provide effective and safe anesthesia care at a reasonable cost to society. The ideal is to provide the highest-quality sedation for patients with the lowest cost.

References

1. Freeman ML. Sedation and monitoring for gastrointestinal endoscopy. In: Yamada T, ed. *Textbook of gastroenterology*. 4th ed. Philadelphia: Lippincott Williams & Wilkins; 2003:2818–2820.
2. American Society of Anesthesiologists. Continuum of depth of sedation: definition of general anesthesia and levels of sedation/analgesia. Approved by ASA House of Delegates on October 13, 1999, and amended on October 27, 2004.
3. Zuccaro Jr G. Sedation and analgesia for GI endoscopy. *Gastrointest Endosc*. 2006;63:95–96.
4. Patel S, Vargo JJ, Khandwala F, et al. Deep sedation occurs frequently during elective endoscopy with meperidine and midazolam. *Am J Gastroenterol*. 2005;100:2689–2695.
5. Cohen LB, Wecsler JS, Gaetano JN, et al. Endoscopic sedation in the United States: results from a nationwide survey. *Am J Gastroenterol*. 2006;01:967–974.
6. Tan G, Irwin MG. Recent advances in using propofol by nonanesthesiologists. *F1000 Med Rep*. 2010;2:79.
7. Lazzaroni M, Bianchi Porro G. Preparation, premedication and surveillance. *Endoscopy*. 1998;30:53–60.
8. Froelich F, Harris JK, Wietlisbach V, et al. Current sedation and monitoring practice for colonoscopy: an international observational study (EPAGE). *Endoscopy*. 2006;38:461–469.
9. Ladas SD, Satake Y, Mostafa I, Morse J. Sedation practices for gastrointestinal endoscopy in Europe, North America, Asia, Africa and Australia. *Digestion*. 2010;82:74–76.
10. Reves JG, Glass P, Lubarsky DA, et al. Intravenous anesthetics. In: Miller RD, ed. *Miller's anesthesia*. 7th ed. Orlando, Fla: Churchill Livingstone; 2009.
11. DeWitt J, McGreevy K, Sherman S, Imperiale TF. Nurse-administered propofol sedation compared with midazolam and meperidine for EUS: a prospective, randomized trial. *Gastrointest Endosc*. 2008;68: 499–509.
12. Nayar DS, Guthrie WG, Goodman A, et al. Comparison of propofol deep sedation versus moderate sedation during endosonography. *Dig Dis Sci*. 2010;55:2537–2544.
13. Cohen LB, Hightower CD, Wood DA, et al. Moderate level sedation during endoscopy: a prospective study using low-dose propofol, meperidine/fentanyl, and midazolam. *Gastrointest Endosc*. 2004;59:795–803.
14. Sipe BW, Rex DK, Latinovich D, et al. Propofol versus midazolam/meperidine for outpatient colonoscopy; administration by nurses supervised by endoscopists. *Gastrointest Endosc*. 2002;55:815–825.
15. Ulmer BJ, Hansen JJ, Overley CA, et al. Propofol versus midazolam/fentanyl for outpatient colonoscopy: administration by nurses supervised by endoscopists. *Clin Gastroenterol Hepatol*. 2003;1:425–432.
16. Cohen LB. Redefining quality in endoscopic sedation. *Dig Dis Sci*. 2010;55:2425–2427.
17. Cote GA, Hovis RM, Ansstas MA, et al. Incidence of sedation-related complications with propofol use during advanced endoscopic procedures. *Clin Gastroenterol and Hepatol*. 2010;8:137–142.
18. McQuaid KR, Laine L. A systematic review and meta-analysis of randomized, controlled trials of moderate sedation for routine endoscopic procedures. *Gastrointest Endosc*. 2008;67:910–923.
19. Singh H, Poluha W, Cheung M, et al. Propofol for sedation during colonoscopy. *Cochrane Database Syst Rev*. 2008;(4):CD006268.
20. Sharma VK, Nguyen CC, Cromwell MD, et al. A national study of cardiopulmonary unplanned events after GI endoscopy. *Gastrointest Endosc*. 2007;66:27–34.
21. Rex DK, Deenadayalu VP, Eid E, et al. Endoscopist-directed administration of propofol: a worldwide safety experience. *Gastroenterology*. 2009;137:1229–1237.
22. Wehrmann T, Riphaus A. Sedation with propofol for interventional endoscopic procedures: a risk factor analysis. *Scand J Gastroenterol*. 2008;43:368–374.
23. Rex DK. Endoscopist-directed propofol. *Techn Gastrointest Endosc*. 2009;11:177–180.
24. van Natta ME, Rex DK. Propofol alone titrated to deep sedation versus propofol in combination with opioids and/or benzodiazepines and titrated to moderate sedation for colonoscopy. *Am J Gastroenterol*. 2006;101:2209–2217.
25. Clarke AC, Chiragakis L, Hillman LC, Kaye GL. Sedation for endoscopy: the safe use of propofol by general practitioner sedationists. *Med J Aust*. 2002;76:158–161.
26. Repici A, Pagano N, Hassan C, et al. Balanced propofol sedation administration by nonanesthesiologists: the first Italian experience. *World J Gastroenterol*. 2011;17:3818–3823.
27. Heuss LT, Froehlich F, Beglinger C. Nonanesthesiologist-administered propofol sedation: from the exception to standard practice—sedation and monitoring trends over 20 years. *Endoscopy*. 2012;44:504–511.
28. Sayfo S, Vakil KP, Alqaqa'a A, et al. A retrospective analysis of proceduralist-directed, nurse-administered propofol sedation for implantable cardioverter-defibrillator procedures. *Heart Rhythm*. 2012;9:342–346.

29. Kottkamp H, Hindricks G, Eitel C, et al. deep sedation for catheter ablation of atrial fibrillation: a prospective study in 650 consecutive patients. *J Cardiovasc Electrophysiol.* 2011;22:1339–1343.

30. Poincloux L, Laquiere A, Baxin JE, et al. A randomized controlled trial of endoscopist vs anaesthetist-administered sedation for colonoscopy. *Dig Liver Dis.* 2011;43:553–558.

31. Trummel JM, Surgenor SD, Cravero JP, et al. Comparison of differing sedation practice for upper endoscopic ultrasound using expert observational analysis of the procedural sedation. *J Pat Safety.* 2009;5:153–159.

32. Khiani VS, Soulos P, Gancayco J, et al. Anesthesiologist involvement in screening colonoscopy: temporal trends and cost implications in the Medicare population. *Clin Gastroenterol Hepatol.* 2012;10:58–64.

33. Liu H, Waxman DA, Main R, Mattke S. Utilization of anesthesia services during outpatient endoscopies and colonoscopies and associated spending in 2003-2009. *JAMA.* 2012;307:1178–1184.

34. Rex DK. Effect of the Centers for Medicare & Medicaid Services policy about deep sedation on use of propofol. *Ann Int Med.* 2011;154:622–626.

35. Hassan C, Rex DK, Cooper GS, et al. Endoscopist-directed propofol administration versus anesthesiologist assistance for colorectal cancer screening: a cost-effectiveness analysis. *Endoscopy.* 2012;44:456–464.

36. American Society of Anesthesiologists. Statement on safe use of propofol. Approved by ASA House of Delegates on October 27, 2004, and amended on October 21, 2009.

37. American Society of Anesthesiologists. Statement on granting privileges to nonanesthesiologist practitioners for personally administering deep sedation or supervising deep sedation by individuals who are not anesthesia professionals. Approved by the ASA House of Delegates on October 18, 2006

38. Vargo JJ, Cohen LB, Rex DK, et al. Position statement: nonanesthesiologist administration of propofol for GI endoscopy. *Gastroenterology.* 2009;137:2161–2167.

39. Centers for Medicare & Medicaid Services. Revised appendix A: interpretive guidelines for hospitals. Revision date December 2, 2011. Publication no. 100–07, Baltimore, Md: Centers for Medicare and Medicaid Services.

40. Dumonceau JM, Riphaus A, Aparicio JR, et al. European Society of Gastrointestinal Endoscopy, European Society of Gastroenterology and Endoscopy Nurses and Associates, and the European Society of Anesthesiology Guideline: Non-anesthesiologist administration of propofol for GI endoscopy. *Endoscopy.* 2010;42:960–974.

41. Pelosi P. Retraction of endorsement—European Society of Gastrointestinal Endoscopy, European Society of Gastroenterology and Endoscopy Nurses and Associates, and the European Society of Anesthesiology guideline: non-anesthesiologist administration of propofol for GI endoscopy. *Endoscopy.* 2012;44:302.

42. Jalowiecki P, Rudner R, Gonciarz M, et al. Sole use of dexmedetomidine has limited utility for conscious sedation during outpatient colonoscopy. *Anesthesiology.* 2005;103:269–273.

43. Green SM, Klooster M, Harris T, et al. Ketamine sedation for pediatric gastroenterology procedures. *J Pediatr Gastroenterol Nutr.* 2001;32:26–33.

44. Gilger MA, Spearman RS, Dietrich CL, et al. Safety and effectiveness of ketamine as a sedative agent for pediatric GI endoscopy. *Gastrointest Endosc.* 2004;59:659–663.

45. Brecelj J, Kamhi Trop T, Orel R. Ketamine with and without midazolam for gastrointestinal endoscopies in children. *J Pediatr Gastrenterol Nutr.* 2012;54:748–752.

46. Tosun Z, Aksu R, Guler G, et al. Propofol-ketamine vs propofol-fentanyl for sedation during pediatric upper gastrointestinal endoscopy. *Pediatr Anesth.* 2007;17:983–988.

47. Moerman AT, Foubert LA, Herregods LL, et al. Propofol versus remifentanil for monitored anaesthesia care during colonoscopy. *Eur J Anaesth.* 2003;20:461–466.

48. Akcaboy ZN, Akcaboy EY, Albayrak D, et al. Can Remifentanil be a better choice than propofol for colonoscopy during monitored anesthesia care? *Acta Anaesthesiol Scand.* 2006;50:736–741.

49. Hirsch I, Vaissler A, Chernin J, et al. Fentanyl or tramadol, with midazolam, for outpatient colonoscopy: analgesia, sedation, and safety. *Dig Dis Sci.* 2006;51:1946–1951.

50. Tu RH, Grewall P, Leung JW, et al. Diphenhydramine as an adjunct to sedation for colonoscopy: a double-blind randomized, placebo-controlled study. *Gastrointest Endosc.* 2006;63:87–94.

51. Bhananker SM, Posner KL, Cheney FW, et al. Injury and liability associated with monitored anesthesia care. *Anesthesiology.* 2006;104:228–234.

52. Thomson A, Andrew G, Jones DB. Optimal sedation for gastrointestinal endoscopy: review and recommendations. *J Gastroenterol Hepatol.* 2010;25:469–478.

53. Conlong P, Rees W. The use of hypnosis in gastroscopy: a comparison with intravenous sedation. *Postgrad Med J.* 1999;75:223–225.

54. Evans LT, Saberi S, Kim HM, et al. Pharyngeal anesthesia during sedated EGDs: is "the spray" beneficial? A meta-analysis and systematic review. *Gastrointest Endosc.* 2006;63:761–766.

55. Rudin D, Kiss A, Wetz RV, et al. Music in the endoscopy suite: a meta-analysis of randomized controlled studies. *Endoscopy.* 2007;39:507–510.

56. Axon AE. The use of propofol by gastroenterologists: medico-legal issues. *Digestion.* 2010;82:110–112.

SECTION 5

The Future of Non–Operating Room Anesthesia

SECTION OUTLINE

23 *Development of Future Systems*

24 *Novel Staffing Coverage for Anesthesia Outside the Operating Room*

23 Development of Future Systems

LARRY LINDENBAUM

Anesthetizing patients is a complex business. The number of tasks to perform on a daily basis has increased dramatically, and the number of locations in which they are performed also has risen. Effectively monitoring a patient, charting the patient's progress, anticipating changes in the surgical field, and adapting the anesthesia care requires a substantial amount of multitasking. Further, delivery of anesthesia care outside the operating room is complicated by variability of locations, workspaces, monitoring equipment, and other medical devices, in addition to the myriad cables and connectors required to keep things running. This often results in suboptimal physical arrangements in the non–operating room anesthesia (NORA) suite.

The introduction of the electronic medical record (EMR) and anesthesia record-keeping systems would, on the surface, seem to help alleviate some of the complexity and multitasking involved in the care of the patient during a procedure. However, that industry remains immature. A lack of standards for device integration further complicates the adoption of these systems with truly automatic functioning. Additionally, because a true wireless monitoring system is not available to the anesthesiologist, this integration comes at the cost of additional cables in the work space, making things even more difficult for a practitioner to function effectively.

Coupled with the difficulties described is the increasing need for anesthesiologists in non–operating room settings. The use of diagnostic endoscopy for the evaluation of upper and lower gastrointestinal disorders has dramatically increased in the last decade.[1,2] This rise in performed procedures comes with a concomitant increase in the use of trained anesthesia providers to administer sedation for these patients.[2] Further, the proportion of low-risk patients (American Society of Anesthesiologists [ASA] class 1 or 2) receiving sedation services from an anesthesiologist or certified registered nurse anesthetist has grown out of proportion to the overall number of procedures performed in the gastrointestinal suite.[2] In this same period, the cost of anesthesia services has increased. One study estimates that the cost of anesthesia services for these procedures in the United States amounted to $1.1 billion in 2009.[3] Another study shows that participation by anesthesia personnel in these procedures is expected to increase to greater than 50% by 2015.[4]

The escalating costs and use of an already limited resource naturally leads to the discussion of exactly which services are being offered and whether a safer, more economical way exists to provide these services. This discussion is complicated by the fact that it is increasingly commonplace for North American patients to request general anesthesia or at least deeper levels of sedation than are typically provided

for procedures of this type,[5,6] although at the same time proceduralists would prefer to use medications such as propofol but are afraid to do so because of the risks involved.[7,8] A review of the literature through 2009 shows at least 460,000 cases of nonanesthesiologist-administered propofol sedation for endoscopy.[9] The majority of those cases involved administration of propofol sedation by nurses. Three deaths were recorded in this group, occurring during or after esophagogastroduodenoscopy (EGD).[10]

The provision of anesthesia consists of several components: unconsciousness or anesthetic depth, analgesia, and neuromuscular blockade. Each of these associated components requires careful monitoring. New monitors are available to assist in the anesthetic management of the patient. These recently introduced monitors provide improvements in patient safety by using new physiological monitoring systems purported to aid in assessment of anesthesia depth. Automatic delivery systems, most commonly in the form of target-controlled infusion (TCI, or open-loop systems) pumps also have made an appearance in some markets.

A TCI is an infusion controlled to enable a user-defined drug concentration in a tissue of interest. Kruger-Thiemer[11] first suggested this concept in 1968, but it was not until the 1980s that pharmacokinetic models and equations were incorporated into computer-controlled devices. The first TCI pump introduced to clinical practice was the Diprifusor in 1996 (Figure 23-1).[12-14] Pumps and pharmacokinetic models have continued to evolve since that time.

These advances, when taken together, have opened the door for the creation of fully closed-loop systems. These closed-loop systems are designed to not just deliver a drug in a controlled fashion but to also monitor the patient for a parameter appropriate to the particular medication in use—for example, monitoring respiratory rate and end-tidal carbon dioxide ($ETCO_2$) as a feedback mechanism while infusing remifentanil. The introduction of decision support systems has paralleled these developments (more commonly in the military and critical care setting) to further help personnel make appropriate decisions.

The medical device industry has worked to develop automated systems for delivery of anesthesia care as it applies to the healthiest patients having the least complicated procedures. The focus of this chapter is the current state of automated or computer-assisted systems and those known to be in development. Although these devices are not yet routinely available in the United States, the SEDASYS System (Ethicon Endo-Surgery, Cincinnati, Ohio) was recently approved by the U.S. Food and Drug Administration (FDA) (on May 3, 2013). Canada and several European countries allow use of the SEDASYS System.

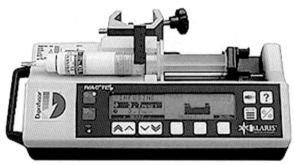

Figure 23-1 Diprifusor pump. (Courtesy of Carefusion, San Diego, CA.)

Evolution of Automated or Computer-Assisted Systems

Traditionally, automated anesthesia delivery systems have been broken down into closed- or open-loop systems; however, that nomenclature does not accurately reflect the reality of the systems currently under development because these systems often share characteristics of both. No matter how these devices are classified in the future, it is important to understand how the current open-loop, or TCI-based, devices function for comparison.

TCI devices were originally presented for clinical use in 1990[15] and are designed for the delivery of hypnotic or analgesic agents using a pharmacokinetic algorithm. The algorithms are based on commonly used three-compartment models of distribution and elimination. These models are based on population studies correlating drug blood concentrations with target site concentrations. They do not measure any actual effect of the drug and are thus considered open-loop devices. These devices have become relatively popular in Europe, with a prevalence of use in 10% to 25% of all total intravenous anesthesia cases[16]; however, only one device is currently available in North America.

A review of current TCI systems demonstrated that the main advantage of these systems over manual infusion is a reduction in the number of manual interventions needed to maintain anesthesia at a particular clinical end point.[17] The same review showed a small increase in total propofol consumption but no advantage in terms of induction speed, recovery time, or intraoperative movement. A different study revealed superior hemodynamics and more efficient dosing of remifentanil by TCI than by manual administration.[18]

Although TCI systems were initially built to infuse opioids or propofol, the idea of using TCI methods for volatile anesthetics has more recently emerged with both the Zeus (Dräger, Lübeck, Germany) and Felix (Taema, Antony, France) anesthesia workstations. These systems take advantage of closed-circuit ventilation and use feedback to control direct injection of anesthetic vapor into the breathing circle.

The successful creation of these devices has spurred the development of closed-loop systems, which represent the next step in the evolution of automated anesthesia systems. These newer systems are designed to automatically administer anesthesia by monitoring the effects of the medications in use and using patient response as a feedback mechanism for the system. The currently available closed-loop systems comprise three parts: a computerized operating system programmed with delivery algorithms, a drug delivery system, and an effect monitor. To be effective, these new systems must have a suitable effect that can be precisely measured for the feedback loop of each component of anesthesia being delivered.

A complete anesthesia delivery system has three effects that must be reliably monitored: depth of anesthesia, neuromuscular blockade, and pain control. Neuromuscular blockade is the easiest of the three effects to monitor in clinical practice. Multiple devices on the market take advantage of several mechanisms for measuring neuromuscular blockade. The major problems with many of the current devices are the relative lack of user-friendliness and difficulty in setting up for routine use. By contrast, twitch monitors are simple to use, easy to configure, and provide reliable information when set up appropriately.

Monitoring depth of anesthesia—or level of sedation—has grown in popularity over the last 10 to 15 years. The current devices use proprietary techniques for monitoring spontaneous electroencephalograph activity while displaying a synthesized number that purportedly reflects the patient's relative depth of sedation (typically on a scale of 1-100). Although controversy exists on the precise utility of these systems and the actual meaning of the numbers displayed, some studies have demonstrated the successful use of these systems as closed-loop systems, not just in efficacy but also in outperforming the manual administration of sedative-hypnotic medications.[19-21] As additional safeguards, these systems may also measure pulse oximetry and respiratory rate, especially when used for nonsurgical sedation.

Pain control, the third effect monitored, is more difficult to assess because the patient may be heavily sedated, under general anesthesia, or otherwise unable to communicate directly to personnel in the non–operating room location. Several studies have shown that hemodynamic parameters can be useful in the dosing of opioids.[22] Hemmerling et al[23] successfully demonstrated the utility of a scoring system in providing successful feedback control in a closed-loop system, although this was a very small study. Further work is necessary to validate these results.

MCSLEEPY

Researchers at McGill University in Montreal, Canada, developed the world's first completely automatic anesthesia delivery system, named McSleepy. As a complete anesthesia delivery system, McSleepy monitors the patient's depth of consciousness, muscle movements, and level of pain and stimulation during surgery. This information is fed back into the system's brain to adjust administration of the appropriate medication.

McSleepy is relatively simple to use.[24] After an intravenous cannula is placed, sensors are applied to measure the patient's muscle movement. Height, weight, age, and gender information, as well as the type of surgery being performed, are entered into the main console. McSleepy then allows the anesthesiologist to specify preferences regarding the drug dosages to be used before medication administration and monitoring of the patient. The system monitors data and adjusts dosing every minute while displaying all relevant data on a screen.[10,25]

SADASYS SYSTEM

Although McSleepy was the first closed-loop system introduced, the first computer-assisted system to aggressively pursue regulatory approval was designed for gastroenterologists. The SEDASYS System is a sedation delivery system designed to enable nonanesthesiologists to administer propofol in the endoscopy laboratory. Reasons for the focus on endoscopy for the SEDASYS System include the increasing number of procedures in the endoscopy suite, especially to help accommodate the demand for early colon cancer screening,[26] and noted advantages to sedation with propofol over benzodiazepine and opioid combinations in terms of turnover time and patient satisfaction.[27]

Originally endorsed by the FDA's Anesthesiology and Respiratory Therapy Devices Advisory Committee in 2009, the SEDASYS System was rejected by the FDA in 2010, an unusual occurrence because the FDA typically follows the advice of its advisory committees. Ethicon Endo-Surgery (a division of Johnson & Johnson) appealed the decision, and FDA Commissioner Margaret Hamburg, MD, granted a hearing scheduled for December 2011. However, in November 2011, Ethicon Endo-Surgery announced that it had withdrawn its request for appeal because it had reached a settlement with the FDA's Center for Devices and Radiologic Health "to settle the company's appeal" of its previous denial.

The FDA accordingly agreed to reopen the premarket approval application and "review it expeditiously." The SEDASYS System was approved by the FDA in May of 2013 for the delivery of propofol for minimal-to-moderate sedation during colonoscopy and EGD procedures. The device is also currently approved for sale in Canada for sedation of patients undergoing colonoscopy and in Australia for patients undergoing colonoscopy and EGD. It was granted the mark of approval in the European Union for use during routine colonoscopy and EGD in May of 2010.[28,29] In the United States, the device carries the following caveats: The device is restricted for use by health care professionals that have the types of training defined in the labeling, and to settings where an anesthesia professional is immediately available for assistance or consultation. Also, the SEDASYS System should not be used in:

- Patients with known hypersensitivity to 1% propofol injectable emulsion or its components
- Patients with allergies to eggs, egg products, soybeans, or soy products
- Patients with a known hypersensitivity to fentanyl
- Pregnant or lactating women
- Delivery of any drug other than 1% propofol injectable emulsion
- Patients with a full stomach

The SEDASYS System initiates sedation with a loading dose based on the patient's weight and the maintenance infusion rate selected by the physician, delivered over 3 minutes. The maximum initial maintenance rate the physician can select is 75 mcg/kg/min, which yields a 0.5 mg/kg loading dose. After the loading dose is delivered, the SEDASYS System delivers the infusion rate selected by the physician. Detection of oversedation is determined by several mechanisms, including falling oxygen saturation,

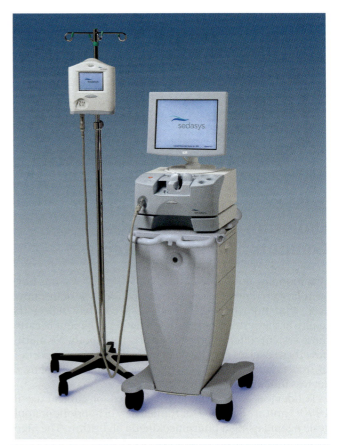

Figure 23-2 The SEDASYS System. (Courtesy of Ethicon Endo-Surgery, Inc., Cincinnati, Ohio.)

depressed respiratory rate, and failure of detection of the $ETCO_2$ curve. If any of these signals occur, the propofol infusion is automatically stopped. Further, the machine adds an additional layer of monitoring by talking to the patient at varied intervals and asking the patient to squeeze a handset. If the patient fails to comply, the propofol infusion is automatically reduced.

Unlike McSleepy, the SEDASYS System is designed to deliver only propofol. The computer-assisted delivery mechanism is integrated with the patient monitoring as part of a feedback loop. The SEDASYS System is equipped with standard ASA monitors, including $ETCO_2$. The device is physically made of two primary subunits, a bedside monitoring unit and a procedure room unit (Figure 23-2). The mobile bedside monitoring unit is attached to the patient and moves with the patient throughout the perioperative environment. It has a port for attachment of an oronasal cannula for oxygen delivery, and it monitors and displays oxygen saturation, noninvasive blood pressure, and electrocardiogram. This unit also houses the automated responsiveness monitor, designed to assess patient responsiveness.

The approval of the device comes primarily from Ethicon's study of 1000 adults in ASA class 1 to 3 undergoing routine EGD or colonoscopy.[30] In this study, patients were randomized into two groups, one for sedation with the SEDASYS System and one for sedation with each site's current standard of care for these procedures. Of note is that the standard of care at each of these facilities was a benzodiazepine and opioid combination, not propofol.

The results of this study showed that the area under the curve of oxygen desaturation was significantly lower for the SEDASYS System than it was for the benzodiazepine and opioid group. Further, the SEDASYS System patients were said to be significantly more satisfied, as were the clinicians involved. The SEDASYS System group was shown to recover faster, and the incidence of adverse effects was slightly but not significantly lower.

Although the studies described are worth noting, the larger question is whether the use of the SEDASYS System to administer propofol can prevent the progression of sedation to unintended depths. The SEDASYS System should be used by physicians trained in the management of the cardiorespiratory effects of propofol, including propofol pharmacology, identification of high-risk patients, recognition of progression of levels of sedation and the actions necessary to return the patient to intended levels, determination of adequate ventilation, and management of airway obstruction and hypoventilation.

Propofol has a narrow therapeutic index and a very large interpatient variability between drug clearance and anesthetic requirements.[33,34] The precise variability is, at present, completely unknown but most likely multifactorial. Age, weight, circulation time, body fat percentage, and genetic polymorphisms may influence the variable effect of propofol. The algorithm in use by the SEDASYS System is not publicly known, further increasing the anxiety surrounding the possibility of a medication administration error.

Conclusion

In spite of the controversy and concerns, the use of propofol by endoscopists without the supervision of trained anesthesiology professionals is on the rise. Given the current health care environment, the challenge remains to balance patient safety, cost effectiveness, and overall efficiency. Anesthesiology as a profession has demonstrated impressive improvements in safety over the last few decades, largely through the use of new technology. The development of these automated and computer-assisted anesthesia delivery systems is a natural direction for the specialty. Close collaboration between anesthesiologists and procedural specialists is necessary to ensure the safe care of patients, regardless of the developments that evolve.

References

1. Harewood GC, Lieberman DA. Colonoscopy practice patterns since introduction of Medicare coverage for average-risk screening. *Clin Gastroenterol Hepatol.* 2004;2(1):72–77.
2. Liu H, Waxman DA, Main R, Mattke S. Utilization of anesthesia services during outpatient endoscopies and colonoscopies and associated spending in 2003-2009. *JAMA.* 2012;307(11):1178–1184.
3. Smith MJ. Use, cost of anesthesia for endoscopy increasing. *Gastroenterol Endosc News.* 2012;63:5.
4. Inadomi JM, Gunnarsson CL, Rizzo JA, Fang H. Projected increased growth rate of anesthesia professional-delivered sedation for colonoscopy and EGD in the United States: 2009 to 2015. *Gastrointest Endosc.* 2010;72(3):580–586.
5. Chanpong B, Haas DA, Locker D. Need and demand for sedation or general anesthesia in dentistry: a national survey of the Canadian population. *Anesth Prog.* 2005;52(1):3–11.
6. Jamieson J. Anesthesia and sedation in the endoscopy suite? (influences and options). *Curr Opin Anaesthesiol.* 1999;12(4):417–423.
7. McQuaid KR, Laine L. A systematic review and meta-analysis of randomized, controlled trials of moderate sedation for routine endoscopic procedures. *Gastrointest Endosc.* 2008;67(6):910–923.
8. Cohen LB, DeLegge M, Kochman M, et al. AGA institute review on endoscopic sedation. *Gastroenterology.* 2007;133(2):675–701.
9. Vargo JJ, Cohen LB, Rex DK, Kwo PY. Position statement: nonanesthesiologist administration of propofol for GI endoscopy. *Am J Gastroenterol.* 2009;104(12):2886–2892. Sedation guidelines update: http://www.asge.org/assets/0/71542/71544/4a572112-29a4-4313-8ab8-b7801e8f84e2.pdf.
10. Deenadayalu VP, Eid EF, Gotf JS, et al. Non-anesthesiologist administered propofol sedation for endoscopic procedures: a worldwide safety review [abstr]. *Gastrointest Endosc.* 2008;67:AB107.
11. Kruger-Thiemer E. Continuous intravenous infusion and multicompartmental accumulation. *Eur J Pharmacol.* 1968;4(3):317–324.
12. White M, Kenny GN. Intravenous propofol anaesthesia using a computerized infusion system. *Anaesthesia.* 1990;45(3):204–209.
13. Kenny GN, White M. A portable target controlled propofol infusion system. *Int J Clin Monit Comput.* 1992;9(3):179–182.
14. Gray JM, Kenny GNC. Development of the technology for the 'Diprifusor' TCI systems. *Anaesthesia.* 1998;53(suppl 1):22–27.
15. Schwilden H, Schuttler J. The determination of an effective therapeutic infusion rate for intravenous anesthetics using feedback-controlled dosages. *Anaesthetist.* 1990;39(11):603–606.
16. Schwilden H, Schuttler J. Target controlled anaesthetic drug dosing. *Handb Exp Pharmacol.* 2008;182:425–450.
17. Leslie K, Clavisi O, Hargrove J. Target-controlled infusion versus manually-controlled infusion of propofol for general anesthesia or sedation in adults. *Cochrane Database Syst Rev.* 2008;(3):CD006059.
18. De Castro V, Godet G, Mencia G, et al. Target-controlled infusion for remifentanil in vascular patients improves hemodynamics and decreases remifentanil requirement. *Anesth Analg.* 2003;96(1):33–38.
19. Struys MM, De Smet T, Versichelen LF, et al. Comparison of closed-loop controlled administration of propofol using bispectral index as the controlled variable versus "standard practice" controlled administration. *Anesthesiology.* 2001;95(1):6–17.
20. Hemmerling TM, Charabati S, Zaouter C, Minardi C, Mathieu PA. A randomized controlled trial demonstrates that a novel closed-loop propofol system performs better hypnosis control than manual administration. *Can J Anaesthesiol.* 2010;57(8):725–735.
21. De Smet T, Struys M, Neckebroek M, Van den Hauwe K, Bonte S, Mortier E. The accuracy and clinical feasibility of a new Bayesian-based closed-loop control system for propofol administration using the bispectral index as a controlled variable. *Anesth Analg.* 2008;107(4):1200–1210.
22. Gentilini A, Schaniel C, Morari M, et al. A new paradigm for the closed-loop intraoperative administration of analgesics in humans. *IEEE Trans Biomed Eng.* 2002;49(4):289–299.
23. Hemmerling ZTM, Charabati S, Salhab E, et al. The Analgoscore: a novel score to monitor intraoperative nociception and its use for closed-loop application of remifentanil. *J Comput.* 2009;4:311–318.
24. Hemmerling TM. Automated anesthesia. *Curr Opin Anaesthesiol.* 2009;22:757–763.
25. Hemmerling TM, Charabati S, Mathieu PA. McSleepy: a completely automatic anesthesia delivery system [abstr S46]. *STA Meeting.* January, 2009.
26. Seeff L, Nadel M, Blackman D. Colorectal cancer test use among persons aged >50 years: United States, 2001. *Morbid Mortal Wkly Rep.* 2003;52:193–196.
27. Sipe BW, Rex DK, Latinovich D, et al. Propofol versus midazolam/meperidine for outpatient colonoscopy: administration by nurses supervised by endoscopists. *Gastrointest Endosc.* 2002;55:815–825.
28. Public summary for ARTG entry for SEDASYS System in Australia. https://www.ebs.tga.gov.au/servlet/xmlmillr?dbidebs/PublicHTML/pdfStore.nsf&docid175411&agid(PrintDetailsPublic)&actionid1.
29. Ethicon Endo-Surgery SEDASYS System receives approval in Canada and CE mark in European Union. http://www.investor.jnj.com/releasedetail.cfm?ReleaseID=465904.

30. Pambianco DJ, Vargo JJ, Pruitt RE, Hardi R, Martin JF. Computer-assisted personalized sedation for upper endoscopy and colonoscopy: a comparative, multicenter randomized study. *Gastrointest Endosc.* 2001;73:765–772.
31. Deleted in page proofs.
32. Deleted in page proofs.
33. Iohom G, Ni CM, O'Brien JK, et al. An investigation of potential genetic determinants of propofol requirements and recovery from anaesthesia. *Eur J Anaesthesiol.* 2007;24:912–919.
34. Ortolani O, Conti A, Ngumi ZW, et al. Ethnic differences in propofol and fentanyl response: a comparison among Caucasians, Kenyan Africans and Brazilians. *Eur J Anaesthesiol.* 2004;21:314–319.

24 Novel Staffing Coverage for Anesthesia Outside the Operating Room

MARY ELLEN WARNER, LINDSAY L. WARNER, and NAFISSEH S. WARNER

The demand for non–operating room anesthesia (NORA) services is expanding rapidly and for diverse reasons. NORA procedures are often less invasive; many of these minimally or even noninvasive procedures are either no longer adaptable or not able to be performed in traditional operating rooms, or they do not need to be performed in expensive and highly staffed operating rooms. The growth in procedures that no longer routinely need to be performed in operating rooms encompasses practices ranging from radiology (e.g., radiofrequency tumor ablation, radiation seed implantation, transhepatic biliary duct stent placement) to gastroenterology (e.g., endoscopic placement of biliary stents, closed gastric stapling) to interventional cardiology (e.g., transfemoral aortic valve replacement). Many simple procedures may be performed in relatively spartan procedure rooms or even at the bedside, such as dressing and pack changes. Regardless of the location of the patient's procedural care, a pain-free, safe, and relatively inexpensive experience is the primary desired outcome for both the patient and proceduralist. New anesthesia and sedation care models are needed to support the new procedural practices that are NORA cases.

The main goal of anesthesia delivery in any setting is to ensure safe, high-quality care. This can be challenging in operating settings where resources are often readily available and support staff and colleagues are nearby. It can be even more challenging outside the operating room environment. In best-case scenarios, distance from extra knowledgeable hands and resources requires additional planning and raises concerns. In worst-case scenarios, anesthesia providers may be unfamiliar with the environment and procedural issues, have very limited or minimal resources, and lack support if unanticipated complications or extraordinary needs arise.

Complexity as the Norm

Unless institutional processes and facilities are specifically adapted to support NORA, the delivery of safe anesthesia care is both administratively and medically difficult. Preplanning and standardization reduce complexity and the risks inherent in one-off activities. If sufficient numbers of non–operating room procedures are to be done, it may be possible to group them into specific locations. These locations can then be appropriately resourced with personnel, supplies, and emergency equipment. Standardized processes of care can be implemented and metrics of their success tracked as in other surgical or procedural environments. For example, sufficient numbers of unique gastroenterological endoscopy procedures may be done in a facility to support standard practices. These would include scheduling systems, quality-improvement processes, specific recovery areas, and staff who are trained and knowledgeable about the many procedures that take place in such facilities. In settings that allow consolidation of typical NORA procedures, care within the context of healthy patients undergoing complex procedures or medically compromised patients undergoing simple procedures can be fairly routine. This care becomes more challenging when medically compromised patients undergo complex procedures.

Administrative difficulties arise, however, when it is not possible to develop consolidated practice areas for typical and atypical procedures outside the operating room. For example, in many settings the provision of anesthesia care for patients undergoing radiation therapy is infrequent and inconsistent. This scenario requires deliberate review and planning. Radiation therapy environments are often distant from regular operating room settings and thus isolate anesthesia providers from colleagues. Many providers are not comfortable caring for seriously ill patients or providing care to medically complex patients in emergency rooms or isolated interventional radiology or endoscopy sites. These locations all require careful planning and creation of myriad well-defined collaborative arrangements among services and staff to ensure cooperation and patient safety. These agreements need to be written, readily available, and reviewed periodically so that providers involved in these experiences understand their roles and responsibilities when working in isolated non–operating room sites. Box 24-1 lists examples of the issues to be identified and documented.

Medical complexity is a major challenge for many non–operating room procedures. Anesthesia personnel are typically requested when a patient's condition is medically challenging, a procedure is complex, or both. Patients who are sick or compromised clearly increase periprocedural risks. Metzner et al[1] reviewed the American Society of Anesthesiologists (ASA) Closed Claims database entries from 1990 to 2009 and found that non–operating room locations were more likely to involve older and sicker patients ($p < 0.01$) undergoing emergency procedures than were operating rooms. Not surprisingly, monitored anesthesia care was eight times more likely to be the anesthesia technique used rather than general anesthesia in the operating room setting. The severity of injuries in these remote locations was greater, with a significant increase in death in contrast

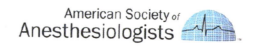

American Society of
Anesthesiologists

STATEMENT ON GRANTING PRIVILEGES FOR ADMINISTRATION OF MODERATE SEDATION TO PRACTITIONERS WHO ARE NOT ANESTHESIA PROFESSIONALS

Practice Guidelines for Sedation and Analgesia by Nonanesthesiologists (Approved by ASA House of Delegates on October 25, 1995, and last amended on October 17, 2001)

Continuum of Depth of Sedation – Definition of General Anesthesia and Levels of Sedation/Analgesia (Approved by ASA House of Delegates on October 13, 1999, and last amended on October 21, 2009)

Practice Guidelines for Preoperative Fasting and the Use of Pharmacologic Agents to Reduce the Risk of Pulmonary Aspiration: Application to Healthy Patients Undergoing Elective Procedures (Approved by ASA House of Delegates on October 21, 1998, and effective January 1, 1999)

The Ad Hoc Committee on Sedation Credentialing Guidelines for Nonanesthesiologists took the contents of the above documents into consideration when developing this statement.

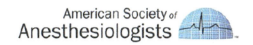

American Society of
Anesthesiologists

STATEMENT ON GRANTING PRIVILEGES FOR ADMINISTRATION OF MODERATE SEDATION TO PRACTITIONERS WHO ARE NOT ANESTHESIA PROFESSIONALS

DEFINITIONS

Anesthesia Professional: An anesthesiologist, certified registered nurse anesthetist (CRNA) or anesthesiologist assistant (AA).

Nonanesthesiologist Sedation Practitioner: A licensed physician (allopathic or osteopathic), dentist or podiatrist who has not completed postgraduate training in anesthesiology but is specifically trained to personally administer or supervise the administration of moderate sedation.

Supervised Sedation Professional: A licensed registered nurse, advanced practice nurse or physician assistant who is trained to administer medications and monitor patients during moderate sedation **under the direct supervision of a nonanesthesiologist sedation practitioner or an anesthesiologist.**

Credentialing: The process of documenting and reviewing a practitioner's credentials.

Credentials: The professional qualifications of a practitioner including education, training, experience and performance.

Privileges: The clinical activities within a health care organization that a practitioner is permitted to perform based on the practitioner's credentials.

Guidelines: A set of recommended practices that should be considered but permit discretion by the user as to whether they should be applied under any particular set of circumstances.

* Moderate Sedation: "Moderate Sedation/Analgesia ("Conscious Sedation") is a drug-induced depression of consciousness during which patients respond purposefully to verbal commands, either alone or accompanied by light tactile stimulation. No interventions are required to maintain a patent airway, and spontaneous ventilation is adequate. Cardiovascular function is usually maintained."

* Deep Sedation: "Deep Sedation/Analgesia is a drug-induced depression of consciousness during which patients cannot be easily aroused but respond purposefully following repeated or painful stimulation. The ability to independently maintain ventilatory function may be impaired. Patients may require assistance in maintaining a patent airway, and spontaneous ventilation may be inadequate. Cardiovascular function is usually maintained."

* Rescue: "Rescue of a patient from a deeper level of sedation than intended is an intervention by a practitioner proficient in airway management and advanced life support. The qualified practitioner corrects adverse physiologic consequences of the deeper-than intended level of sedation (such as hypoventilation, hypoxia and hypotension) and returns the patient to the originally intended level of sedation."

* General Anesthesia: "General Anesthesia is a drug-induced loss of consciousness during which patients are not arousable, even by painful stimulation. The ability to independently

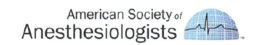

**STATEMENT ON GRANTING PRIVILEGES FOR
ADMINISTRATION OF MODERATE SEDATION TO PRACTITIONERS
WHO ARE NOT ANESTHESIA PROFESSIONALS**

maintain ventilatory function is often impaired. Patients often require assistance in maintaining a patent airway, and positive pressure ventilation may be required because of depressed spontaneous ventilation or drug-induced depression of neuromuscular function. Cardiovascular function may be impaired."

---

*The definitions marked with an asterisk are extracted verbatim from "Continuum of Depth of Sedation – Definition of General Anesthesia and Levels of Sedation/Analgesia" (Approved by ASA House of Delegates on October 13, 1999, and amended on October 27, 2004).

American Society *of*
Anesthesiologists

STATEMENT ON GRANTING PRIVILEGES FOR
ADMINISTRATION OF MODERATE SEDATION TO PRACTITIONERS
WHO ARE NOT ANESTHESIA PROFESSIONALS

STATEMENT

The following statement is designed to assist health care organizations develop a program for the delineation of clinical privileges for practitioners who are not anesthesia professionals to administer sedative and analgesic drugs to establish a level of moderate sedation. (Moderate sedation is also known as "conscious sedation.") The statement is written to apply to every setting in which an internal or external credentialing process is required for granting privileges to administer sedative and analgesic drugs to establish a level of moderate sedation (e.g., hospital, freestanding procedure center, ambulatory surgery center, physician's, dentist's or podiatrist's office, etc.). The statement is not intended nor should it be applied to the granting of privileges to administer deep sedation or general anesthesia.

The granting, reappraisal and revision of clinical privileges should be awarded on a time-limited basis in accordance with rules and regulations of the health care organization, its medical staff, organizations accrediting the health care organization and relevant local, state and federal governmental agencies.

I. NONANESTHESIOLOGIST SEDATION PRACTITIONERS

Only physicians, dentists or podiatrists who are qualified by education, training and licensure to administer moderate sedation should supervise the administration of moderate sedation. Nonanesthesiologist sedation practitioners may directly supervise patient monitoring and the administration of sedative and analgesic medications by a **supervised sedation professional**. Alternatively, they may personally perform these functions, with the proviso that the individual monitoring the patient should be distinct from the individual performing the diagnostic or therapeutic procedure (see *ASA Guidelines for Sedation and Analgesia by Nonanesthesiologists*).

A. Education and Training

The nonanesthesiologist sedation practitioner who is to supervise or personally administer medications for moderate sedation should have satisfactorily completed a formal training program in: (1) the safe administration of sedative and analgesic drugs used to establish a level of moderate sedation, and (2) rescue of patients who exhibit adverse physiologic consequences of a deeper-than-intended level of sedation. This training may be a part of a recently completed residency or fellowship training (e.g., within two years), or may be a separate educational program. A knowledge-based test may be used to verify the practitioner's understanding of these concepts.[**] The following subject areas should be included:

1. Contents of the following ASA documents that should be understood by practitioners who administer sedative and analgesic drugs to establish a level of moderate sedation:

    •   *Practice Guidelines for Sedation and Analgesia by Nonanesthesiologists*

[**]The post-test included with the ASA Sedation/Analgesia by Nonanesthesiologists videotape (ASA Document #30503-10PPV) may be considered for this purpose.

STATEMENT ON GRANTING PRIVILEGES FOR ADMINISTRATION OF MODERATE SEDATION TO PRACTITIONERS WHO ARE NOT ANESTHESIA PROFESSIONALS

- *Continuum of Depth of Sedation – Definition of General Anesthesia and Levels of Sedation/Analgesia*

2. Appropriate methods for obtaining informed consent through pre-procedure counseling of patients regarding risks, benefits and alternatives to the administration of sedative and analgesic drugs to establish a level of moderate sedation.

3. Skills for obtaining the patient's medical history and performing a physical examination to assess risks and co-morbidities, including assessment of the airway for anatomic and mobility characteristics suggestive of potentially difficult airway management. The nonanesthesiologist sedation practitioner should be able to recognize those patients whose medical condition suggests that sedation should be provided by an anesthesia professional.

4. Assessment of the patient's risk for aspiration of gastric contents as described in the *ASA Practice Guidelines for Preoperative Fasting*: "In urgent, emergent or other situations where gastric emptying is impaired, the potential for pulmonary aspiration of gastric contents must be considered in determining (1) the target level of sedation, (2) whether the procedure should be delayed or (3) whether the trachea should be protected by intubation."

5. The pharmacology of (1) all sedative and analgesic drugs the practitioner requests privileges to administer to establish a level of moderate sedation, (2) pharmacological antagonists to the sedative and analgesic drugs and (3) vasoactive drugs and antiarrhythmics.

6. The benefits and risks of supplemental oxygen.

7. Proficiency of airway management with facemask and positive pressure ventilation. This training should include appropriately supervised experience in managing the airways of patients, or qualified instruction on an airway simulator (or both).

8. Monitoring of physiologic variables, including the following:
   a. Blood pressure
   b. Respiratory rate
   c. Oxygen saturation by pulse oximetry
   d. Electrocardiographic monitoring. Education in electrocardiographic (EKG) monitoring should include instruction in the most common arrhythmias seen during sedation and anesthesia, their causes and their potential clinical implications (e.g., hypercapnia), as well as electrocardiographic signs of cardiac ischemia.
   e. Depth of sedation. The depth of sedation should be based on the ASA definitions of "moderate sedation" and "deep sedation." (See above)
   f. Capnography– During moderate sedation the adequacy of ventilation shall be evaluated by continual observation of qualitative clinical signs and monitoring for the

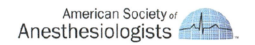

American Society *of*
Anesthesiologists

STATEMENT ON GRANTING PRIVILEGES FOR ADMINISTRATION OF MODERATE SEDATION TO PRACTITIONERS WHO ARE NOT ANESTHESIA PROFESSIONALS

presence of exhaled carbon dioxide unless precluded or invalidated by the nature of the patient, procedure, or equipment.

9. The importance of continuous use of appropriately set audible alarms on physiologic monitoring equipment.

10. Documenting the drugs and fluids administered, the patient's physiologic condition and the depth of sedation at regular intervals throughout the period of sedation and analgesia, using a graphical, tabular or automated record.

11. Regardless of the availability of a "code team" or the equivalent, the non-anesthesiologist sedation practitioner will have advanced life support skills and current certificate such as those required for Advanced Cardiac Life Support (ACLS). When granting privileges to administer moderate sedation to pediatric patients, the non-anesthesiologist practitioner will have advanced life support skills and current certificate such as those required for Pediatric Advanced Life Support (PALS). Initial ACLS and PALS training and subsequent retraining shall be obtained from the American Heart Association or another vendor that includes "hands-on" training and skills demonstration of airway management and automated external defibrillator (AED) use.

When the practitioner is being granted privileges to administer sedative and analgesic drugs to pediatric patients to establish a level of moderate sedation, the education and training requirements enumerated in #1-9 above should be appropriately tailored to qualify the practitioner to administer sedative and analgesic drugs to pediatric patients.

B. Licensure

1. The nonanesthesiologist sedation practitioner should have a current active, unrestricted medical, osteopathic, dental or podiatric license in the state, district or territory of practice. (Exception: practitioners employed by the federal government may have a current active license in any U.S. state, district or territory.)

2. The nonanesthesiologist sedation practitioner should have a current unrestricted Drug Enforcement Administration (DEA) registration (schedules II-V).

3. The credentialing process should require disclosure of any disciplinary action (final judgments) against any medical, osteopathic or podiatric license by any state, district or territory of practice and of any sanctions by any federal agency, including Medicare/Medicaid, in the last five years.

4. Before granting or renewing privileges to administer or supervise the administration of sedative and analgesic drugs to establish a level of moderate sedation, the health care organization should search for any disciplinary action recorded in the National Practitioner Data Bank (NPDB) and take appropriate action regarding any Adverse Action Reports.

American Society of
Anesthesiologists

STATEMENT ON GRANTING PRIVILEGES FOR ADMINISTRATION OF MODERATE SEDATION TO PRACTITIONERS WHO ARE NOT ANESTHESIA PROFESSIONALS

C. Practice Pattern

1. Before granting initial privileges to administer or supervise administration of sedative and analgesic drugs to establish a level of moderate sedation, a process should be

   developed to evaluate the practitioner's performance. For recent graduates (e.g., within two years), this may be accomplished through letters of recommendation from directors of residency or fellowship training programs which include moderate sedation as part of the curriculum. For those who have been in practice since completion of their training, this may be accomplished through communication with department heads or supervisors at the institution where the individual holds privileges to administer moderate sedation. Alternatively, the nonanesthesiologist sedation practitioner could be proctored or supervised by a physician, dentist or podiatrist who is currently privileged to administer sedative and analgesic agents to provide moderate sedation. The facility should establish an appropriate number of procedures to be supervised.

2. Before granting ongoing privileges to administer or supervise administration of sedative and analgesic drugs to establish a level of moderate sedation, a process should be developed to re-evaluate the practitioner's performance at regular intervals. For example, the practitioner's performance could be reviewed by an anesthesiologist or a nonanesthesiologist sedation practitioner who is currently privileged to administer sedative and analgesic agents to provide moderate sedation. The facility should establish an appropriate number of procedures that will be reviewed.

D. Performance Improvement

Credentialing in the administration of sedative and analgesic drugs to establish a level of moderate sedation should require active participation in an ongoing process that evaluates the practitioner's clinical performance and patient care outcomes through a formal program of continuous performance improvement.

1. The organization in which the practitioner practices should conduct peer review of its clinicians.
2. The performance improvement process should assess up-to-date knowledge as well as ongoing competence in the skills outlined in the educational and training requirements described above.
3. The performance improvement process should monitor and evaluate patient outcomes and adverse events.

II. SUPERVISED SEDATION PROFESSIONAL

A. Education and Training

The supervised sedation professional who is granted privileges to administer sedative and analgesic drugs under supervision of a nonanesthesiologist sedation practitioner or anesthesiologist and to monitor patients during moderate sedation can be a registered

American Society of
Anesthesiologists

STATEMENT ON GRANTING PRIVILEGES FOR
ADMINISTRATION OF MODERATE SEDATION TO PRACTITIONERS
WHO ARE NOT ANESTHESIA PROFESSIONALS

nurse who has graduated from a qualified school of nursing or a physician assistant who has graduated from an accredited physician assistant program. They may only administer sedative and analgesic medications on the order of an anesthesiologist or nonanesthesiologist sedation practitioner. They should have satisfactorily completed a formal training program in 1) the safe administration of sedative and analgesic drugs used to establish a level of moderate sedation, 2) use of reversal agents for opioids and

benzodiazepines, 3) monitoring of patients' physiologic parameters during sedation, and 4) recognition of abnormalities in monitored variables that require intervention by the nonanesthesiologist sedation practitioner or anesthesiologist. Training should include the following:

1. Contents of the following ASA documents:

    - *Practice Guidelines for Sedation and Analgesia by Nonanesthesiologists*
    - *Continuum of Depth of Sedation –*
      Definition of General Anesthesia and Levels of Sedation/Analgesia

2. The pharmacology of (1) all sedative and analgesic drugs the practitioner requests privileges to administer to establish a level of moderate sedation, and (2) pharmacological antagonists to the sedative and analgesic drugs.

3. The benefits and risks of supplemental oxygen.

4. Airway management with facemask and positive pressure ventilation.

5. Monitoring and recognizing abnormalities of physiologic variables, including the following:
    a. Blood pressure
    b. Respiratory rate
    c. Oxygen saturation by pulse oximetry
    d. Electrocardiographic monitoring
    e. Depth of sedation. The depth of sedation should be based on the ASA definitions of "moderate sedation" and "deep sedation." (See above)
    f. Capnography–if moderate sedation is to be administered unless precluded or invalidated by the nature of the patient, procedure, or equipment.

6. The importance of continuous use of appropriately set audible alarms on all physiologic monitors.

7. Documenting the drugs administered, the patient's physiologic condition and the depth of sedation at regular intervals throughout the period of sedation and analgesia, using a graphical, tabular or automated record.

B. Licensure

1. The supervised sedation professional should have a current active nursing license or physician assistant license or certification, in the U.S. state, district or territory of

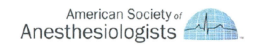
American Society of
Anesthesiologists

STATEMENT ON GRANTING PRIVILEGES FOR
ADMINISTRATION OF MODERATE SEDATION TO PRACTITIONERS
WHO ARE NOT ANESTHESIA PROFESSIONALS

practice. (Exception: practitioners employed by the federal government may have a current active license in any U.S. state, district or territory.)

2. Before granting or renewing privileges for a supervised sedation professional to administer sedative and analgesic drugs and to monitor patients during moderate sedation, the health care organization should search for any disciplinary action recorded in the National Practitioner Data Bank (NPDB) and take appropriate action regarding any Adverse Action Reports.

C. Practice Pattern

1. Before granting ongoing privileges to administer sedative and analgesic drugs to establish a level of moderate sedation, a process should be developed to re-evaluate the supervised sedation professional's performance. The facility should establish performance criteria and an appropriate number of procedures to be reviewed.

D. Performance Improvement

Credentialing of supervised sedation professionals in the administration of sedative and analgesic drugs and monitoring patients during moderate sedation should require active participation in an ongoing process that evaluates the health care professional's clinical performance and patient care outcomes through a formal program of continuous performance improvement.

1. The organization in which the practitioner practices should conduct peer review of its supervised sedation professionals.

2. The performance improvement process should assess up-to-date knowledge as well as ongoing competence in the skills outlined in the educational and training requirements described above.

ADVISORY ON GRANTING PRIVILEGES FOR DEEP SEDATION TO NON-ANESTHESIOLOGIST SEDATION PRACTITIONERS

Committee of Origin: *Ad Hoc* on Non-Anesthesiologist Privileging

(Approved by the ASA House of Delegates on October 20, 2010)

1. INTRODUCTION

The American Society of Anesthesiologists is vitally interested in the safe administration of all anesthesia services including moderate and deep sedation. As such, it has concern for any system or set of practices, used either by its members or the members of other disciplines that would adversely affect the safety of anesthesia or sedation administration. It has genuine concern that individuals, however well intentioned, who are not anesthesia professionals may not recognize that sedation and general anesthesia are on a continuum, and thus deliver levels of sedation that may, in fact, be general anesthesia without having the training and experience to respond appropriately.

ASA believes that anesthesiologist participation in all deep sedation is the best means to achieve the safest care. ASA acknowledges, however, that Medicare regulations permit some non-anesthesiologists to administer or supervise the administration of deep sedation. This advisory should not be considered as an endorsement, or absolute condemnation, of this practice by ASA but rather to serve as a potential guide to its members who may be called upon by administrators or others to provide input in this process. This document provides a framework to identify those physicians, dentists, oral surgeons or podiatrists who may potentially qualify to administer or supervise the administration of deep sedation.

This document applies only to the care of patients undergoing procedural sedation, and it may not be construed as privileges to intentionally administer general anesthesia. Unrestricted general anesthesia shall only be administered by anesthesia professionals within their scope of practice (anesthesiologists, certified registered nurse anesthetists and anesthesiologist assistants). If the patient loses consciousness and the ability to respond purposefully, the anesthesia care is a general anesthetic, irrespective of whether airway instrumentation is required.

When deep sedation is intended, there is a significant risk that patients may slip into a state of general anesthesia (from which they cannot be aroused by painful or repeated stimulation). Therefore, individuals requesting privileges to administer deep sedation must demonstrate their ability to (1) recognize that a patient has entered a state of general anesthesia and (2) maintain a patient's vital functions until the patient has been returned to an appropriate level of sedation.

Definitions of terms appear at the end of this document. Of special note, for purposes of this document the following definitions are relevant:

1.1 Anesthesia Professional: An anesthesiologist, anesthesiologist assistant (AA), or certified registered nurse anesthetist (CRNA).

1.2 Non-anesthesiologist Sedation Practitioner: A licensed physician (allopathic or osteopathic); or dentist, oral surgeon, or podiatrist who is qualified to administer anesthesia under State law; who has not completed postgraduate training in anesthesiology but is specifically trained to administer personally or to supervise the administration of deep sedation.

ADVISORY ON GRANTING PRIVILEGES FOR DEEP SEDATION TO NON-ANESTHESIOLOGIST SEDATION PRACTITIONERS

2. ADVISORY

This advisory is designed to assist health care facilities in developing a program for the delineation of clinical privileges for practitioners who are not anesthesia professionals to administer sedative and analgesic drugs to establish a level of deep sedation. They are written to apply to every setting in which an internal or external privileging process is required for granting privileges to administer sedative and analgesic drugs to establish a level of deep sedation (e.g., hospital, freestanding procedure center, ambulatory surgery center, physician's or dentist's office, etc.). These recommendations do not lead to the granting of privileges to administer general anesthesia.

The granting, reappraisal and revision of clinical privileges will be awarded on a time-limited basis in accordance with rules and regulations of the health care facility, its medical staff, organizations accrediting the health care facility, and relevant local, state and federal governmental agencies.

NON-ANESTHESIOLOGIST SEDATION PRACTITIONERS

> Note: The *Hospital Anesthesia Services Condition of Participation 42 CFR 482.52(a)* limits the administration of deep sedation to "qualified anesthesia professionals" within their scope of practice. CMS defines these personnel specifically as an anesthesiologist; non-anesthesiologist MD or DO; dentist, oral surgeon, or podiatrist who is qualified to administer anesthesia under State law; CRNA, and AA. See also the *Ambulatory Surgery Center Condition for Coverage 42 CFR 416.42(b)*.

Only physicians and other practitioners specifically permitted by CMS, above, who are qualified by education, training and licensure to administer deep sedation may administer deep sedation or supervise the administration of deep sedation when administered by CRNAs. Because training is procedure specific, the type and complexity of procedures for which the practitioner may administer or supervise deep sedation must be specified in the privileges granted.

Any professional who administers and monitors deep sedation must be dedicated to that task. Therefore, the non-anesthesiologist sedation practitioner who administers and monitors deep sedation must be different from the individual performing the diagnostic or therapeutic procedure (see ASA Guidelines for Sedation and Analgesia by Non-anesthesiologists).

3. EDUCATION AND TRAINING

The non-anesthesiologist sedation practitioner will have satisfactorily completed a formal training program in (1) the safe administration of sedative and analgesic drugs used to establish a level of deep sedation, and (2) rescue of patients who exhibit adverse physiologic consequences of a deeper-than-intended level of sedation. This training may be a formally recognized part of a recently completed Accreditation Council for Graduate Medical Education (ACGME) residency or fellowship training (e.g., within two years), or may be a separate deep sedation educational program that is accredited by Accreditation Council for Continuing Medical Education (ACCME) or equivalent providers recognized for dental, oral surgical and podiatric continuing education, and that includes the didactic and performance concepts below. A knowledge-based test is necessary to objectively demonstrate the knowledge of concepts required to obtain privileges. The following subject areas will be included:

ADVISORY ON GRANTING PRIVILEGES FOR DEEP SEDATION TO NON-ANESTHESIOLOGIST SEDATION PRACTITIONERS

3.1   Contents of the following ASA documents (or their more current version if subsequently modified) that will be understood by practitioners who administer sedative and analgesic drugs to establish a level of deep sedation

     3.1.1   Practice Guidelines for Sedation and Analgesia by Non-Anesthesiologists. Anesthesiology 2002: 96; 1004-1017.

     3.1.2   Continuum of Depth of Sedation; Definition of General Anesthesia and Levels of Sedation/Analgesia (ASA HOD 2004, amended 2009)

     3.1.3   Standards for Basic Anesthetic Monitoring (Approved by the ASA House of Delegates on October 21, 1986, and last amended on October 25, 2005)

     3.1.4   Practice Guidelines for Preoperative Fasting and the Use of Pharmacologic Agents to Reduce the Risk of Pulmonary Aspiration: Application to Healthy Patients Undergoing Elective Procedures (Approved by ASA House of Delegates on October 21, 1998, and effective January 1, 1999)

3.2   Appropriate methods for obtaining informed consent through pre-procedure counseling of patients regarding risks, benefits and alternatives to the administration of sedative and analgesic drugs to establish a level of deep sedation.

3.3   Skills for obtaining the patient's medical history and performing a physical examination to assess risks and co-morbidities, including assessment of the airway for anatomic and mobility characteristics suggestive of potentially difficult airway management. The non-anesthesiologist sedation practitioner will be able to recognize those patients whose medical condition requires that sedation needs to be provided by an anesthesia professional, such as morbidly obese patients, elderly patients, pregnant patients, patients with severe systemic disease, patients with obstructive sleep apnea, or patients with delayed gastric emptying.

3.4   Assessment of the patient's risk for aspiration of gastric contents as described in the ASA Practice Guidelines for Preoperative Fasting. In urgent, emergent or other situations where gastric emptying is impaired, the potential for pulmonary aspiration of gastric contents must be considered in determining

     3.4.1   The target level of sedation

     3.4.2   Whether the procedure should be delayed

     3.4.3   Whether the sedation care should be transferred to an anesthesia professional for the delivery of general anesthesia with endotracheal intubation.

3.5   The pharmacology of

     3.5.1   All sedative and analgesic drugs the practitioner requests privileges to administer to establish a level of deep sedation

     3.5.2   Pharmacological antagonists to the sedative and analgesic drugs

ADVISORY ON GRANTING PRIVILEGES FOR DEEP SEDATION TO NON-ANESTHESIOLOGIST SEDATION PRACTITIONERS

     3.5.3 Vasoactive drugs and antiarrhythmics.

3.6   The benefits and risks of supplemental oxygen.

3.7   Recognition of adequacy of ventilatory function: This will include experience with patients whose ventilatory drive is depressed by sedative and analgesic drugs as well as patients whose airways become obstructed during sedation. This will also include the ability to perform capnography and understand the results of such monitoring. Non-anesthesiologist practitioners will demonstrate competency in managing patients during deep sedation, and understanding of the clinical manifestations of general anesthesia so that they can ascertain when a patient has entered a state of general anesthesia and rescue the patient appropriately.

3.8   Proficiency in advanced airway management for rescue: This training will include appropriately supervised experience to demonstrate competency in managing the airways of patients during deep sedation, and airway management using airway models as well as using high-fidelity patient simulators. The non-anesthesiologist practitioner must demonstrate the ability to reliably perform the following:

    3.8.1. Bag-valve-mask ventilation

    3.8.2 Insertion and use of oro- and nasopharyngeal airways

    3.8.3 Insertion and ventilation through a laryngeal mask airway

    3.8.4 Direct laryngoscopy and endotracheal intubation

    This will include clinical experience on no less than 35 patients or equivalent simulator experience (See ACGME reference). The facility with oversight by the Director of Anesthesia Services will determine the number of cases needed to demonstrate these competencies, and may increase beyond the minimum recommended.

3.9   Monitoring of physiologic variables, including the following:

    3.9.1 Blood pressure.

    3.9.2 Respiratory rate.

    3.9.3 Oxygen saturation by pulse oximetry with audible variable pitch pulse tone.

    3.9.4 Capnographic monitoring. The non-anesthesiologist practitioner shall be familiar with the use and interpretation of capnographic waveforms to determine the adequacy of ventilation during deep sedation.

    3.9.5 Electrocardiographic monitoring. Education in electrocardiographic (EKG) monitoring will include instruction in the most common dysrhythmias seen during sedation and anesthesia, their causes and their potential clinical implications (e.g., hypercapnia), as well as electrocardiographic signs of cardiac ischemia.

ADVISORY ON GRANTING PRIVILEGES FOR DEEP SEDATION TO NON-ANESTHESIOLOGIST SEDATION PRACTITIONERS

    3.9.6 Depth of sedation. The depth of sedation will be based on the ASA definitions of "deep sedation" and "general anesthesia." (See below).

3.10 The importance of continuous use of appropriately set audible alarms on physiologic monitoring equipment.

3.11 Documenting the drugs administered, the patient's physiologic condition and the depth of sedation at five-minute intervals throughout the period of sedation and analgesia, using a graphical, tabular or automated record which documents all the monitored parameters including capnographic monitoring.

3.12 The importance of monitoring the patient through the recovery period and the inclusion of specific discharge criteria for the patient receiving sedation.

3.13 Regardless of the availability of a "code team" or the equivalent, the non-anesthesiologist practitioner will have advanced life support skills and current certificate such as those required for Advanced Cardiac Life Support (ACLS). When granting privileges to administer deep sedation to pediatric patients, the non-anesthesiologist practitioner will have advanced life support skills and current certificate such as those required for Pediatric Advanced Life Support (PALS). Initial ACLS and PALS training and subsequent retraining shall be obtained from the American Heart Association or another vendor that includes "hands-on" training and skills demonstration of airway management and automated external defibrillator (AED) use.

3.14 Required participation in a quality assurance system to track adverse outcomes and unusual events including respiratory arrests, use of reversal agents, prolonged sedation in recovery process, larger than expected medication doses, and occurrence of general anesthesia, with oversight by the Director of Anesthesia services or their designee.

3.15 Knowledge of the current CMS Conditions of Participation regulations and their interpretive guidelines pertaining to deep sedation, including requirements for the pre-anesthesia evaluation, anesthesia intra-operative record, and post-anesthesia evaluation.

Separate privileging is required for the care of pediatric patients. When the non-anesthesiologist practitioner is granted privileges to administer sedative and analgesic drugs to pediatric patients to establish a level of deep sedation, the education and training requirements enumerated in #1-15 above will be specifically defined to qualify the practitioner to administer sedative and analgesic drugs to pediatric patients.

4. LICENSURE

4.1 The non-anesthesiologist sedation practitioner will have a current active, unrestricted medical, osteopathic, or dental license in the state, district or territory of practice. (Exception: practitioners employed by the federal government may have a current active license in any U.S. state, district or territory.)

4.2 The non-anesthesiologist sedation practitioner will have a current unrestricted Drug Enforcement Administration (DEA) registration (schedules II-V).

ADVISORY ON GRANTING PRIVILEGES FOR DEEP SEDATION TO NON-ANESTHESIOLOGIST SEDATION PRACTITIONERS

4.3   The privileging process will require disclosure of any disciplinary action (final judgments) against any medical, osteopathic or dental license by any state, district or territory of practice and of any sanctions by any federal agency, including Medicare/Medicaid, in the last five years.

4.4   Before granting or renewing privileges to administer or supervise the administration of sedative and analgesic drugs to establish a level of deep sedation, the health care organization shall search for any disciplinary action recorded in the National Practitioner Data Bank (NPDB) and take appropriate action regarding any Adverse Action Reports.

5. PERFORMANCE EVALUATION

5.1   Before granting initial privileges to administer or supervise administration of sedative and analgesic drugs to establish a level of deep sedation, a process will be developed to evaluate the practitioner's performance and competency. For recent graduates (e.g., within two years), this may be accomplished through letters of recommendation from directors of residency or fellowship training programs that include deep sedation as part of the curriculum. For those who have been in practice since completion of their training, performance evaluation may be accomplished through specific documentation of performance evaluation data transmitted from department heads or supervisors at the institution where the individual previously held privileges to administer deep sedation. Alternatively, the non-anesthesiologist sedation practitioner could be proctored or supervised by a physician or dentist who is currently privileged to administer sedative and analgesic agents to provide deep sedation. The Director of Anesthesia Services with oversight by the facility governing body will determine the number of cases that need to be performed in order to determine independent competency in deep sedation.

5.2   Before granting ongoing privileges to administer or supervise administration of sedative and analgesic drugs to establish a level of deep sedation, a process will be developed to re-evaluate the practitioner's performance at regular intervals. Re-evaluation of competency in airway management will be part of this performance evaluation. For example, the practitioner's performance could be reviewed by an anesthesiologist or a non-anesthesiologist sedation practitioner who is currently privileged to administer deep sedation. The facility will establish an appropriate number of procedures that will be reviewed.

6. PERFORMANCE IMPROVEMENT

Privileging in the administration of sedative and analgesic drugs to establish a level of deep sedation will require active participation in an ongoing process that evaluates the practitioner's clinical performance and patient care outcomes through a formal facility program of continuous performance improvement. The facility's deep sedation performance improvement program will be developed with advice from and with outcome review by the Director of Anesthesia Services.

6.1   The organization in which the practitioner practices will conduct peer review of its clinicians.

6.2   The performance improvement program will assess up-to-date knowledge as well as

ADVISORY ON GRANTING PRIVILEGES FOR DEEP SEDATION TO NON-ANESTHESIOLOGIST SEDATION PRACTITIONERS

ongoing competence in the skills outlined in the educational and training requirements described above.

6.3   Continuing medical education in the delivery of anesthesia services is required for renewal of privileges.

6.4   The performance improvement program will monitor and evaluate patient outcomes and adverse or unusual events.

6.5   Any of the following events will be referred to the facility quality assurance committee for evaluation and performance evaluation:

   6.5.1 Unplanned admission

   6.5.2 Cardiac arrest

   6.5.3 Use of reversal agents

   6.5.4 Use of assistance with ventilation requiring bag-valve-mask ventilation or laryngeal or endotracheal airways.

   6.5.5 Prolonged periods of oxygen desaturation (<85% for 3 minutes)

   6.5.6 Failure of the patient to return to 20% of pre-procedure vital signs

7. DEFINITIONS

Anesthesia Professional: An anesthesiologist, anesthesiologist assistant (AA), or certified registered nurse anesthetist (CRNA).

Non-anesthesiologist Sedation Practitioner: A licensed physician (allopathic or osteopathic); or dentist, oral surgeon, or podiatrist who is qualified to administer anesthesia under State law; who has not completed postgraduate training in anesthesiology but is specifically trained to administer personally or to supervise the administration of deep sedation.

Privileges: The clinical activities within a health care organization that a practitioner is permitted to perform.

Privileging: The process of granting permission to perform certain clinical activities based on credentials, experience, and demonstrated performance

Credentials: The professional qualifications of a practitioner including education, training, experience and performance

Credentialing: The process of obtaining, verifying, and assessing the qualifications of a practitioner to provide care or services in or for a healthcare organization.

Procedural sedation: The administration of sedative and analgesic drugs for a non-surgical diagnostic or therapeutic procedure.

ADVISORY ON GRANTING PRIVILEGES FOR DEEP SEDATION TO NON-ANESTHESIOLOGIST SEDATION PRACTITIONERS

Definitions of the continuum of sedation:
* Moderate Sedation: "Moderate Sedation/Analgesia ("Conscious Sedation") is a drug- induced depression of consciousness during which patients respond purposefully to verbal commands, either alone or accompanied by light tactile stimulation. No interventions are required to maintain a patent airway, and spontaneous ventilation is adequate. Cardiovascular function is usually maintained."

* Deep Sedation: "Deep Sedation/Analgesia is a drug-induced depression of consciousness during which patients cannot be easily aroused but respond purposefully following repeated or painful stimulation. The ability to independently maintain ventilatory function may be impaired. Patients may require assistance in maintaining a patent airway, and spontaneous ventilation may be inadequate. Cardiovascular function is usually maintained."

* Rescue: "Rescue of a patient from a deeper level of sedation than intended is an intervention by a practitioner proficient in airway management and advanced life support. The qualified practitioner corrects adverse physiologic consequences of the deeper-than-intended level of sedation (such as hypoventilation, hypoxia and hypotension) and returns the patient to the originally intended level of sedation. It is not appropriate to continue the procedure at an unintended level of sedation."

* General Anesthesia: "General Anesthesia is a drug-induced loss of consciousness during which patients are not arousable, even by painful stimulation. The ability to independently maintain ventilatory function is often impaired. Patients often require assistance in maintaining a patent airway, and positive pressure ventilation may be required because of depressed spontaneous ventilation or drug-induced depression of neuromuscular function. Cardiovascular function may be impaired."

*The definitions marked with an asterisk are extracted verbatim from "Continuum of Depth of Sedation – Definition of General Anesthesia and Levels of Sedation/Analgesia" (Approved by ASA House of Delegates on October 13, 1999, and amended on October 21, 2009).
Expanded definitions of moderate and deep sedation can be found in the CMS Interpretive Guidelines.

8. REFERENCES

The American Society of Anesthesiologists has produced many documents over the years related to the topic addressed by this advisory, among them the following (in alphabetical order):

AANA-ASA Joint Statement Regarding Propofol Administration (April 14, 2004)

<u>Continuum of Depth of Sedation – Definition of General Anesthesia and Levels of Sedation/Analgesia</u> (Approved by ASA House of Delegates on October 13, 1999, and last amended on October 21, 2009).

<u>Distinguishing Monitored Anesthesia Care ("MAC") from Moderate Sedation/Analgesia (Conscious Sedation)</u>. (Approved by the ASA House of Delegates on October 27, 2004 and last amended on October 21, 2009)

<u>Guidelines for Ambulatory Anesthesia and Surgery</u> (Approved by ASA House of Delegates on October 11, 1973, and last amended on October 22, 2008)

ADVISORY ON GRANTING PRIVILEGES FOR DEEP SEDATION TO NON-ANESTHESIOLOGIST SEDATION PRACTITIONERS

Guidelines for Delineation of Clinical Privileges in Anesthesiology (Approved by ASA House of Delegates on October 15, 1975, and last amended on October 22, 2008)

Guidelines for Office-Based Anesthesia and Surgery (Approved by ASA House of Delegates on October 13, 1999, and last affirmed on October 21, 2009)

Outcome Indicators for Office-Based and Ambulatory Surgery (ASA Committee on Ambulatory Surgical Care and Task Force on Office-Based Anesthesia, April 2003)

Practice Guidelines for Preoperative Fasting and the Use of Pharmacologic Agents to Reduce the Risk of Pulmonary Aspiration: Application to Healthy Patients Undergoing Elective Procedures. Anesthesiology 1999; 90: 896-905.

Practice Guidelines for Sedation and Analgesia by Non-anesthesiologists. Anesthesiology 2002: 96; 1004-1017.

Standards for Basic Anesthetic Monitoring (Approved by the ASA House of Delegates on October 21, 1986, and last amended on October 20, 2010)

Statement on Granting Privileges for Administration of Moderate Sedation to Practitioners Who Are Not Anesthesia Professionals (Approved by the ASA House of Delegates on October 25, 2005, and last amended on October 18, 2006)

Statement on Qualifications of Anesthesia Providers in the Office-Based Setting (Approved by ASA House of Delegates on October 13, 1999, and last amended on October 21, 2009)

Statement on Safe Use of Propofol (Approved by ASA House of Delegates on October 27, 2004 and amended on October 21, 2009)

In addition the following references may be considered:

ACGME Emergency Medicine residency program guidelines for number of intubations needed:
http://www.acgme.org/acWebsite/RRC_110/110_guidelines.asp#res

American Academy of Pediatrics, American Academy of Pediatric Dentistry, Cote CJ, Wilson S, and the Workgroup on Sedation. Guidelines for Monitoring and Management of Pediatric Patients During and After Sedation for Diagnostic and Therapeutic Procedures: An Update. Pediatrics 2006; 118: 2587-2602.

Centers for Medicare and Medicaid Services Revisions to Interpretive Guidelines for Hospital Condition of Participation, December 11, 2009.
http://www.cms.gov/surveycertificationgeninfo/pmsr/itemdetail.asp?itemid=CMS1231690

Centers for Medicare and Medicaid Services Revisions to Interpretive Guidelines for Ambulatory Surgery Centers Condition for Coverage, December 30, 2009.
https://www.cms.gov/transmittals/downloads/R56SOMA.pdf

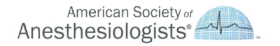

American Society of
Anesthesiologists®

GUIDELINES FOR AMBULATORY ANESTHESIA AND SURGERY

Committee of Origin: Ambulatory Surgical Care

(Approved by the ASA House of Delegates on October 15, 2003, last amended on October 22, 2008, and reaffirmed on October 16, 2013)

The American Society of Anesthesiologists (ASA) endorses and supports the concept of Ambulatory Anesthesia and Surgery. ASA encourages the anesthesiologist to play a leadership role as the perioperative physician in all hospitals, ambulatory surgical facilities and office-based settings, and to participate in facility accreditation as a means for standardization and improving the quality of patient care.

These guidelines apply to all care involving anesthesiology personnel administering ambulatory anesthesia in all settings. These are minimal guidelines which may be exceeded at any time based on the judgment of the involved anesthesia personnel. These guidelines encourage high quality patient care, but observing them cannot guarantee any specific patient outcome. These guidelines are subject to periodic revision, as warranted by the evolution of technology and practice.

I. ASA Standards, Guidelines and Policies should be adhered to in all settings except where they are not applicable to outpatient care.

II. A licensed physician should be in attendance in the facility, or in the case of overnight care, immediately available by telephone, at all times during patient treatment and recovery and until the patients are medically discharged.

III. The facility must be established, constructed, equipped and operated in accordance with applicable local, state and federal laws and regulations. At a minimum, all settings should have a reliable source of oxygen, suction, resuscitation equipment and emergency drugs. Specific reference is made to the ASA *"Statement on Nonoperating Room Anesthetizing Locations."*

IV. Staff should be adequate to meet patient and facility needs for all procedures performed in the setting, and should consist of:

    A. Professional Staff

        1. Physicians and other practitioners who hold a valid license or certificate are duly qualified.

        2. Nurses who are duly licensed and qualified.

    B. Administrative Staff

    C. Housekeeping and Maintenance Staff

V. Physicians providing medical care in the facility should assume responsibility for credentials review, delineation of privileges, quality assurance and peer review.

VI. Qualified personnel and equipment should be on hand to manage emergencies. There should be established policies and procedures to respond to emergencies and unanticipated patient transfer to an acute care facility.

VII. Minimal patient care should include:

    A. Preoperative instructions and preparation.

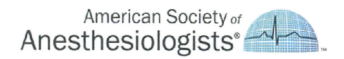

American Society *of*
Anesthesiologists®

B. An appropriate pre-anesthesia evaluation and examination by an anesthesiologist, prior to anesthesia and surgery. In the event that nonphysician personnel are utilized in the process, the anesthesiologist must verify the information and repeat and record essential key elements of the evaluation.

C. Preoperative studies and consultations as medically indicated.

D. An anesthesia plan developed by an anesthesiologist, discussed with and accepted by the patient and documented.

E. Administration of anesthesia by anesthesiologists, other qualified physicians or nonphysician anesthesia personnel medically directed by an anesthesiologist. Non-anesthesiologist physicians who are administering or supervising the administration of the continuum of anesthesia must be qualified by education, training, licensure, and appropriately credentialed by the facility.

F. Discharge of the patient is a physician responsibility.

G. Patients who receive other than unsupplemented local anesthesia must be discharged with a responsible adult.

H. Written postoperative and follow-up care instructions.

I. Accurate, confidential and current medical records.

GUIDELINES FOR OFFICE-BASED ANESTHESIA

Committee of Origin: Ambulatory Surgical Care

(Approved by the ASA House of Delegates on October 13, 1999, and last affirmed on October 21, 2009)

These guidelines are intended to assist ASA members who are considering the practice of ambulatory anesthesia in the office setting: office-based anesthesia (OBA). These recommendations focus on quality anesthesia care and patient safety in the office. These are minimal guidelines and may be exceeded at any time based on the judgment of the involved anesthesia personnel. Compliance with these guidelines cannot guarantee any specific outcome. These guidelines are subject to periodic revision as warranted by the evolution of federal, state and local laws as well as technology and practice.

ASA recognizes the unique needs of this growing practice and the increased requests for ASA members to provide OBA for health care practitioners* who have developed their own office operatories. Since OBA is a subset of ambulatory anesthesia, the ASA "Guidelines for Ambulatory Anesthesia and Surgery" should be followed in the office setting as well as all other ASA standards and guidelines that are applicable.

There are special problems that ASA members must recognize when administering anesthesia in the office setting. Compared with acute care hospitals and licensed ambulatory surgical facilities, office operatories currently have little or no regulation, oversight or control by federal, state or local laws. Therefore, ASA members must satisfactorily investigate areas taken for granted in the hospital or ambulatory surgical facility such as governance, organization, construction and equipment, as well as policies and procedures, including fire, safety, drugs, emergencies, staffing, training and unanticipated patient transfers.

ASA members should be confident that the following issues are addressed in an office setting to provide patient safety and to reduce risk and liability to the anesthesiologist.

Administration and Facility

Quality of Care

- The facility should have a medical director or governing body that establishes policy and is responsible for the activities of the facility and its staff. The medical director or governing body is responsible for ensuring that facilities and personnel are adequate and appropriate for the type of procedures performed.

- Policies and procedures should be written for the orderly conduct of the facility and reviewed on an annual basis.

- The medical director or governing body should ensure that all applicable local, state and federal regulations are observed.

- All health care practitioners* and nurses should hold a valid license or certificate to perform their assigned duties.

- All operating room personnel who provide clinical care in the office should be qualified to perform services commensurate with appropriate levels of education, training and experience.

*defined herein as physicians, dentists and podiatrists

GUIDELINES FOR OFFICE-BASED ANESTHESIA

- The anesthesiologist should participate in ongoing continuous quality improvement and risk management activities.
- The medical director or governing body should recognize the basic human rights of its patients, and a written document that describes this policy should be available for patients to review.

Facility and Safety

- Facilities should comply with all applicable federal, state and local laws, codes and regulations pertaining to fire prevention, building construction and occupancy, accommodations for the disabled, occupational safety and health, and disposal of medical waste and hazardous waste.
- Policies and procedures should comply with laws and regulations pertaining to controlled drug supply, storage and administration.

Clinical Care

Patient and Procedure Selection

- The anesthesiologist should be satisfied that the procedure to be undertaken is within the scope of practice of the health care practitioners and the capabilities of the facility.
- The procedure should be of a duration and degree of complexity that will permit the patient to recover and be discharged from the facility.
- Patients who by reason of pre-existing medical or other conditions may be at undue risk for complications should be referred to an appropriate facility for performance of the procedure and the administration of anesthesia.

Perioperative Care

- The anesthesiologist should adhere to the "Basic Standards for Preanesthesia Care," "Standards for Basic Anesthetic Monitoring," "Standards for Postanesthesia Care" and "Guidelines for Ambulatory Anesthesia and Surgery" as currently promulgated by the American Society of Anesthesiologists.
- The anesthesiologist should be physically present during the intraoperative period and immediately available until the patient has been discharged from anesthesia care.
- Discharge of the patient is a physician responsibility. This decision should be documented in the medical record.
- Personnel with training in advanced resuscitative techniques (e.g., ACLS, PALS) should be immediately available until all patients are discharged home.

Monitoring and Equipment

- At a minimum, all facilities should have a reliable source of oxygen, suction, resuscitation equipment and emergency drugs. Specific reference is made to the ASA "Statement on Nonoperating Room Anesthetizing Locations."
- There should be sufficient space to accommodate all necessary equipment and personnel and to allow for expeditious access to the patient, anesthesia machine (when present) and all monitoring equipment.
- All equipment should be maintained, tested and inspected according to the manufacturer's specifications.

GUIDELINES FOR OFFICE-BASED ANESTHESIA

- Back-up power sufficient to ensure patient protection in the event of an emergency should be available.

- In any location in which anesthesia is administered, there should be appropriate anesthesia apparatus and equipment which allow monitoring consistent with ASA "Standards for Basic Anesthetic Monitoring" and documentation of regular preventive maintenance as recommended by the manufacturer.

- In an office where anesthesia services are to be provided to infants and children, the required equipment, medication and resuscitative capabilities should be appropriately sized for a pediatric population.

Emergencies and Transfers

- All facility personnel should be appropriately trained in and regularly review the facility's written emergency protocols.

- There should be written protocols for cardiopulmonary emergencies and other internal and external disasters such as fire.

- The facility should have medications, equipment and written protocols available to treat malignant hyperthermia when triggering agents are used.

- The facility should have a written protocol in place for the safe and timely transfer of patients to a prespecified alternate care facility when extended or emergency services are needed to protect the health or well-being of the patient.

STATEMENT ON QUALIFICATIONS OF ANESTHESIA PROVIDERS IN THE OFFICE-BASED SETTING

Committee of Origin: Ambulatory Surgical Care

(Approved by the ASA House of Delegates on October 13, 1999, and last amended on October 21, 2009)

ASA policy documents, including the "Guidelines for Ambulatory Anesthesia and Surgery," and "Statement on the Anesthesia Care Team" state that all anesthetics should be delivered by or under the medical direction of an anesthesiologist. ASA acknowledges, however, that Medicare regulations and the laws or regulations of virtually all states recognize that where anesthesiologist participation is not practical, nonphysician anesthesia providers must at a minimum be medically supervised by a licensed physician.

ASA believes that anesthesiologist participation in all office-based surgery is the best means to achieve the safest anesthesia care. It does not oppose, however, regulatory requirements that, where necessary, speak merely in terms of "physician" medical supervision. Those requirements should, however, require that the medically supervising physician be specifically trained in sedation, anesthesia and rescue techniques appropriate to the type of sedation or anesthesia being provided and to the office-based surgery being performed.

ASA believes that specific anesthesia training for medically supervising, while important in all anesthetizing locations, is especially critical in connection with office-based surgery where normal institutional back-up or emergency facilities and capacities are often not available.

This statement should be read in conjunction with ASA's Guidelines for Office-Based Anesthesia, adopted by its House of Delegates in October 2004.

Statement on Qualifications of Anesthesia Providers in the Office-Based Setting (2009) is reprinted with permission of the American Society of Anesthesiologists, 520 N. Northwest Highway, Park Ridge, IL 60068-2573.

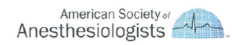

American Society of
Anesthesiologists

CONTINUUM OF DEPTH OF SEDATION:
DEFINITION OF GENERAL ANESTHESIA AND LEVELS OF SEDATION/ANALGESIA *

Committee of Origin: Quality Management and Departmental Administration

**(Approved by the ASA House of Delegates on October 13, 1999, and amended on
October 21, 2009)**

	Minimal Sedation Anxiolysis	*Moderate Sedation/ Analgesia* ("Conscious Sedation")	*Deep Sedation/ Analgesia*	*General Anesthesia*
Responsiveness	Normal response to verbal stimulation	Purposeful** response to verbal or tactile stimulation	Purposeful** response following repeated or painful stimulation	Unarousable even with painful stimulus
Airway	Unaffected	No intervention required	Intervention may be required	Intervention often required
Spontaneous Ventilation	Unaffected	Adequate	May be inadequate	Frequently inadequate
Cardiovascular Function	Unaffected	Usually maintained	Usually maintained	May be impaired

Minimal Sedation (Anxiolysis) is a drug-induced state during which patients respond normally to verbal commands. Although cognitive function and physical coordination may be impaired, airway reflexes, and ventilatory and cardiovascular functions are unaffected.

Moderate Sedation/Analgesia ("Conscious Sedation") is a drug-induced depression of consciousness during which patients respond purposefully** to verbal commands, either alone or accompanied by light tactile stimulation. No interventions are required to maintain a patent airway, and spontaneous ventilation is adequate. Cardiovascular function is usually maintained.

*   Monitored Anesthesia Care does not describe the continuum of depth of sedation, rather it describes "a specific anesthesia service in which an anesthesiologist has been requested to participate in the care of a patient undergoing a diagnostic or therapeutic procedure."

** Reflex withdrawal from a painful stimulus is NOT considered a purposeful response.

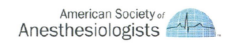

American Society *of*
Anesthesiologists

CONTINUUM OF DEPTH OF SEDATION:
DEFINITION OF GENERAL ANESTHESIA AND LEVELS OF SEDATION/ANALGESIA

Deep Sedation/Analgesia is a drug-induced depression of consciousness during which patients cannot be easily aroused but respond purposefully** following repeated or painful stimulation. The ability to independently maintain ventilatory function may be impaired. Patients may require assistance in maintaining a patent airway, and spontaneous ventilation may be inadequate. Cardiovascular function is usually maintained.

General Anesthesia is a drug-induced loss of consciousness during which patients are not arousable, even by painful stimulation. The ability to independently maintain ventilatory function is often impaired. Patients often require assistance in maintaining a patent airway, and positive pressure ventilation may be required because of depressed spontaneous ventilation or drug-induced depression of neuromuscular function. Cardiovascular function may be impaired.

Because sedation is a continuum, it is not always possible to predict how an individual patient will respond. Hence, practitioners intending to produce a given level of sedation should be able to rescue*** patients whose level of sedation becomes deeper than initially intended. Individuals administering Moderate Sedation/Analgesia ("Conscious Sedation") should be able to rescue*** patients who enter a state of Deep Sedation/Analgesia, while those administering Deep Sedation/Analgesia should be able to rescue*** patients who enter a state of General Anesthesia.

**   Reflex withdrawal from a painful stimulus is NOT considered a purposeful response.

***   Rescue of a patient from a deeper level of sedation than intended is an intervention by a practitioner proficient in airway management and advanced life support. The qualified practitioner corrects adverse physiologic consequences of the deeper-than-intended level of sedation (such as hypoventilation, hypoxia and hypotension) and returns the patient to the originally intended level of sedation. It is not appropriate to continue the procedure at an unintended level of sedation.

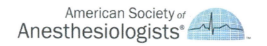

American Society *of*
Anesthesiologists®

DISTINGUISHING MONITORED ANESTHESIA CARE ("MAC") FROM MODERATE SEDATION/ANALGESIA (CONSCIOUS SEDATION)

Committee of Origin: Economics

(Approved by the ASA House of Delegates on October 27, 2004, last amended on October 21, 2009, and reaffirmed on October 16, 2013)

Moderate Sedation/Analgesia (Conscious Sedation; hereinafter known as Moderate Sedation) is a physician service recognized in the CPT procedural coding system. During Moderate Sedation, a physician supervises or personally administers sedative and/or analgesic medications that can allay patient anxiety and control pain during a diagnostic or therapeutic procedure. Such drug-induced depression of a patient's level of consciousness to a "moderate" level of sedation, as defined in the Joint Commission (TJC) standards, is intended to facilitate the successful performance of the diagnostic or therapeutic procedure while providing patient comfort and cooperation. Physicians providing moderate sedation must be qualified to recognize "deep" sedation, manage its consequences and adjust the level of sedation to a "moderate" or lesser level. The continual assessment of the effects of sedative or analgesic medications on the level of consciousness and on cardiac and respiratory function is an integral element of this service.

The American Society of Anesthesiologists has defined Monitored Anesthesia Care (*see Position on Monitored Anesthesia Care, updated on October 16, 2013*). This physician service can be distinguished from Moderate Sedation in several ways. An essential component of MAC is the anesthesia assessment and management of a patient's actual or anticipated physiological derangements or medical problems that may occur during a diagnostic or therapeutic procedure. While Monitored Anesthesia Care may include the administration of sedatives and/or analgesics often used for Moderate Sedation, the provider of MAC must be prepared and qualified to convert to general anesthesia when necessary. Additionally, a provider's ability to intervene to rescue a patient's airway from any sedation-induced compromise is a prerequisite to the qualifications to provide Monitored Anesthesia Care. By contrast, Moderate Sedation is not expected to induce depths of sedation that would impair the patient's own ability to maintain the integrity of his or her airway. These components of Monitored Anesthesia Care are unique aspects of an anesthesia service that are not part of Moderate Sedation.

The administration of sedatives, hypnotics, analgesics, as well as anesthetic drugs commonly used for the induction and maintenance of general anesthesia is often, but not always, a part of Monitored Anesthesia Care. In some patients who may require only minimal sedation, MAC is often indicated because even small doses of these medications could precipitate adverse physiologic responses that would necessitate acute clinical interventions and resuscitation. If a patient's condition and/or a procedural requirement is likely to require sedation to a "deep" level or even to a transient period of general anesthesia, only a practitioner privileged to provide anesthesia services should be allowed to manage the sedation. Due to the strong likelihood that "deep" sedation may, with or without intention, transition to general anesthesia, the skills of an anesthesia provider are necessary to manage the effects of general anesthesia on the patient as well as to return the patient quickly to a state of "deep" or lesser sedation.

Like all anesthesia services, Monitored Anesthesia Care includes an array of post-procedure responsibilities beyond the expectations of practitioners providing Moderate Sedation, including

Distinguishing Monitored Analgesia Care ("MAC") from Moderate Sedation/ Analgesia (Conscious Sedation) (2009) is reprinted with permission of the American Society of Anesthesiologists, 520 N. Northwest Highway, Park Ridge, IL 60068-2573.

American Society *of*
Anesthesiologists®

assuring a return to full consciousness, relief of pain, management of adverse physiological responses or side effects from medications administered during the procedure, as well as the diagnosis and treatment of co-existing medical problems.

Monitored Anesthesia Care allows for the safe administration of a maximal depth of sedation in excess of that provided during Moderate Sedation. The ability to adjust the sedation level from full consciousness to general anesthesia during the course of a procedure provides maximal flexibility in matching sedation level to patient needs and procedural requirements. In situations where the procedure is more invasive or when the patient is especially fragile, optimizing sedation level is necessary to achieve ideal procedural conditions.

In summary, Monitored Anesthesia Care is a physician service that is clearly distinct from Moderate Sedation due to the expectations and qualifications of the provider who must be able to utilize all anesthesia resources to support life and to provide patient comfort and safety during a diagnostic or therapeutic procedure.

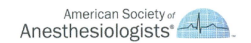

American Society of
Anesthesiologists®

POSITION ON MONITORED ANESTHESIA CARE

Committee of Origin: Economics

(Approved by the House of Delegates on October 25, 2005, and last amended on October 16, 2013)

Monitored anesthesia care is a specific anesthesia service for a diagnostic or therapeutic procedure. Indications for monitored anesthesia care include the nature of the procedure, the patient's clinical condition and/or the potential need to convert to a general or regional anesthetic.

Monitored anesthesia care includes all aspects of anesthesia care – a preprocedure visit, intraprocedure care and postprocedure anesthesia management. During monitored anesthesia care, the anesthesiologist provides or medically directs a number of specific services, including but not limited to:

- Diagnosis and treatment of clinical problems that occur during the procedure
- Support of vital functions
- Administration of sedatives, analgesics, hypnotics, anesthetic agents or other medications as necessary for patient safety
- Psychological support and physical comfort
- Provision of other medical services as needed to complete the procedure safely.

Monitored anesthesia care may include varying levels of sedation, analgesia and anxiolysis as necessary. The provider of monitored anesthesia care must be prepared and qualified to convert to general anesthesia when necessary. If the patient loses consciousness and the ability to respond purposefully, the anesthesia care is a general anesthetic, irrespective of whether airway instrumentation is required.

Monitored anesthesia care is a physician service provided to an individual patient. It should be subject to the same level of payment as general or regional anesthesia. Accordingly, the ASA Relative Value Guide® provides for the use of proper base units, time and any appropriate modifier units as the basis for determining payment.

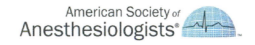

STATEMENT ON THE INTEROPERABILITY OF MEDICAL DEVICES

Committee of Origin: Equipment and Facilities

(Approved by the ASA House of Delegates on October 22, 2008 and reaffirmed on October 16, 2013)

ASA believes that intercommunication and interoperability of electronic medical devices could lead to important advances in patient safety and patient care, and that the standards and protocols to allow such seamless intercommunication should be developed fully with these advances in mind. ASA also recognizes that, as in all technological advances, interoperability poses safety and medico legal challenges as well. The development of standards and production of interoperable equipment protocols should strike the proper balance to achieve maximum patient safety, efficiency, and outcome benefit.

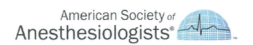

American Society of
Anesthesiologists®

STATEMENT ON NONOPERATING ROOM ANESTHETIZING LOCATIONS

Committee of Origin: Standards and Practice Parameters

(Approved by the ASA House of Delegates on October 19, 1994, and last amended on October 16, 2013)

These guidelines apply to all anesthesia care involving anesthesiology personnel for procedures intended to be per-formed in locations outside an operating room. These are minimal guidelines which may be exceeded at any time based on the judgment of the involved anesthesia personnel. These guidelines encourage quality patient care but observing them cannot guarantee any specific patient outcome. These guidelines are subject to revision from time to time, as warranted by the evolution of technology and practice. ASA Standards, Guidelines and Policies should be adhered to in all nonoperating room settings except where they are not applicable to the individual patient or care setting.

1. There should be in each location a reliable source of oxygen adequate for the length of the procedure. There should also be a backup supply. Prior to administering any anesthetic, the anesthesiologist should consider the capabilities, limitations and accessibility of both the primary and backup oxygen sources. Oxygen piped from a central source, meeting applicable codes, is strongly encouraged. The backup system should include the equivalent of at least a full E cylinder.

2. There should be in each location an adequate and reliable source of suction. Suction apparatus that meets operating room standards is strongly encouraged.

3. In any location in which inhalation anesthetics are administered, there should be an adequate and reliable system for scavenging waste anesthetic gases.

4. There should be in each location: (a) a self-inflating hand resuscitator bag capable of administering at least 90 percent oxygen as a means to deliver positive pressure ventilation; (b) adequate anesthesia drugs, supplies and equipment for the intended anesthesia care; and (c) adequate monitoring equipment to allow adherence to the "Standards for Basic Anesthetic Monitoring." In any location in which inhalation anesthesia is to be administered, there should be an anesthesia machine equivalent in function to that employed in operating rooms and maintained to current operating room standards.

5. There should be in each location, sufficient electrical outlets to satisfy anesthesia machine and monitoring equipment requirements, including clearly labeled outlets connected to an emergency power supply. In any anesthetizing location determined by the health care facility to be a "wet location" (e.g., for cystoscopy or arthroscopy or a birthing room in labor and delivery), either isolated electric power or electric circuits with ground fault circuit interrupters should be provided.*

6. There should be in each location, provision for adequate illumination of the patient, anesthesia machine (when present) and monitoring equipment. In addition, a form of battery-powered illumination other than a laryngoscope should be immediately available.

7. There should be in each location, sufficient space to accommodate necessary equipment and personnel and to allow expeditious access to the patient, anesthesia machine (when present) and monitoring equipment.

American Society of
Anesthesiologists®

8. There should be immediately available in each location, an emergency cart with a defibrillator, emergency drugs and other equipment adequate to provide cardiopulmonary resuscitation

9. There should be in each location adequate staff trained to support the anesthesiologist. There should be immediately available in each location, a reliable means of two-way communication to request assistance.

10. For each location, all applicable building and safety codes and facility standards, where they exist, should be observed

11. Appropriate postanesthesia management should be provided (see Standards for Postanesthesia Care). In addition to the anesthesiologist, adequate numbers of trained staff and appropriate equipment should be available to safely transport the patient to a postanesthsia care unit.

*See National Fire Protection Association. Health Care Facilities Code 99; Quincy, MA: NFPA, 2012.

STATEMENT ON RESPIRATORY MONITORING DURING ENDOSCOPIC PROCEDURES
Committee of Origin: Ambulatory Surgical Care
(Approved by the ASA House of Delegates on October 21, 2009)

Monitoring for exhaled carbon dioxide should be considered during endoscopic procedures in which sedation is provided with propofol alone or in combination with opioids and/or benzodiazepines, and especially during these procedures on the upper gastrointestinal tract. Careful attention to airway management must be provided during endoscopic retrograde cholangiopancreaticography (ERCP) procedures performed in the prone position where ventilatory monitoring, airway maintenance, and resuscitation may be especially difficult.

Statement on Respiratory Monitoring During Endoscopic Procedures (2009) is reprinted with permission of the American Society of Anesthesiologists, 520 N. Northwest Highway, Park Ridge, IL 60068-2573.

Index

A

Ablation
catheter-based, 102–107
anesthesia protocols for, 104b
atrial fibrillation, 102–104, 102f–103f
challenges, isoproterol, 104
challenges, other drugs, 104
complications of, 105–106, 106t
hybrid convergent procedures, 105, 105f
for other dysrhythmias, 106–107
laser, 138
radiofrequency (RFA), 139
Acarbose, 79
ACC. See American College of Cardiology (ACC).
Accountability structures, 6
ACE inhibitors. See Angiotensin-converting enzyme (ACE) inhibitors.
ACLS protocols. See Advanced Cardiac Life Support (ACLS) protocols.
Action potentials, 96–97, 97f
modulation, 97
phase 0 (depolarization), 96
phase 1 (early repolarization), 96
phase 2 (plateau), 96–97
phase 3 (repolarization), 97
phase 4 (resting), 97
Active errors, 39–40
Additional call positions, 182
Adjustment, risk, 6
Admission provisions, unplanned, 5. See also Reactive approaches.
Advanced Cardiac Life Support (ACLS) protocols, 115
Adverse events
as learning opportunities, 6–7
reporting guidelines for, 38
responses to, 5–6. See also Reactive approaches.
Agressive blood pressure lowering, 75
AHA. See American Heart Association (AHA) recommendations.
AIMS. See Anesthesia information management systems (AIMS).
Air bubble precautions, 92, 93b
Air-conditioning and heat systems, 10–11
Air embolization, systemic, 92, 93b
Airway management
airway bleeding, 147
airway loss, 148
for bronchoscopy, 143–145
bilevel positive airway pressure (BiPAP), 145
continuous positive airway pressure (CPAP), 145
criteria for, 143
endotracheal tubes, 145
no airway, 143–145
noninvasive ventilation (NIV), 145
rigid bronchoscopy, 145
supraglottic airways (SGAs), 143–145, 143b, 144t
central airway obstructions amnd, 138
central airway obstructions and, 138
for electrophysiology procedures, 93–94, 94f

Airway management (Continued)
examinations, 70–72, 73b
reflex supression, 141
stenting, 138–139
supplies checklists, 24, 24b
for upper gastrointestinal (GI) endoscopy, 128–129, 129f
ALARA principle. See Low As Reasonably Achievable (ALARA) principle.
Alerts, automated, 42
Alfieri edge-to-edge repairs, 88, 89f
Allergic reactions, 28, 28b
American College of Cardiology (ACC)
stent recommendations, 74–75, 75b
testing and revascularization recommendations, 73, 73f
American College of Chest Physicians, 140
American College of Emergency Physicians, 30–31
American College of Radiology recommendations, 21
American Heart Association (AHA)
recommendations, 74, 74b
revascularization, 73, 73f
testing, 73, 73f
American Society of Anesthesiologists (ASA)
guidelines
definitions and standards, 211
Continuum of Depth of Sedation: Definition of General Anesthesia and Levels of Sedation/Analgesia (2009), 211, 238f–240f
Distinguishing Monitored Anesthesia Care ("MAC") from Moderate Sedation/Analgesia (Conscious Sedation), 211, 240f–242f
Position on Monitored Anesthesia Care (2005, 2013), 211, 242f
Statement on the Interoperability of Medical Devices (2008, 2013), 211, 243f
monitoing and equipment, 211
Statement on Nonoperating Room Anesthetizing Locations (2013), 211, 244f–246f
Statement on Respiratory Monitoring During Endoscopic Procedures (2009), 211, 246f
personnel, priviledges, and credentials, 211
Advisory in Granting Privileges for Deep Sedation to Non-Anesthesiologist Sedation Practitioners (2010), 211, 223f–232f
Guidelines for Ambulatory Anesthesia and Surgery (2013), 41–42, 211, 232f–234f
Guidelines for Office-Based Anesthesia (2009), 41–42, 211, 234f–237f
Statement on Granting Privileges for Administration of Moderate Sedation to Practitioners Who Are Not Anesthesia Professionals (2011), 211, 213f–223f
Statement on Qualifications of Anesthesia Providers in the Office-Based Setting (2009), 211, 237f
American Society of Testing Materials (ASTM)
guidelines, 22

Analyses
Closed Claims, 31
failure mode and analysis (FMEA), 4–5
finanacial vs. operational, 183–189
health care failure mode and analysis (HFMEA), 4–5
human factor (HFAs), 40–41
profit, 186, 186f
root cause (RCAs), 5–6, 39–40. See also Reactive approaches.
Anaphylactic reactions, 28, 28b
Ancillary support, 187–188
Anemia, 77
Anesthesia care (non-operating room)
financial considerations for
analyses, financial vs. operational, 183–189
competitive strategies, 190–198
scheduling services, 177–182
future considerations for
staffing coverage, novel, 205–210
systems development, 199–204
management principles for
bronchoscopy suites, 137–150
colonoscopy suites, 132–136
continuous quality improvement (CQI), 35–42
endoscopy, upper gastrointestinal, 126–131
high-frequency ventilation (HFV), 117–125
intravenous (IV) anesthesia and sedation, 50–60
magnetic resonance imaging (MRI) environments, 171–176
monitoring issues, critical, 43–49
radiology suites, 151–160
radiology suites, pediatric, 161–170
practices and principles for
cardioversion procedures, 113–116
catheterization laboratory procedures, 82–90
electrophysiology procedures, 91–112
practice procedures, 61–69
preoperative evaluations, 70–81
respiratory immobilization procedures, 113–116
preparation activites for
anesthesiologist roles in, 30–34
excellence criteria, design, 8–17
excellence criteria, engineering, 1–7
medications, critical, 18–29
room set-ups, 18–29
standards, safety and engineering, 8–17
supplies, critical, 18–29
Anesthesia information management systems (AIMS), 41–42
Anesthesia kits, 33
Anesthesia Quality Institute (AQI), Recommended Quality Indicators, 37–38, 39t
Anesthesiologist roles, 30–34
in anesthesia and sedation levels, 31–32
in equipment selection criteria, 33
future perspectives of, 30, 34
historical perspectives of, 30
importance of, 34
in monitored anesthesia care (MAC), 31–32
in nil per os (NPO) standards, 30–31

Page numbers followed by *b*, *t*, and *f* indicate boxes, tables, and figures, respectively.

Anesthesiologist roles *(Continued)*
    oversight roles, 30–31
    with pediatric patients, 30
    personnel-related, 33–34
    in propofol credentialing, 30–31
    recent changes in, 30
    in safe practice organization, 32–33
Anesthetic records, 113
Angiotensin-converting enzyme (ACE) inhibitors, 78
Antacids, 140
Antibiotic prophylaxis, 74
Anticholinergics, 140
Anticoagulant therapy, 74–75, 79, 113–114
Antiemetics, 140
Antihypertensives, 78
Antiplatelet therapy, 75b, 78–79
Anxiolysis, 62
Aortic regurgitation, 86–87
Aortic stenosis, 83
Aortic valve replacement (AVR), 83–85
APC. *See* Argon plasma coagulation (APC).
Apnea physiology, 76, 124
Apron, lead glass, 178
AQI. *See* Anesthesia Quality Institute (AQI),
        Recommended Quality Indicators.
Area-specific units, 180
Argon plasma coagulation (APC), 138
Arrhythmias, cardiac, 100–102, 100b
    bradyarrhythmias, 100–102, 100b
    comparisons of, 100b
    tachyarrhythmias, 100–102, 100b
ASA guidelines. *See* American Society of
        Anesthesiologists (ASA) guidelines.
Aspirin, 78–79
Atrial fibrillation ablation, 102–104, 102f–103f. *See
        also* Ablation.
Attending level discussions, 180
Automated alerts, 42
Auto-positive end-expiratory pressure
        (auto-PEEP), 122–123, 123f
AVR. *See* Aortic valve replacement (AVR).
Axial dispersion, 121, 121f

B
Backup support, 5
Balloon
    dilation, bronchoscopic, 139
    mitral valvuloplasty, 82
Bar code use, 42
Barotrauma, 147
Barriers, entry, 185
Basic economics, 185–186
Beat-to-beat blood pressure, 82–83
Benchmarking, 42
Benzocaine spray, 28–29
Benzodiazepines, 80, 99–100
Best practices principle, 36
Beta-andrenergic blockers, 73, 78
Bias, perception, 38
Bilevel positive airway pressure (BiPAP), 145
Billing, 185–186
BiPAP. *See* Bilevel positive airway pressure (BiPAP).
Bleeding, airway, 147
Block
    heart, 87
    schedules, 179–182
BMI. *See* Body mass index (BMI).
Body mass index (BMI), 76
Booking, cases, 179
Bradyarrhythmias, 100–102, 100b. *See also* Cardiac
        arrhythmias.
Breath stacking, 122–123, 123f. *See also* High-
        frequency ventilation (HFV).
Brief deep sedation, 30–31

Bronchial theroplasty, 139
Bronchodilators, 140–141
Bronchoscopic balloon dilation, 139
Bronchoscopic lung volume reduction, 139
Bronchoscopy suites, 137–150
    airway choices, 143–145
        bilevel positive airway pressure (BiPAP), 145
        continuous positive airway pressure (CPAP), 145
        criteria for, 143
        endotracheal tubes, 145
        no airway, 143–145
        nonivasive ventilation (NIV), 145
        rigid bronchoscopy, 145
        supraglottic airways (SGAs), 143–145, 143b, 144t
    anesthesia management, 140–142
        airway reflex supression and, 141
        antacids, 140
        anticholinergics, 140
        antiemetics, 140
        bronchodilators, 140–141
        gastrokinetics, 140
        local anesthetics, 141
        moderate sedation, 141–142
        nasal anesthesia, 141
        for posterior oropharynx, 141
        premedications, 140–141
        sedatives, 140
        steroids, 140
        for upper airways, 141
    complications management, 147–148
        airway bleeding, 147
        airway loss, 148
        barotrauma, 147
        emergency cricothyroidotomy, 148, 148b
        fire, 147–148
        hypoxia, 147
        pneumocardium, 147
        pneumomediastinum, 147
        pneumoperitoneum, 147
        pneumopthorax, 147
        subcutaneous emphysema, 147
        tracheal laceration/rupture, 148
    emergence, 146–147
    extubation, 146–147
    fluid management, 146–147
    future directions for, 148
    general anesthesia, 142–143
        induction, 142–143
        maintenenace, 142
        muscle relaxation, 142–143
    interventional bronchoscopic techniques, 137–139
        airway stenting, 138–139
        anesthesia for, 137, 138t
        bronchial theroplasty, 139
        bronchoscopic balloon dilation, 139
        bronchoscopic lung volume reduction, 139
        for central airway obstructions, 138
        electromagnetic navigational bronchoscopy
                (ENB), 137–138
        endobrachial ultrasound with transbronchial
                needle aspiration (EBUS-TBNA), 137
        radiofrequency ablation (RFA), 139
    monitoring, 146
    oxygenation, 145–146
    postoperative management, 147
    preoperative evaluations, 139–140
        histories, 139–140
        preprocedure studies, 140
        systems reviews, 139–140
    resources for, 148
    ventilation techniques, 145–146
        jet ventilation, 146
        jet ventilation, high-frequency (HFJV), 146
        jet ventilation, low-frequency (LFJV), 146
        positive-pressure ventilation, 145–146

Bubble precautions, 92, 93b
Bundled payments, 182
Bypass grafting, 73

C
CABG. *See* Coronary artery.
CAD. *See* Coronary artery.
Calcific aortic stenosis, 83
Call positions, additional, 182
Cannulation
    femoral artery, 82–83
    radial arterial, 82–83
Carbon dioxide elimination, 122. *See also* High-
        frequency ventilation (HFV).
    catheter position, 122
    driving pressure, 122
    inspiratory fraction, 122
    mechanical load, 122
    respiratory rates, 122
Cardiac arrhythmias, 100–102, 100b
    bradyarrhythmias, 100–102, 100b
    comparisons of, 100b
    tachyarrhythmias, 100–102, 100b
Cardiac conduction, 97
Cardiac evaluation algorithms, 73, 73f
Cardiovascular medications, 78
Cardiovascular recovery rooms (CVRRs), 180
Cardioversion procedures, 113–116
    Advanced Cardiac Life Support (ACLS) protocols, 115
    cardioversion, definition of, 113
    historical perspectives of, 113
    intraoperative management, 114–115
    oucomes for, 115
    post operative care, 115
    preoperative assessments for, 113–114
        anesthetic records, 113
        anticoagulation regimen compliance, 113–114
        detailed medical histories, 114
        laboratory data reviews, 114
        medication reviews, 114
        prior cardioversion attempts, 113
    protocols for, 3–4, 4b
    resources for, 115
Cardioverterdefibrillators, 75, 75b
Care improvements, 36. *See also* Continuous quality
        improvement (CQI).
Care reimbursement, 185–186
Case
    booking, 179
    ranking, 179
Catheter-based ablation, 102–107. *See also* Ablation.
    anesthesia protocols for, 104b
    atrial fibrillation, 102–104, 102f–103f
    challenges
        isoproterol, 104
        other drugs, 104
    complications of, 105–106, 106t
    hybrid convergent procedures, 105, 105f
    for other dysrhythmias, 106–107
Catheter-delivered closure devices, 87–88
Catheterization laboratory procedures, 82–90
    balloon mitral valvuloplasty, 82
    diagnostic catheterizations, 82
    guidelines for, 82
    interventional cardiology catheterization
            laboratories (ICCLs), 82
    percutaneous coronary interventions, 82
    valves and devices, 82–90
        future directions for, 88
        hemodynamic monitoring, 82–83
        left atrial appendage (LAA) closure devices,
                84f, 88
        mitral prosthesis paravalvular regurgitation,
                transapical closure of, 87–88, 88f

Catheterization laboratory procedures *(Continued)*
  mitral valve edge-to-edge clip repairs, 85f, 88
  resources for, 90
  transcatheter aortic valve replacement (TAVR),
    83–85. *See also* Transcatheter aortic valve
    replacement (TAVR).
  transesophageal echocardiography (TEE), 82
Centers for Medicaid and Medicare Service (CMS), 30
Central airway obstructions, 138
Challenges
  isoproterol, 104
  other drugs, 104
Checklists, 3–4, 3t, 4b
  presurgical, 3–4, 3t
  for quality models, 36, 37t
Chest radiographs, preoperative, 78
Chronic conditions
  anticoagulation, 79
  chronic obstructive pulmonary disease (COPD),
    140
Clear accountability structures, 6
Clinical
  coverge contracts, 179–180, 181f
  decision support systems, 42
  outcomes indicators, 37–38, 39t. *See also*
    Indicators.
  support backup, 5
Clopidogrel (Plavix), 78–79
Closed Claims analyses, 31, 38. *See also* Analyses.
Closure devices
  catheter-delivered, 87–88
  left atrial appendage (LAA), 84f, 88
C-Mac emergency airway equipment,
    178
CMS. *See* Centers for Medicaid and Medicare Service
    (CMS).
Coexisting diseases, 73–78
  antibiotic prophylaxis for, 74
  anticoagulant therapy and, 74–75
  coronary artery disease (CAD), 73
  diabetes, 76
  heart failure, 73
  heart murmurs, 73–74
  hypertension, 75
  implantable cardioverterdefibrillators (ICDs) and,
    75, 75b
  increased risks with, 73
  obesity, 76
  obstructive sleep apnea (OSA), 76
  percutaneous coronary interventions (PCIs) and,
    74–75
  pregnancy, 77–78
  pulmonary disease, 75–76
  reneal disease, 76–77
  sichemic heart disease, 73
  stents and, 74–75
"Cold" therapies, 138
Colonoscopy procedures, 132–136
  anesthesiology assistance guidelines, 132, 132b
  anesthetic choices, 133–135, 133t
    sedation levels, 133–134
    sedative medications, 133–135, 134t
  complications of, 135
  difficult intubation predictors, 133b
  difficult mask ventilation predictors, 133b
  historical perspectives of, 132
  monitoring, 133
  patient positioning, 133
  resources for, 135
Color-coded
  floor lines, 14
  systems, 3, 31–32
Color flow Doppler assessments, 82
Combination insulin, 79. *See also* Insulin.
Comfirmation metrics, 37

Communication considerations, 10
Comorbidities, 73–78
  antibiotic prophylaxis and, 74
  anticoagulant therapy and, 74–75
  coexisting diseases
    heart murmurs, 73–74
  coronary artery disease (CAD), 73
  diabetes, 76
  heart failure, 73
  hypertension, 75
  implantable cardioverterdefibrillators (ICDs) and,
    75, 75b
  increased risks with, 73
  obesity, 76
  obstructive sleep apnea (OSA), 76
  percutaneous coronary interventions (PCIs) and,
    74–75
  pregnancy, 77–78
  pulmonary disease, 75–76
  reneal disease, 76–77
  stents and, 74–75
Competitive strategies, 190–198. *See also* Financial
    considerations.
  alternative and additional modalities, 196
  depth of sedation continuum, 190, 191t
  economic considerations, 194–195
  entry barriers, 185
  future directions for, 197
  moderate sedation, 196
  practice patterns, 190–191
  propofol use
    guidelines for, 195–196
    by nonanesthesiologists, 191–192
    policy considerations for, 195–196
    safety considerations for, 192–194
Competitive landscapes, 184–185
Competitors, 184
Complete
  anesthesia kits, 33
  heart block, 101
Complex procedure scheduling, 182
Complications
  of bronchoscopy, 147–148
  of catheter-based ablations, 105–106, 106t
  of lead extractions, 108
  of stenting, 139
  of transcatheter aortic valve replacement (TAVR),
    85–87
    aortic regurgitation, 86–87
Conduction, cardiac, 97
Conscious sedation, 62
Continuous invasive arterial pressure measurement,
    82–83
Continuous positive airway pressure (CPAP), 76,
    139, 145
Continuous quality improvement (CQI), 35–42
  analyses. *See also* Analyses.
    human factor (HFAs), 40–41
    root cause (RCAs), 39–40
  definition of, 36
  electronic medical records (EMRs) and, 41
  future directions for, 41
    anesthesia information management systems
      (AIMS), 41–42
    automated alerts, 42
    bar code use, 42
    clinical decision support systems, 42
    electronic medical records (EMRs), 41
    health information technologies (HITs), 41
  importance of, 42
  indicator selection criteria, 36–37
    best practices principle and, 36
    Donabedian clinical indicators as basis of, 36
    outcomes, 37
    process, 36

Continuous quality improvement *(Continued)*
    quality-of-care indicators, 38
    structural, 36
  indicator validation, 37–38
    Anesthesia Quality Institute (AQI),
      Recommended Quality Indicators, 37–38,
      39t
    benchmarking to national standards, 42
    comfirmation metrics for, 37
    limitations of, 36
    patient satisfaction surveys and, 38, 40f
    validity, definition of, 37
  Institute of Medicine (IOM) achievement areas, 36
  models, 36, 38
    checklists for, 36, 37t
    definition of, 36
    descriptions of, 38
    Donabedian Quality-of-Care Framework, 36
    plan-do-study-act approaches, 36, 37f
  quality in health care, definition of, 36
  reporting guidelines
    for adverse events, 38
    for critical incidents, 38
    for sentinel events, 38
  surveillance processes for, 41–42
  Universal Protocol and, 41
Contracts, 179–180, 181f
Contrast
  administration protocols, 76–77
  nephropathy, contrast-induced, 28
Controlled substances, 80
Convection, 121
Convergent hybrid procedures, 105, 105f. *See also*
    Catheter-based ablation.
"Cookbook medicine" concept, 3
COPD. *See* Chronic conditions.
Coronary artery
  bypass grafting (CABG), 73
  disease (CAD), 73
  obstructions, 87
Coronary interventions, percutaneous. *See*
    Percutaneous coronary interventions (PCIs).
Cost
  accounting, 185f, 185–186
  total, 185f, 185–186
  variable, 185f, 185–186
  volume profit analyses, 186, 186f. *See also*
    Analyses.
Coverge contracts, 179–180, 181f
CPAP. *See* Continuous positive airway pressure
    (CPAP).
CQI. *See* Continuous quality improvement (CQI).
Credentialing, 30–31
Cricothyroidotomy, 148, 148b
Critical incidents
  reporting guidelines for, 38
Critical materials and procedures
  medications, 26–28
    allergic reactions and, 28
    benzocaine spray, 28–29
    dantrolene, 29
    dexmedetomide, 27
    on emergency carts, 26
    ketamine, 27–28
    low-light situations and, 26
    for malignant hyperthermia, 29
    methemoglobinemia and, 28–29
    midazolam, 26–27
    propofol, 27
    tackle box transporation of, 26, 26f
  monitoring, 43–49
  supplies, 24, 24b
Crossing the Quality Chasm report (Institute of
    Medicine), 2
Cultural interactions, 4

Customers, new, 183
CVRRs. *See* Cardiovascular recovery rooms (CVRRs)
Cyanosis, 28–29
CyberKnife procedures, 20–21

D

Dabigartran (Pradaxa), 79
Daily
    huddles, 5
    schedules, 179–182, 180t. *See also* Scheduling
        services.
        area-specific postanesthesia care units, 180
        block, 179–182
        case rankings, 179
        clinical coverge contracts, 179–180, 181f
        fixed, 179–182
        imaging technique incorporation, 180–182
        night and weekend procedures, 180
Dantrolene, 29
Debridement, mechanical, 138
Decision support systems, 42
Deep sedation, 62
Depolarization phase, 96. *See also* Action potentials.
Design excellence, 8–17
    for communication, 10
    for electrical power, 11
    ergonomics, 9–10
    evaculation routes, 10
    guidelines for, 8–9
    humidity control, 12
    hybrid operating rooms, 14–15. *See also* Hybrid
        operating rooms.
    infection control, 12
    intraoperative suites
        angiography (IA), 16f, 11
        magnetic resonance (MRI), 14–15, 14t, 15f
    lighting, 10
    magnetic resonance imaging (MRI), areas, 13–14,
        13f, 14t
    materials management, 12
    medical gases management, 11–12
    minimum size guidelines, 9, 9t
    movement-related considerations, 10
    noise control, 10
    post-anesthesia care units (PACUs), 9
    power management, 11–12
    radiation therapy areas, 12–13
    simulations and, 10
    temperature control, 10–11
    timelines for, 17t
    ventilation, 12
Detailed medical histories, 114
Development, systems, 199–204
Device selection criteria, 3
Dexmedetomidine, 27, 100, 134t, 135
Diabetes, 76
Diagnostic catheterizations, 82
Difficult airways, 24, 178
Diffusion, 121
Dilation, balloon, 139
Dispersion, axial, 121, 121f
Dissociative sedation, 30–31
Distribution-workload optimization, 187, 187f
Diuretics, 78
DLTs. *See* Double-lumen endotraheal tubes (DLTs).
Donabedian
    clinical indicators, 36
    Quality-of-Care Framework, 36
Door sizes, 178
Double-lumen endotraheal tubes (DLTs), 139
Driving pressure, 122
Dual-frequency jet ventilators, 118, 119f. *See also*
    High-frequency ventilation (HFV).
Dysrhythmias, 106–107

E

Early repolarization phase, 96. *See also* Action
    potentials.
EBUS-TBNA. *See* Endobrachial ultrasound with
    transbronchial needle aspiration (EBUS-TBNA).
ECGs. *See* Electrocardiograms (ECGs).
Echocardiography, transesophageal (TEE), 73–74
Economics, basic, 185–186
Edwards SAPIEN valves, 83
Effectiveness, 36
Efficiency, 36
EGD. *See* Esophagogastroduodenoscopy (EGD).
Electrically-controlled ventilator devices, 118f, 121.
    See also High-frequency ventilation (HFV).
Electrical outlet numbers, 178
Electrical power, 11
Electrocardiograms (ECGs), 78
Electrocautery, 138
Electromagnetic navigational bronchoscopy (ENB),
    137–138
Electronic medical records (EMRs), 41
Electronic schedulers, 188, 189t
Electrophysiology procedures, 91–112
    action potentials, 96–97, 97f
    air bubble precautions for, 92, 93b
    airway management for, 93–94, 94f
    anesthesiologist roles in, 91, 92f
    anesthetic management for, 93
    cardiac arrhythmias, 100–102, 100b
        bradyarrhythmias, 100–102, 100b
        comparisons of, 100b
        tachyarrhythmias, 100–102, 100b
    catheter-based ablations, 102–107
        anesthesia protocols for, 104b
        atrial fibrillation, 102–104, 102f–103f
        challenges, isoproterol, 104
        challenges, other drugs, 104
        complications of, 105–106, 106t
        hybrid convergent procedures, 105, 105f
        for other dysrhythmias, 106–107
    common cases, 91, 92t
    communication considerations for, 95, 96f
    device implantation, 107–108
        complications of, 108
        indications for, 107
        protocols for, 107
    environmental factors for, 95
    fluid management for, 95
    future directions for, 110
    lead extractions, 108–109
        complications of, 108
        indications for, 108
        protocols for, 108–109b
    monitoring for, 94–95
    noninvasive programmed stimulation (NIPS), 109
        indications for, 109
        protocols for, 109b
    padding for, 94, 94f
    pain management for, 109
    pharmacopeia for, 95, 96t
        action potentials, 96–97, 97f
        anesthetic drug effects, 97–98
        benzodiazepines, 99–100
        cardiac conduction and, 97
        dexmedetomidine, 100
        drug effects, basic, 95
        environmental effects, 97
        etomidate, 100
        humoral effects, 97
        inhalation agents, 98
        neuromuscular blockers, 100
        opioids, 99
        parasympathetic nervous system effects of, 97
        propofol, 98–99
        sympathetic nervous system effects of, 97

Electrophysiology procedures (*Continued*)
    positioning for, 94
    postoperative care, 109
    preprocedure testing for, 92–100, 93b
    resources for, 110
    teamwork considerations for, 95
    temperature control for, 95
Embolization, systemic air, 92, 93b
Emergency
    airway equipment, 178
    carts, 26
    cricothyroidotomy, 148, 148b
    help availbility, 179
Emphysema, subcutaneous, 147
EMRs. *See* Electronic medical records (EMRs).
ENB. *See* Electromagnetic navigational bronchoscopy
    (ENB).
Endobrachial ultrasound with transbronchial needle
    aspiration (EBUS-TBNA), 137
Endocarditis prophylaxis indications, 74, 74b
Endoscopic retrograde cholangiopancreatography
    (ERCP), 126. *See also* Upper gastrointestinal (GI)
    endoscopy.
Endoscopy, upper gastrointestinal (GI), 126–131
Endotracheal tubes, 145
Engineering
    excellence criteria, 1–7
        accountability structures, clear, 6
        future perspectives of, 6–7
        historical perspectives of, 2
        importance of, 2
        organizational approaches to, 6
        patient-centered care, 6
        performance measurements, 6
        proactive *vs.* reactive approaches to, 3
        standards, 8–17
Enterococcus spp., 41
Entrainment, 121–122, 122f. *See also* High-frequency
    ventilation (HFV).
Entry barriers, 185
Equipment
    infrastructure, 187–188
    selection criteria, 33
Equitable care, 36
Equivalents, metabolic (METs), 70, 72t, 73
ERCP. *See* Endoscopic retrograde
    cholangiopancreatography (ERCP).
Ergonomics, 9–10
Errors, active, 39–40
Esophagogastroduodenoscopy (EGD), 126. *See also*
    Upper gastrointestinal (GI) endoscopy.
Etomidate, 100
Evacuation routes, 10
Evaluations, preoperative, 70–81
Event reporting systems, 5
Example profit analyses, 186–187. *See also* Analyses.
Excellence criteria
    design, 8–17
        American Society of Anesthesiologists (ASA)
            guidelines for, 8–9
        communication, 10
        electrical power, 11
        ergonomics, 9–10
        evacuation routes, 10
        humidity control, 12
        hybrid operating rooms, 14–15. *See also* Hybrid
            operating rooms.
        infection control, 12
        initial planning processes, 8–9
        intraoperative suites, angiography (IA), 16f, 11
        intraoperative suites, magnetic resonance (MRI),
            14–15, 14t, 15f
        lighting, 10
        magnetic resonance imaging (MRI), areas,
            13–14, 13f, 14t

Excellence criteria *(Continued)*
    materials management, 12
    medical gases management, 11–12
    minimum size guidelines, 9, 9t
    movement-related considerations, 10
    noice control, 10
    post-anesthesia care units (PACUs), 9
    power management, 11–12
    radiation therapy areas, 12–13
    simulations and, 10
    tasks, 10
    temperature control, 10–11
    timelines for, 17t
    ventilation, 12
  engineering, 1–7
    accountability structures, clear, 6
    future perspectives of, 6–7
    historical perspectives of, 2
    importance of, 2
    organizational approaches to, 6
    patient-centered care, 6
    performance measurements, 6
    proactive *vs.* reactive approaches to, 3
  organizational, 6
Extractions, lead, 108–109
  complications of, 108
  protocols for, 108b–109b
Extubation, 146–147
Eyewear, lead, 178

F
Facility Guidelines Institute, 8
Failure mode and analysis (FMEA), 4–5. *See also*
    Analyses.
Fall and trip risks, 24–25
Fasting guidelines, 80
FDA approvals. *See* Food and Drug Administration
    (FDA) approvals.
Femoral artery cannulation, 82–83. *See also*
    Cannulation.
Fentanyl, 134, 134t
FEV$_1$. *See* Forced expiratory volume in 1 second
    (FEV$_1$).
FiO$_2$ management, 145
Fiberoptic difficult airway cart, 178
Financial considerations
  analyses, 183–189. *See also* Analyses.
    billing, 185–186
    comparative advantages, 185
    competitive landscapes, 184–185
    cost accounting, 185f, 185–186
    cost volume profit, 186, 186f
    economic basics, 185–186
    examples of, 186–187
    market analyses, 183–184. *See also* Market
      analyses.
    operational intrastructure, 187–188
    reimbursement, 185–186
    revenue, 186
  competitive strategies, 190–198
  scheduling services, 177–182
Fire risks, 147–148
First-degree heart block, 101
Fixed
  communication designs, 10
  costs, 185f, 185–186
  schedules, 179–182
Fluid management
  for bronchoscopy preocedures, 146–147
  for electrophysiology procedures,
    95
FMEA. *See* Failure mode and analysis (FMEA).
Food and Drug Administration (FDA) approvals, 82,
    88

Forced air warming systems, 20
Forced expiratory volume in 1 second (FEV$_1$),
    139–140
Full-dose aspirin, 78–79
Funcational capacity, 70, 72t, 73

G
Gamma knife procedures, 20–21, 32
Garlic supplements, 79
Gases management, 11–12
Gastrointestinal (GI) endoscopic procedures
  colonoscopy, 132–136. *See also* Colonoscopy
    procedures.
    anesthesiology assistance guidelines, 132,
      132b
    anesthetic choices, 133–135, 133t
    complications of, 135
    monitoring, 133
    patient positioning, 133
    resources for, 135
  historical perspectives of, 132
  upper, 126–131. *See also* Upper gastrointestinal
    (GI) endoscopy.
    airway management for, 128–129, 129f
    anesthetic drugs for, 127–128, 128t
    complications of, 130, 130b
    future directions for, 130–131
    indications for, 129–130, 130b
    monitoring for, 130
    patient populations presenting for, 126
    preprocedure evaluations for, 126–127
    resources for, 131
Gastrokinetics, 140
Gawande, Atul, 3
General anesthesia, 62
General management principles
  continuous quality inprovement (CQI), 35–42
  intravenous (IV) anesthesia and sedation,
    50–60
  monitoring issues, critical, 43–49
GFRs. *See* Glomerular filtration rates (GFRs).
Gingko supplements, 79
Ginseng supplements, 79
Glargine (Lantus) insulin, 79. *See also* Insulin.
Glidescope emergency airway equipment, 178
Glomerular filtration rates (GFRs), 76–77
Gold standard concept, 6
Grafting, bypass, 73
Guidelines (ASA). *See* American Society of
    Anesthesiologists (ASA) guidelines.

H
Halothane, 98
Health care failure mode and analysis (HFMEA), 4–5.
    See also analyses.
Health information technologies (HITs), 41
Health outcomes, 36. *See also* Continuous quality
    improvement (CQI).
Heart
  block, 87
    complete, 101
    first-degree, 101
    second-degree, 101
    third-degree, 101
  failure, 73
  murmurs, 73–74
Heat and air-conditioning systems, 10–11
Help availbility, 179
Hemisternotomy, 83–84
Hemodynamic
  effects, 124
  instability, persistent, 85–86
  monitoring, 82–83

Hemopericardium, 87
Heparin
  low-molecular-weight (LMWH), 79
  subcutaneous unfractionated, 79
Herbal supplements, 79
HFE. *See* Human factors engineering (HFE).
HFMEA. *See* Health care failure mode and analysis
    (HFMEA).
HFV. *See* High-frequency ventilation (HFV).
High-decible areas, 10
High-frequency devices. *See also* High-frequency
    ventilation (HFV).
  jet ventilators (HFJVs), 118, 118f
  oscillators, 118, 119f
  percussive ventilators, 118, 120f
High-frequency ventilation (HFV), 117–125
  anesthetic management of, 124
  apnea, physiology of, 124
  breath stacking, 122–123, 123f
  carbon dioxide elimination, 122
    catheter position, 122
    driving pressure, 122
    inspiratory fraction, 122
    mechanical load, 122
    respiratory rates, 122
  entrainment, 121–122, 122f
  future directions for, 124
  hemodynamic effects of, 124
  indications for, 117
  inspired gas, humidification of, 124
  monitoring of, 123–124
  physics of, 121, 121f
    axial dispersion, 121, 121f
    convection, 121
    diffusion, 121
    pendelluft, 121, 121f
  positive end-expiratory pressure (PEEP) and, 122
  resources for, 124
  ventilator types, 118–121
    dual-frequency jet, 118, 119f
    electrically-controlled devices, 118f, 121
    fluidic valve devices, 120, 121f
    high-frequency jet, 118, 118f
    high-frequency oscillators, 118, 119f
    high-frequency percussive, 118, 120f
    manually-operated pneumatic devices,
      119–120, 120f
    negative-pressure high frequency oscillators, 119
High lung compliance, 123
High-performing organizations, 6
High-volume areas, 180
His-Purkinje system, 98
Histories, medical, 70, 71f–72f
HITs. *See* Health information technologies (HITs).
"Hot" therapies, 138
Huddles, daily, 5
Human characteristics studies, 40–41
Human factor (HFAs) analyses, 40–41. *See also*
    Analyses.
Human factors engineering (HFE), 3
Humidification, inspired gas, 124
Humidity control, 12
Hybrid convergent procedures, 105, 105f.
    See also Catheter-based ablation.
Hybrid operating rooms, 14–15, 180
  importance of, 14
  intraoperative angiography (IA), 15, 16f
  intraoperative magnetic resonance imaging (IMRI),
    14–15, 14t, 15f
Hypertension, 75
Hyperthermia, malignant, 29
Hypoglycemia, 79
Hypotension, refractory, 78
Hypovolemia, 78
Hypoxia, 147

I

IA. *See* Intraoperative angiography (IA).
IA rooms. *See* Intraoperative angiography (IA) rooms.
ICCLs. *See* Interventional cardiology catheterization laboratories (ICCLs).
ICDs. *See* Implantable cardioverterdefibrillators (ICDs).
Imaging environments. *See* Magnetic resonance imaging (MRI) environments.
Immobilization, respiratory, 113–116
Implantable cardioverterdefibrillators (ICDs), 75, 75b
IMRI. *See* Intraoperative magnetic resonance imaging (IMRI).
Indicators, 6
    selection criteria for, 36–37
        Anesthesia Quality Institute (AQI), Recommended Quality Indicators, 37–38, 39t
        best practices principle and, 36
        Donabedian clinical indicators as basis of, 36
        outcomes, 37
        process, 36
        quality-of-care indicators, 38
        structural, 36
    validation of, 37–38
        Anesthesia Quality Institute (AQI), Recommended Quality Indicators, 37–38, 39t
        benchmarking to national standards, 42
        comfirmation metrics for, 37
        limitations of, 36
        patient satisfaction surveys and, 38, 40f
        validity, definition of, 37
Individual suites, 12–15
    importance of, 12
    magnetic resonance imaging (MRI), 13–14, 13f
    radiation therapy suites, 12–13
Infection control, 12
Infrastructure, operational, 187–188
    ancillary support, 187–188
    equipment, 187–188
    staffing, 187, 187f
    utilization rates, 187
Infusion credentialing, 30–31
Inhalation agents, 91
INR. *See* International normalized ratio (INR).
INR suites. *See* Interventional neuroradiology (INR) suites.
Inspiratory fraction, 122
Inspired gas, humidification of, 124
Institute of Medicine (IOM)
    Crossing the Quality Chasm report, 2
    To Err is Human report, 2
    quality health care aims, 6
    quality in health care definitions, 6, 36
    six areas of achievement, 36
Insulin, 79
    combination, 79
    glargine (Lantus), 79
    intermediate-acting, 79
    lente, 79
    long-acting, 79
    neutral protamine Hagedorn (NPH), 79
    as perioperative medication, 79
    pumps, 79
    sensitizers, 79
Integration, services, 182
Intermediate-acting insulin, 79. *See also* Insulin.
International Normalized Ratio (INR), 79, 113–114
Interventional bronchoscopic techniques, 137–139
    airway stenting, 138–139
    anesthesia for, 137, 138t
    bronchial theroplasty, 139
    bronchoscopic balloon dilation, 139
    bronchoscopic lung volume reduction, 139

Interventional bronchoscopic techniques *(Continued)*
    for central airway obstructions, 138
    electromagnetic navigational bronchoscopy (ENB), 137–138
    endobrachial ultrasound with transbronchial needle aspiration (EBUS-TBNA), 137
    radiofrequency ablation (RFA), 139
Interventional cardiology catheterization laboratories (ICCLs), 82
Interventional neuroradiology (INR) suites, 180
Intraoperative angiography (IA), 15, 16f
Intraoperative angiography (IA) rooms, 11, 16f
Intraoperative magnetic resonance imaging (IMRI), 14–15, 14t, 15f
Intravenous (IV)
    anesthesia and sedation, 50–60
    contrast agent allergies, 28, 28b
    fluid warmers, 20
Invasive arterial pressure measurement, continuous, 82–83
Investigational devices
    for left atrial appendage (LAA) appendage closures, 88
    for mitral valve edge-to-edge clip repairs, 88
IOM. *See* Institute of Medicine (IOM).
Ischemic heart disease, 73
Isoflurane, 98
Isoproterol, 104
IV. *See* Intravenous (IV).

J

The Joint Commission (TJC)
    ambulatory and office-based anesthesia goals, 34
    anesthesiologist requirements, 31
    Sentinel Event Database, 38
    Sentinel Event Policy, 38
    site design guidelines, 8
    web site, 33

K

Kaplan-Meir survival plots, 117, 118f
Ketamine, 27–28, 134–135, 134t
Ketamine/propofol, 28
Kidney disease, 76–77
Kink-resistant cannula, 148
Kits
    anesthesia, 33
    complete *vs.* light, 33
Knowledge of procedures, 179
    case booking, 179
    emergency help availbility, 179
    patient ownership, 179
    Preoperative Evaluation Service (PES), 179

L

Laboratory
    data reviews, 114
    procedures, catheterization, 82–90
Lacerations, tracheal, 148
Landscapes, competitive, 184–185
    competitors, 184
    entry barriers, 184
Lantus insulin, 79. *See also* Insulin.
Lasers
    laser ablation, 138. *See also* Ablation.
    Nd:YAG, 147–148
Latent errors, 39–40
Lead
    extractions, 108–109
        complications of, 108
        protocols for, 108b–109b
    glass sheilds, 25–26, 26f, 178

LED lights. *See* Light-emitting diode (LED) lights.
Lente insulin, 79. *See also* Insulin.
Levels on the Continuum of Sedation statement (ASA), 31–32
Light-emitting diode (LED) lights, 10
Lighting, 10
LMWH. *See* Low-molecular-weight heparin (LMWH).
Long-acting insulin, 79. *See also* Insulin.
Loss, airway, 148. *See also* Airway management.
Low As Reasonably Achievable (ALARA) principle, 25
Low-light challenges, 26
Low-molecular-weight heparin (LMWH), 79
Lung volume reduction surgery (LVRS), 139
LVRS. *See* Lung volume reduction surgery (LVRS).

M

MAC. *See* Monitored anesthesia care (MAC).
Magnetic resonance imaging (MRI) environments, 171–176
    anesthesiologist roles in, 30
    design of, 13–14, 13f, 14t
    intraoperative magnetic resonance imaging (IMRI), 14–15, 14t, 15f
Magnetoencephalography (MEG), 169, 169b
Malignant hyperthermia, 29
Mallampati types, 71–72
Management principles
    bronchoscopy suites, 137–150
    for colonoscopy suites, 132–136
    continuous quality inprovement (CQI), 35–42
    endoscopy, upper gastrointestinal, 126–131
    high-frequency ventilation (HFV), 117–125
    intravenous (IV) anesthesia and sedation, 50–60
    magnetic resonance imaging (MRI) environments, 171–176
    monitoring issues, critical, 43–49
    radiology suites
        adult, 151–160
        pediatric, 161–170
Manually-operated pneumatic ventilators, 119–120, 120f
Mapleson C breathing circuits, 128, 129f
Market analyses, 183–184
    new customers, 183
    opportunities, 184, 184f, 184t
    trends, 183
Materials management, 12
Measurements, performance, 6
Mechanical
    debridement, 138
    load, 122
Medical gases management, 11–12
Medical histories, 70, 71f–72f, 114
Medical records
    electronic (EMRs), 41
    medication reconciliations and, 78
Medications
    critical, 26–28
    for electrophysiology procedures, 95, 96t
    reviews of, 114
Medtronic CoreValve, 83
MEG. *See* Magnetoencephalography (MEG).
Metabolic equivalents (METs), 70, 72t, 73
Metformin, 79
Methcillin-resistant *Staphylococcusa ureus*, 41
Methemoglobinemia, 28–29
Metrics, comfirmation, 37
METs. *See* Metabolic equivalents (METs).
Midazolam, 26–27, 134, 134t
Minimal sedation, 62
Minimum size guidelines, 9, 9t

Mitral valves
  balloon valvuloplasty, 82
  edge-to-edge clip repairs, 88
  mitral prosthesis paravalvular regurgitation,
    transapical closure of, 87–88, 88f
  regurgitation, percutaneous treatments, 88
Mobitz type-1 arrthymias, 101
Models, quality, 36, 38. See also Continuous quality
    improvement (CQI).
  checklists for, 36, 37t
  definition of, 36
  descriptions of, 38
  Donabedian Quality-of-Care Framework, 36
  plan-do-study-act approaches, 36, 37f
Moderate sedation, 62
Modulation, 97
Monitored anesthesia care (MAC), 31–32
Monitoring
  of bronchoscopy procedures, 146
  for electrophysiology procedures, 94–95
  of high-frequency ventilation (HFV), 123–124
  issues, critical, 43–49
Movement-related considerations, 10
MRI environments. See Magnetic resonance imaging
    (MRI) environments.
Multiple-causation principle, 5–6
Multispecialty providers, 30
Murmurs, heart, 73–74
Muscle relaxants, 100
Myocardial stunning, temporary, 115

N

"Name and blame" concept, 39
Nasal anesthesia, 141
National Emphysema Treatment Trial, 139
National Institute for Occupational Safety and Health
    (NIOSH), 25
National standards benchmarking, 42
Nd:YAG lasers. See Neodymium-doped yttrium
    aluminum garnet (Nd:YAG) lasers.
Negative-pressure high-frequency oscillators, 119
Neodymium-doped yttrium aluminum garnet
    (Nd:YAG) lasers, 138, 147–148
Nephrogenic systemic fibrosis, 76–77
Neurological injuries, 87
Neuromuscular blockers, 100
Neutral protamine Hagedorn (NPH) insulin, 79. See
    also Insulin.
New customers, 183
New-onset heart failure, 73
Nicotine replacement therapy, 80
Night and weekend scheduling, 180
Nil per os (NPO) standards, 30–31, 80, 163–164, 163t
NIOSH. See National Institute for Occupational Safety
    and Health (NIOSH).
NIPS. See Noninvasive programmed stimulation
    (NIPS).
Nitrous oxide yolks, 178
NIV. See Nonivasive ventilation (NIV).
No airway choices, 143–145
Noice control, 10
Non-extended moderate sedation, 30–31
Noninvasive programmed stimulation (NIPS), 109
  indications for, 109
  protocols for, 109b
Nonivasive ventilation (NIV), 145
Non-operating room anesthesia (NORA) care
  financial considerations for
    analyses, finanacial vs. operational, 183–189
    competitive strategies, 190–198
    scheduling services, 177–182
  future considerations for
    staffing coverage, novel, 205–210
    systems development, 199–204

Non-operating room anesthesia (NORA) care
    (Continued)
  management principles for
    bronchoscopy suites, 137–150
    colonoscopy suites, 132–136
    continuous quality improvement (CQI), 35–42
    endoscopy, upper gastrointestinal, 126–131
    high-frequency ventilation (HFV), 117–125
    intravenous (IV) anesthesia and sedation, 50–60
    magnetic resonance imaging (MRI)
        environments, 171–176
    monitoring issues, critical, 43–49
    pediatric anesthesia, 161–170
    radiology suites, 151–160
    radiology suites, pediatric, 161–170
  practices and principles for
    cardioversion procedures, 113–116
    catheterization laboratory procedures, 82–90
    electrophysiology procedures, 91–112
    practice procedures, 61–69
    preoperative evaluations, 70–81
    respiratory immobilization procedures, 113–116
  preparation activites for
    anesthesiologist roles in, 30–34
    design excellence criteria, 8–17
    engineering excellence criteria, 1–7
    medications, critical, 18–29
    room set-ups, 18–29
    standards, safety and engineering, 8–17
    supplies, critical, 18–29
NORA care. See Non-operating room anesthesia
    (NORA) care.
Novel staffing coverage, 205–210
NPH insulin. See Neutral protamine Hagedorn (NPH)
    insulin.
NPO standards. See Nil per os (NPO) standards.
Nuclear medicine, 168, 168b

O

Obesity, 76
Obstructions
  central airway, 138
  coronary artery, 87
Obstructive sleep apnea (OSA), 76
Operational
  analyses, 183–189
  infrastructure, 187–188
    ancillary support, 187–188
    equipment, 187–188
    staffing, 187, 187f
    utilization rates, 187
Opioids, 80
  for electrophysiology procedures, 99
Opportunities, 184, 184f, 184t. See also Market
    analyses.
Optimal
  resource utilization, 188
  staffing distributions, 187
Oral diabetes medications, 79
Organizational approaches, 6
Organizational excellence, 6
Oropharynx, posterior, 141
OSA. See Obstructive sleep apnea (OSA).
Oscillators. See also High-frequency ventilation (HFV).
  high-frequency, 118, 119f. See also High-frequency
    ventilation (HFV).
  negative-pressure high-frequency, 119
Outcomes
  improvements, 36. See also Continuous quality
    improvement (CQI).
  indicators, 37. See also Indicators.
Outcomes indicators, 37–38, 39t
Oversedation, 62
Oversight roles, 30–31

Ownership, patient, 179
Oxygenation, 145–146
  FiO$_2$ management, 145
  heliox management, 145
Oxygen saturation (Sao$_2$), 140

P

PACUs. See Post-anesthesia care units (PACUs).
Padding, 94, 94f
Pain management, 109
PALS training, 31
Parasympathetic nervous system, 97
Paravalvular regurgitation, transapical closure of,
    87–88, 88f
Partial information challenges, 72
PARTNER trial, 87–88
Pathogens
  Enterobacteriaceae, 41
  Enterococcus spp., 41
  Staphylococcus spp., 41
Patient-specific issues
  experience indicators, 37–38, 39t
  flow protocols, 32
  outcomes, 36
  ownership, 179
  patient-centered care, 6
    excellence criteria for, 6
    Intitutes of Medicine (IOM) acheivement area, 36
  patient-controlled
    analgesia (PCA) pumps, 67–68
    sedation (PCS) devices, 67–68
  patient-to-nurse ratios, 68
  positioning, 32
  satisfaction surveys, 38, 40f
Patterns, practice, 190–191
Pay-for-performance programs, 42
PCIs. See Percutaneous coronary interventions (PCIs)
Pediatric anesthesia, 161–170
  anestheisologist roles in, 30
  challenges of, 161
  future directions for, 169
  locations for
    radiology suites, 161–170
    remote, 161, 169
  preoperative considerations, 161–164, 162t–163t
    cheeklisto, 166b
    endotracheal tube sizes, 163t
    monitoring, 163–164, 163t
    nil per os (NPO) guidelines, 163–164, 163t
    vital signs, normal ranges for, 162t
  radiologic procedures, 164–169
    computer tomography (CT), 166, 167b
    interventional radiology, 167–168, 168b
    magnetic resonance imaging (MRI), 164–166,
        167b
    magnetoencephalography (MEG), 169, 169b
    nuclear medicine, 168, 168b
    radiation therapy, 166–167, 167b
  resources for, 169
  sentinel events, 167b
Pediatric Sedation Research Consortium, 31, 67
PEEP. See Positive end-expiratory pressure (PEEP).
Pendelluft, 121, 121f
Perception bias, 38
Percussive ventilators, high-frequency, 118, 120f. See
    also High-frequency ventilation (HFV).
Percutaneous coronary interventions (PCIs), 74–75,
    82
Performance measurements, 6
Perioperative medications, 80b
  anticoagulant therapy, 79
  antinypertensive, 78
  antiplatelet, 78–79
  aspirin, 78–79

Perioperative medications (Continued)
  cardiovascular, 78
  controlled substances, 80
  herbal supplements, 79
  insulin, 79. See also Insulin.
  medical record reconciliations and, 78
  oral diabetes, 79
  psychiatric, 79
  steroids, 79
  written instructions for, 78
Peripheral vascular injuries, 87
Persistent hemodynamic instability, 85–86
PES. See Preoperative Evaluation Service (PES).
Pharmacodynamic variability, 127
Pharmacokinetic variability, 127
Phone number lists, 24
Physical
  examinations, 71–72
  space, scheduling and, 178
  status classification, 70–73
Pin-index systems, 3
Pioglitazone, 79
Plan-do-study-act approaches, 36, 37f
Plateau phase, 96–97. See also Action potentials.
Plavix. See Clopidogrel (Plavix).
Pneumatic ventilators, manually-operated, 119–120,
    120f
Pneumocardium, 147
Pneumoperitoneum, 147
Point-of-care laboratory testing, 20
PONV. See Postoperative nausea and vomiting
    (PONV).
Portable vs. fixed communication designs, 10
Positioning
  for electrophysiology procedures, 94
Positive end-expiratory pressure (PEEP), 122,
    145–146
Positive-pressure ventilation, 145–146
Post-anesthesia care units (PACUs), 9
Posterior oropharynx, 141
Postoperative care, 109
Postoperative nausea and vomiting (PONV), 140
Power management, 11–12
Practice patterns, 190–191
Practice procedures, 61–69
  future directions for, 62–63
  patient selection, 62–63
    control of respiratory rate problems, 63
    inability to lie still, 62
    infants, 63
    sedation level problems, 62
    severe claustrophobia problems, 63
    supine position problems, 62
    young children, 63
  pitfalls, 63–65
    distance from main operating room, 63
    distance from monitors, 63, 63f
    distance from patient, 63
    emergency equipment scarcity, 64
    radiation hazards, 64
    renal status problems, 64
    room confirguations, 63–64, 64f
    room temperture, 64
    support staff scarcity, 64
    unfamiliar equipment, 64–65, 65f
  risk factors, 65–67
  safety factors for, 65–67
Practice run simulations, 16
Practices and principles
  cardioversion procedures, 113–116
  catheterization laboratory procedures, 82–90
  electrophysiology procedures, 91–112
  practice procedures, 61–69
  preoperative evaluations, 70–81
  respiratory immobilization procedures, 113–116

Pradaxa. See Dabigartran (Pradaxa).
Pregnancy
  preoperative evaluations and, 77–78
  testing, 78
Premedications, 140–141
  anticholinergics, 140
  antiemetics, 140
  sedatives, 140
  steroids, 140
Preoperative evaluations, 70–81
  anesthetic records, 113
  anticoagulation regimen compliance, 113–114
  for bronchoscopy procedures, 139–140
  Center for Medicare and Medicaid Services
      requirements, 70
  coexisting diseases, 73–78
    anemia, 77
    antibiotic prophylaxis and, 74
    anticoagulant therapy and, 74–75
    coronary artery disease (CAD), 73
    diabetes, 76
    heart failure, 73
    heart murmurs, 73–74
    hypertension, 75
    implantable cardioverterdefibrillators (ICDs) and,
        75, 75b
    increased risks with, 73
    obesity, 76
    obstructive sleep apnea (OSA), 76
    percutaneous coronary interventions (PCIs) and,
        74–75
    pregnancy, 77–78
    pulmonary disease, 75–76
    reneal disease, 76–77
    stents and, 74–75
  components of, 70–73
    airway examinations, 70–72, 73b
    American Society of Anesthesiologists (ASA)
        physical status classification, 70–73
    cardiac evaluation algorithms, 73, 73f
    funcational capacity metabolic equivalents
        (METs), 70, 72t, 73
    medical histories, 70, 71f–72f
    physical examinations, 71–72
    targeted interviews, 70
  detailed medical histories, 114
  fasting guidelines, 80
  future directions for, 80
  laboratory data reviews, 114
  medication reviews, 114
  perioperative medications, 78–80, 80b
    anticoagulant therapy, 79
    antinypertensive, 78
    antiplatelet, 78–79
    aspirin, 78–79
    cardiovascular, 78
    controlled substances, 80
    herbal supplements, 79
    insulin, 79. See also Insulin.
    medical record reconciliations and, 78
    oral diabetes, 79
    psychiatric, 79
    steroids, 79
    written instructions for, 78
  preoperative testing, 78
    advantages vs. disadvantages of, 78
    chest radiographs, 78
    electrocardiograms (ECGs), 78
    pregnancy testing, 78
Preoperative Evaluation Service (PES), 179
Preparation activites
  anesthesiologist roles in, 30–34
  excellence criteria
    design, 8–17
    engineering, 1–7

Preparation activites (Continued)
  medications, critical, 18–29
  room set-ups, 18–29
  standards, safety and engineering, 8–17
  supplies, critical, 18–29
Preprocedure studies, 140
Presurgical checklists, 3–4, 3t
Principles and practices
  cardioversion procedures, 113–116
  catheterization laboratory procedures,
      82–90
  electrophysiology procedures, 91–112
  practice procedures, 61–69
  preoperative evaluations, 70–81
  respiratory immobilization procedures,
      113–116
Proactive approaches. See also Engineering.
  problem anticipation, 3–5
    daily huddles, 5
    guidelines, 4
    health care failure mode and analysis (HFMEA),
        4–5. See also Analyses.
    human factors engineering (HFE), 3
    protocols and checklists, 3–4, 3t, 4b
  vs. reactive approaches, 3
Problem anticipation, 3–5. See also Proactive
      approaches.
  daily huddles, 5
  guidelines, 4
  health care failure mode and analysis (HFMEA),
      4–5
  human factors engineering (HFE), 3
  protocols and checklists, 3–4, 3t, 4b
Procedure knowledge, 179
  case booking, 179
  emergency help availbility, 179
  patient ownership, 179
  Preoperative Evaluation Service (PES), 179
  scheduling services
    Preoperative Evaluation Service (PES), 179
Procedures, practice, 61–69
Process
  indicators, 36–38, 39t. See also indicators.
  surveillance, 41–42
Professional development, 36
Profit analyses, 186, 186f. See also Analyses.
Pronovost, Peter, 3
Prophylaxis, antibiotic, 74
Propofol use
  allergies to, 127
  critical medication status, 27
  for eletrophysiology procedures, 98
  for endoscopic procedures, 134–135, 134t
  guidelines for, 195–196
  infusion credentialing for, 30–31
  by nonanesthesiologists, 191–192
  pharmacodynamic variability of, 127
  pharmacokinetic variability of, 127
  policy considerations for, 195–196
  safety considerations for, 192–194
  for upper gastrointestinal (GI) endoscopy,
      127–128, 128t
Protocols, 3–4, 3t, 4b
Provider-reporting structure relationsips, 4
Psychiatric medications, 79
Psychomimetic reactions, 127–128
Pulmonary disease, 75–76
Pumps, insulin, 79. See also Insulin.

Q

Quality assurance methods, 30–31, 36. See also
    Continuous quality improvement (CQI).
Quality-of-care indicators, 38. See also Indicators.
Quiet environments, 20–21

R

Radial arterial cannulation, 82–83
Radiation
  exposures, 25–26, 26f
  therapy areas, 12–13, 166–167, 167b
Radiofrequency ablation (RFA), 139. *See also* Ablation.
Radiology suites
  adult, 151–160
  pediatric, 161–170
Rapid response teams (RRTs), 5
RCAs. *See* Root cause analyses (RCAs).
Reactive approaches. *See also* Engineering.
  adverse events and, 5–6
  clinical support backup, 5
  event reporting systems, 5
  vs. proactive approaches, 3. *See also* Proactive
    approaches.
  rapid response teams (RRTs), 5
  root cause analyses (RCAs), 5–6. *See also* Analyses.
  unplanned admission provisions, 5
Reason, James, 5–6
Reduction, lung volume, 139
Reflex supression, airway, 141. *See also* Airway
  management.
Refractory hypotension, 78
Regurgitation, aortic, 86–87
Reimbursement, 185–186
Reneal disease, 76–77
Repolarization phase, 97. *See also* Action potentials.
Reporting
  guidelines
    for adverse events, 38
    for critical incidents, 38
    for sentinel events, 38
  structure-provider relationsips, 4
  systems, 5
Resource utilization, 188
Respiratory immobilization, 117–118, 118f
  high-frequency jet ventilation (HFJV), 117–118
  Kaplan-Meir survival plots, 117, 118f
  laryngeal mask airways (LMAs) for, 117
Respiratory immobilization procedures, 113–116
Respiratory rates, 122
Response teams, 5
Resting phase, 97. *See also* Action potentials.
Revascularization and testing recommendations, 73, 73f
Revenue equation, 186
RFA. *See* Radiofrequency ablation (RFA).
Right-to-left blood shunting precautions, 93b
Rigid bronchoscopy, 145
Risk
  adjustment, 6
  indentification, 39
  monitors, 40
Roles, anesthesiologist, 30–34
  in anesthesia and sedation levels, 31–32
  in equipment selection criteria, 33
  future perspectives of, 30, 34
  historical perspectives of, 30
  importance of, 34
  in monitored anesthesia care (MAC), 31–32
Room set-ups, 18–29
  American Society of Anesthesiologists (ASA)
    statements on, 18–24, 18b, 19f
  challenges of, 18, 29
  critical medications for, 26–28, 26f
  critical supplies for, 24, 24b
  in magnetic resonance imaging (MRI) suite zones,
    21–24, 22f–23f
  in radiation therapy, 21
  safety considerations for, 24–26, 25b
Room temperature control, 10–11
Root cause analyses (RCAs), 5–6. *See also* Analyses.
RRTs. *See* Rapid response teams (RRTs).
Ruptures, tracheal, 148

S

Safety standards, 8–17
  anestheiologist roles in, 32–33
  Institute of Medicine (IOM) achievement areas, 36
  As Low As Reasonably Achievable (ALARA)
    principle, 25
  for propofol use, 31, 192–194
  radiation exposure, 25–26, 26f
  for room set-ups, 24–26, 25b. *See also* Room set-ups.
  safe practice organization, 32–33
  Safe Surgery Saves Lives study group, 3
  trace anesthetic gas exposures, 25
  trip and fall risks, 24–25
Sample profit analyses, 186–187. *See also* Analyses.
Sao_2. *See* Oxygen saturation (Sao_2)
SAPIEN valves, 83
Satisfaction surveys, 37f, 38, 40f
Saturation, oxygen. *See* Oxygen saturation (Sao_2)
Schedulers, electronic, 188, 189t
Scheduling services, 177–182
  associated background issues of, 178
    physical space, 178
    standardized equipmennt, 178
  challenges of, 178
  complex procedures and, 182
  daily schedules, 179–182, 180t
    area-specific postanesthesia care units, 180
    block, 179–182
    case rankings, 179
    clinical coverge contracts, 179–180, 181f
    fixed, 179–182
    imaging technique incorporation, 180–182
    night and weekend procedures, 180
  integration with main operating room, 182
  vs. operating room, 178, 182
  procedure knowledge, 179
    case booking, 179
    emergency help availbility, 179
    patient ownership, 179
    Preoperative Evaluation Service (PES), 179
Screens, lead, 178
Second-degree heart block, 101
SEDASYS system, 130–131
Sedation levels, 62
  deep, 62
  minimal, 62
  moderate, 62
Sedatives
  for bronchoscopy procedures, 140
Sensitizers, insulin, 79. *See also* Insulin.
Sentinel events, 38
Serial electrocardiograms (ECGs), 73
Serum electrolyte levels, 76–77
Services scheduling, 177–182
Set-ups, room, 18–29
Sevoflurane
  for eletrophysiology procedures, 98
SGAs. *See* Supraglottic airways (SGAs).
Shields and shielding
  equipment, 178
  lead glass, 25–26, 26f, 178
Short-acting
  bronchodilators, 140–141
  opioids, 127
Significant shortcomings, 6
Simulations, 10
Single-photon emission computed tomography
  (SPECT), 30
Site design, 8–17
Size guidelines, 9, 9t
Sleep apnea, obstructive, 76
SPECT. *See* Single-photon emission computed
  tomography (SPECT).
Spray, benzocaine, 28–29

Stacking, breath, 122–123, 123f. *See also* High-
  frequency ventilation (HFV).
Staffing
  coverage, novel, 205–210
  distribution-workload optimization, 187, 187f
Standardized equipment, 178
Standards, safety and engineering, 8–17
Staphylococcus spp., 41
Status classification, 70–73
Stenosis
  calcific aortic, 83
  tracheal, 123
Stents and stenting, 74–75
  airway, 138–139. *See also* Airway management.
  complications of, 139
Steroids, 79, 140
STOP-BANG questionnaire, 76, 77f
Structural indicators, 36. *See also* Indicators.
Stunning, temporary myocardial, 115
Subcutaneous
  emphysema, 147
  unfractionated heparin, 79
Succinylcholine, 100
Suite settings
  bronchoscopy, 137–150
  colonoscopy, 132–136
  pediatric, radiology, 161–170
  radiology, 151–160
Sulfonyurea agents, 79
Supplements, herbal, 79
Supplies, critical, 18–29, 24, 24b
Support
  ancillary, 187–188
  backup, 5
  clinical, 5
Supraglottic airways (SGAs), 143–145, 143b, 144t.
  See also Airway management.
Surgical Safety Checklist (World Health Organization),
  3, 3t
Surveillance processes, 41–42
Surveys, patient satisfaction, 38, 40f
"Swiss Cheese" error model, 5–6
Sympathetic nervous system, 97
Systemic air embolization, 92, 93b
Systems
  approaches, 36
  development, 199–204
  performance improvements, 36. *See also*
    Continuous quality improvement (CQI).
  reviews, 139–140

T

Tachyarrhythmias, 100–102, 100b. *See also* Cardiac
  arrhythmias.
Tackle box transporation, 26, 26f. *See also*
  Medications.
Target-controlled infusion (TCI), 128
Targeted interviews, 70
TAVR. *See* Transcatheter aortic valve replacement
  (TAVR).
TCI. *See* Target-controlled infusion (TCI)
Teams
  continuous qiality improvement (CQI) and, 36
  for electrophysiology procedures, 95
  rapid response teams (RRTs), 5
TEE. *See* Transesophageal echocardiography (TEE)
Temperature control, 10–11, 95
Temporary myocardial stunning, 115
Testing recommendations, 73, 73f
The Joint Commission (TJC)
  anesthesiologist requirements, 31
  Sentinel Event Database, 38
  Sentinel Event Policy, 38
  site design guidelines, 8

Theroplasty, bronchial, 139
Thienopyridines, 74–75, 78–79
Third-degree heart block, 101
Thyroid protectors, 178
Ticlopidine (Ticlid), 78–79
Timelines, design, 17t. *See also* Design excellence.
Timeliness, 36
TIVA. *See* Total intravenous anesthesia (TIVA).
TJC. *See* The Joint Commission (TJC).
To Err is Human report (Institute of Medicine), 2
Topical benzocaine, 28–29
Total costs, 185f, 185–186
Total intravenous anesthesia (TIVA), 20, 98–99
Trace anesthetic gas exposures, 25
Tracheal
    lacerations, 148
    ruptures, 148
    stenosis, 123
Traditional cost accounting, 185f, 185–186
Tranesophageal cardiography (TEE) probes
    for transcatheter aortic valve replacement (TAVR),
        85, 85f
Transapical closures, 84, 84f, 87–88, 88f
Transcatheter aortic valve replacement (TAVR). *See
    also* Catheterization laboratory procedures.
    anesthetic elements for, 84–85, 86f
    approaches to, 83–85, 84f
        transapical, 84, 84f
        transfemoral, 83–84, 84f
    benefits of, 83
    for calcific aortic stenosis, 83
    complications of, 85–87
        aortic regurgitation, 86–87
        coronary artery obstructions, 87
        heart block, 87
        hemopericardium, 87
        neurological injuries, 87
        peripheral vascular injuries, 87
        persistent hemodynamic instability, 85–86
    Food and Drug Administration (FDA) approvals,
        82, 88
    hemodynamic monitoring for, 82–83
    for high-risk patients, 83
    PARTNER trial of, 87–88
    probes for, 85, 85f
    resources for, 90
Transesophageal echocardiography (TEE), 73–74,
    82, 113
    hemodynamic monitoring for, 82–83
    indications for, 82

Transfemoral transcatheter aortic valve replacement
    (TAVR), 83–84, 84f. *See also* Transcatheter
    aortic valve replacement (TAVR).
Transthoracic echo (TTE), 115
Trends, 183. *See also* Market analyses.
Trip and fall risks, 24–25
TTE. *See* Transthoracic echo (TTE).

U

Ultra-short-acting opioids, 127
Unfamiliar equipment, 64–65, 65f
Unfractionated heparin. subcutaneous, 79
Universal Protocol, 41
Unplanned admission provisions, 5
Upper gastrointestinal (GI) endoscopy, 126–131. *See
    also* Gastrointestinal (GI) endoscopic procedures.
    airway management for, 128–129, 129f
    anesthetic drugs for, 127–128, 128t
        benzodiazepine/midazolam, 127
        benzodiazepine/remifentanil, 127
        comparisons of, 128, 128t
        dexmedetomidine, 128
        etomidate, 127
        ketamine, 127–128
        lidocaine, 127
        propofol, 127–128, 128t
    complications of, 130, 130b
    endoscopic retrograde cholangiopancreatography
        (ERCP), 126
    esophagogastroduodenoscopy (EGD), 126
    future directions for, 130–131
    indications for, 129–130, 130b
    monitoring for, 130
    patient populations presenting for, 126
    preprocedure evaluations for, 126–127
    resources for, 131
Utilization rates, 187

V

Validation
    definition of, 37
    of indicators, 37–38
        Anesthesia Quality Institute (AQI), Recommended
            Quality Indicators, 37–38, 39t
        benchmarking to national standards, 42
        limitations of, 36
        patient satisfaction surveys and, 38, 40f
        validity, definition of, 37

Valvular disease, 73–74
Valvuloplasty, balloon, 82
Variability
    pharmacodynamic, 127
    pharmacokinetic, 127
Variable costs, 185f, 185–186
Vascular injuries, peripheral, 87
Vasculature examinations, 71–72
Ventilation, 12
    techniques, 145–146
        high-frequency (HFV), 117–125
        jet ventilation, 146
        jet ventilation, high-frequency (HFJV), 146
        jet ventilation, low-frequency (LFJV), 146
        positive-pressure ventilation, 145–146
Ventilator types, 118–121. *See also* High-frequency
        ventilation (HFV).
    dual-frequency jet, 118, 119f
    electrically-controlled devices, 118f, 121
    high-frequency jet, 118, 118f
    high-frequency oscillators, 118, 119f
    high-frequency percussive, 118, 120f
    manually-operated pneumatic devices, 119–120,
        120f
    negative-pressure high-frequency oscillators, 119
Venus vasculature examinations, 71–72
Vests, lead glass, 178
Veterans Administration (VA), 4–5
Vital signs, normal ranges, 162t

W

Warming systems, forced air, 20
Weekend and night scheduling, 180
WHO. *See* World Health Organization (WHO).
Wired *vs.* wireless communication designs, 10
Workload-distribution optimization, 187, 187f
World Health Organization (WHO), 3, 3t
Wrong person/site procedures provention, 41

Y

Yolks, nitrous oxide, 178